THE WH

# HA[...]
# AND MARINAS

# THE WHICH? GUIDE TO

# HARBOURS AND MARINAS

## Gill and Basil Heather

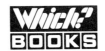

*Published by*
Consumers' Association
and
Hodder & Stoughton

*The Which? Guide to Harbours and Marinas*
was researched by the Cruising Association
for The Association for Consumer Research
and published by Consumers' Association,
2 Marylebone Road, London NW1 4DX and
Hodder and Stoughton, 47 Bedford Square,
London WC1B 3DP

Cover illustration by Moira Huntly
Cover design by Paul Saunders
Typographic design by Dick Vine
Cartography by Jillian Luff

First edition October 1991

Copyright © 1991 Consumers' Association Ltd

*British Library Cataloguing in Publication Data*
Heather, Gill
  The Which? guide to harbours and marinas
  I. Title  II. Heather, Basil
  387.15

ISBN 0–340–52819–2

**Thanks for choosing this book . . .**
If you find it useful, we'd like to hear from you. Even if it doesn't
live up to your expectations or do the job you were expecting,
we'd still like to know. Then we can take your comments into
account when preparing similar titles or, indeed, the next edition
of the book. Address your letter to the Publishing Manager at
Consumers' Association, FREEPOST, 2 Marylebone Road,
London NW1 4DX.
We look forward to hearing from you.

Typeset by Midford Typesetting Limited, London W1
Printed and bound in Great Britain by Richard Clay Limited,
Bungay, Suffolk

# CONTENTS

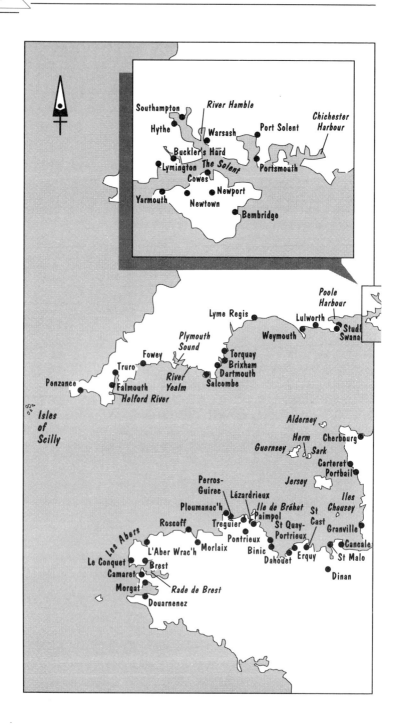

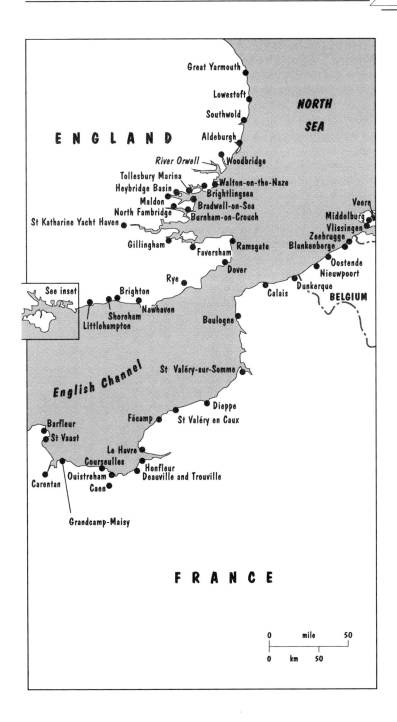

# FOREWORD

## by Libby Purves

*writer, broadcaster and sailor*

There are times, frankly, when any harbour will do and the shelter matters far more than the shopping. 'Any port in a storm,' we mutter as the clouds blacken and the sea heaves warningly beneath us. We may have planned on Chichester, but the sight of Newhaven pierhead unmans us and we shoot between the friendly breakwaters like a frightened mouse into its hole. We may be meeting friends at Bembridge, but the tide turned and we appear to be tied up in East Cowes, where we have never been nor particularly intended to go. And we are glad of it: a boat, any boat, is not a motor-caravan on water. It takes you out into an alien element and there will be times when you are greatly relieved to be back on dry land. The fact that you set out for Barfleur and got magnetically drawn into Cherbourg Marina is neither here nor there. At least the water beneath you is now flat, and the wind rattling your rigging no longer has any power to harm you. And tomorrow, as Scarlett O'Hara said, is another day.

So, on the face of it, why have a book which guides you to harbours and yet keeps silent on the subject of lights and buoys and shelter, concentrating instead on services, shopping-malls, pubs and fun-fairs? Surely, when a sailor talks about 'getting to know the Mudport-on-Sea Bar', he should be referring to the submerged sandbank at the entrance over which the tide rips, and not to the cosy little dive up Herring Road where they generally have a jazz pianist? Surely, when a sailor says 'fair', he should mean the setting on his barometer, not a god-sent opportunity to quell the children's rebellion with candyfloss and dodgems? Surely, in short, this book is a shocking new departure and will outrage the yachting purist?

Well, maybe. But who needs purists? In a way, it is the very uncertainties of cruising which make the guide so commendably useful. If you are up the Deben when you meant to be up the Alde, or rolling uneasily in Dover Harbour when the family think you are in Rye, there is all the more reason to find – with the minimum of fuss and friction – a telephone, a shower, a bank, a bread shop and somewhere to detoxify that unsavoury set of thermal underwear which has not seen soap since somewhere east of Oostende. It is also pleasant, when landing in an utterly strange place with a couple of grumpy children, to know roughly which way to walk along the rainswept quay in order to end up among toyshops and chip shops. It is even better to land in the sunshine and be able to say confidently, after a long passage, 'There's a beach here!' Too often, the exigencies of space in pilot-books mean that the symbol for beach is used geologically rather than recreationally: in other words, what you hoped from the diagram would be a fine sandy strand turns out to be a strip of sharp stones and rusty cans bisected by a slimy green outfall pipe. No longer need this happen: from the Scillies to Great Yarmouth, from Holland to Brittany, this book gives brief, plain, invaluable accounts of life as seen from shoreside. The boat is tied up, the harbour dues are paid, the restorative whisky has been downed in the damp cabin: now for a spell of shore leave – better-informed, better-tempered shore leave than usual. Pipe all hands to dance and skylark, for here, hooray, is a good fish restaurant, a bracing walk and a cinema for the wet evenings.

Of course, the pleasure of exploring new places 'cold' is a great one; but it can still be enjoyed even if you have cheated your conscience by ascertaining briefly that there is, indeed, a launderette. Or that the local yacht club is of the kind which warmly welcomes visitors. Or that Deauville is the posh side, where the price of a cup of coffee will make you reel, whereas Trouville is financially survivable and twice as interesting. A smattering of local history doesn't hurt either: if ever I end up in Caen, now I shall be able to tell the children, with an authority that will astonish them, that Beau Brummel was once the British consul in the town. Not a lot of pilot books tell you that.

Cruising is all about taking life as it comes, one day at a time. The weather is so variable, these northern coasts so demanding of concentration and respect, that it is impossible to plan a cruise in detail. I have sailed with a dozen or more skippers in the days when I was a roving crew, and I wish I had a pound for every time one of them has shouted, 'How do I know? I'm not running a bus service!' when one of the crew demanded an ETA, or a graph of probability about how many days it would take to reach Penzance. Often, let's face it, we end up spending a quite unscheduled three days somewhere having the alternator fixed or waiting for the wind to drop. And taking each day as it comes, good-humouredly, is made a great deal easier if there is a book to hand which introduces the port around you, outlines its possibilities and gives you a clue as to whether it might be worth struggling the next few miles along the coast in a brief lull to somewhere prettier, handier, or (in the last resort) somewhere with a railway station in it.

But use it to plan, as well – if you must. Many a pleasant winter's evening can be devoted to choreographing a neat and tidy tour of the West Country, or the French ports, or the Dutch and Belgian coasts. We can all dream: only it is nicer to dream if you know that wherever you get blown, the guide will get blown with you, tactfully murmuring its practical advice.

One word of warning, though, about what this book is not. It is not a navigational aid. The presence of a building society and a chip shop, as all seasoned cruising people know to their disgust, is no guarantee of decent all-weather shelter. I remember a crewman saying bitterly to his skipper as they cleared out of a rolling anchorage in a sudden onshore wind, 'I really thought we'd be all right, so near the Midland Bank!' In this book, all navigational and pilotage information has been deliberately left out, and nobody should be tempted to skimp on charts, tide tables and specialist pilot books. The *Cruising Association Handbook* – or one of a plethora of others – will get you in safely. What this guide will do is to take over once you have stepped ashore and show you a good time. The odds are that you've earned it.

# INTRODUCTION

Most books about harbours are written from the point of view of the skipper or navigator, who is concerned with tides and currents, rocks and hazards, and the sort of mooring arrangements a harbour provides. The skipper is also, of course, interested in fuelling facilities and possibly in repairs, but it is usually assumed that once these needs have been met a pint of beer and a yarn at the club or pub, followed by a plate of sausages and chips, will fortify the crew and send them to an early bed, ready for a dawn start the next day.

Now that cruising is no longer the preserve of such latter-day Captain Ahabs, sailors need to know more about what to expect ashore. The eighties boom in boating led to a great upsurge in families sailing together, especially on cruising holidays, and more than 2.5 million people now participate in boating activities.

The information in *The Which? Guide to Harbours and Marinas* has been chosen from the point of view of the entire crew. What is a place like? Is it welcoming? Are there showers, toilets, a launderette? Are there good places for food and drink? And if you stay for a day or so, what is there to do ashore in the immediate vicinity and further afield? Last but not least, what public transport is available should you need to leave the boat?

This information has been collected by cruising people, nearly all of them members of the Cruising Association, and is based on personal experience of the harbours described. We are very grateful to these 30 individuals and have made full use of their reports. It says much for the standards of the places listed that there have been hardly any reports of unhelpful or unwelcoming harbours.

## Mooring charges

There has, however, been one area of growing complaint: the rapid spread of high mooring charges, especially in the UK. These charges have been rising ahead of inflation. A widely alleged reason for this is that one company, Marina Developments plc, has been acquiring many existing marinas and building new ones, and so has a near-monopoly.

Complaints to the Office of Fair Trading with a request for referral to the Monopolies and Mergers Commission have brought the reply that

---

**Note**

In this guide there is no navigational or pilotage information – the information you need for that is provided in the *Cruising Association Handbook* which is a comprehensive pilot to all the waters of northern and western Europe. It is the only cruising pilot book for these waters for which annual corrections are published.

the provision of marina berths may be outside the scope of laws governing fair trading. The Royal Yachting Association (RYA) and the Cruising Association are challenging these rulings and trying to have the laws amended by Parliament. The Secretary of State for Trade is currently awaiting the report of the Director General of Fair Trading before deciding whether to refer the matter to the Monopolies and Mergers Commission.

*1992 and all that*
There has been much speculation about the effect on the sailing

---

# *FOREIGN FACTS*

## Medical care

International reciprocal agreements give UK residents on holiday the right to medical assistance in the Netherlands, Belgium and France when care cannot be delayed and they can provide the doctor, dentist, chemist or hospital with an international insurance form (E111), or copy. Remember to get your form, from any main post office, before you leave the UK.

## NETHERLANDS

### Tourist information

Tourist offices will be found in the larger towns. They display the triangular 'VVV' sign and the familiar *i* sign, too. They will provide information about recreational facilities, events, sights and attractions for the whole country as well as all bus, train, underground and boat connections. Ask them, too, where to go if you need medical or similar advice.

In general VVV offices are open weekdays 0900–1700 and Saturdays 1000–1200. During the summer they are often open in the evening.

### Bicycle hire

Special Railstar bicycles can be hired from most stations for the day. The cost is very low, but you will be asked for a refundable deposit and proof of identification.

### Business hours

**Banks** Open weekdays 0900–1600/1700 (sometimes also on late shopping evenings)
**Post offices** Open weekdays 0900–1230 and 1330–1600
**Shops** Open weekdays 0830/0900–1730/1800 (Saturdays until 1600/1700). Some shops shut in the lunch hour and many close for one half or whole day a week

community of the European internal market which is due to come into operation on 1 January 1993. At the time of writing many details remain to be settled, and some changes may take several years. One long-term possibility is that 'Duty Free' will disappear, so that you will not be able to buy ships' stores untaxed unless you propose to voyage outside the European Community (EC). You would, however, be able to buy wine, for example, at a good price in a French shop and bring it home without restriction on quantity. Agreements on harmonising VAT levels and specific duties are still some way off, but it seems likely that the purchase of boat equipment, or even a whole new boat, would not

## Telephoning

To call the Netherlands from the UK, dial 010-31 followed by the town code, minus the initial 0, and the number.

To call the UK from the Netherlands, dial 09 (wait for the tone to change), then 44, then the area code minus the initial 0, followed by the number.

**Phone cards** Many payphones now take cards.

## Public holidays

| | |
|---|---|
| March/April | Good Friday and Easter Monday |
| April 30 | Queen's Birthday |
| May 5 | Liberation Day |
| April/May | Hemelvaarts Dag – Ascension Day |
| May/June | Pinksteren – Whit Sunday and Monday |

With the exception of Good Friday most shops are closed on these days.

# BELGIUM

## Tourist information

You should have no language difficulties in Belgium; English is understood and spoken almost everywhere. Tourist offices (called Dienst voor Toerisme or Syndicat d'Initiatif) can be found in most ports. They will provide information about local attractions and are usually helpful with travel or car or bicycle hire problems. Ask them, too, where to go if you need medical or similar advice.

There are no long-distance or inter-city bus services in Belgium. Buses are used mainly to serve outlying villages or to supplement inadequate train services.

Bicycles can be hired at most railway stations.

attract tax on importation provided that it had already been paid at approximately the same rate in another EC country.

Other possible effects of EC rulings refer to the registration of boats and qualifications for skippers. Again, no details are known, but it is likely that the British Small Ships Register and the RYA qualifications will be acceptable.

Pollution is another subject for future controls. It is already accepted practice not to use sea-water toilets in harbour, but legislation may lead to holding tanks becoming compulsory. Such a development may not be too onerous but one needs to be sure that the receiving authority does

---

# *FOREIGN FACTS*

### Business hours

**Banks** Open weekdays 0900–1200 and 1400–1600 (some remain open at midday)
**Post offices** Open weekdays 0900–1700. Larger offices also open on Saturdays 0900–1200
**Shops** Open (in general) weekdays 0900–1800 (in the main cities till 2100 on Fridays)

### Telephoning

To call Belgium from the UK, dial 010-32 followed by the town code, minus the initial 0, and the number.

To call the UK from Belgium, dial 00 (wait for the tone to change), then 44, then the area code, minus the initial 0, followed by the number.
**Phone cards** Many payphones take cards.

### Public holidays

| | |
|---|---|
| March/April | Easter Monday (but not Good Friday) |
| May 1 | May Day |
| April/May | Ascension Day |
| May/June | Whit Monday |
| July 21 | National Holiday |
| August 15 | Assumption Day |

## FRANCE

### Tourist information

Tourist offices (Office de Tourisme, sometimes called Syndicat d'Initiatif) can be found in almost every port. They provide information on local attractions and are usually helpful with

not pump the arisings straight back into the sea!

EC legislation on the subject of pollution is likely to cover other aspects, from noise to oil spillage and rubbish. The first is a matter of consideration for others – music and the noise of an outboard motor in the small hours can both be disturbing. Oil spillage must be prevented at all costs, and the best advice on what may be thrown overboard is – nothing.

Other rules governing the importation of fresh meat, plants and animals will remain unchanged, and there will continue to be customs and immigration between the UK and the rest of the EC.

travel or car or bicycle hire problems. Ask them, too, where to go if you need medical or similar advice.

## Business hours

**Banks** Open weekdays 0900–1200 and 1400–1600/1630 (in small towns they usually shut on Mondays and sometimes on other days as well)
**Post offices** Open weekdays 0800–1200, 1400–1700 (closed on Saturday afternoons)
**Shops** Open (in general) 0900–1200, 1400–1900. Closed on Sundays and Mondays (or Monday mornings). Food shops usually open an hour earlier and some may operate on a Sunday morning (especially bakers). Hypermarkets tend to stay open much later than town shops, sometimes until 2100 or even later.

## Telephoning

To call France from the UK, dial 010-33 followed by the eight-digit number.

To call the UK from France, dial 19 (wait for the tone to change), then 44, then the area code minus the initial 0, followed by the number.
**Phone cards** Phone booths taking phone cards outnumber the coin-operated ones in some places. The Télécarte (50 or 120 units) can be bought from post offices, railway stations and newsagents.

## Public holidays

| | |
|---|---|
| March/April | Easter Monday (but not Good Friday) |
| May | 1 (Labour Day), 8 (VE Day), Ascension Day |
| June | Whit Monday |
| July 14 | Bastille Day |
| August 15 | Assumption Day |

# HOW TO USE THIS BOOK

The purpose of this book is to take over from the navigator when you have tied up and are about to step ashore. We aim to tell you what a place is like, what sort of welcome you can expect and what facilities, diversions and entertainments there are. The entries are in geographical order: west to east along the English coast and back again along the continent. The map on pages 6 and 7 shows all but the smallest places described. Factual information for each harbour and marina is given below the information about the town or river in which it is located.

Suggestions are made for interesting places to visit and things to do if you want a break from sailing or the weather imposes one. Information has been given about travel, car hire and bicycle hire for your expeditions ashore. Relevant walks are included from the *Holiday Which? Good Walks Guide* and the *Holiday Which? Town and Country Walks Guide* (both published by Consumers' Association and Hodder & Stoughton). Taxi, bus, train, plane and ferry services for crew changes or returns home in mid-cruise are also given.

We tell you when security is good, so that you can feel confident about leaving the boat, although we cannot guarantee the safety of your boat or possessions in any harbour or marina.

## Maps
Simple maps have been provided to show you which way to go for shops, banks, post office, restaurants, beach and railway station. A key to the symbols is inside the front cover. We have used some symbols sparingly, so that, for example, in a marina, where water and electricity can be assumed to exist, symbols have been used only where these things are difficult to locate.

## VHF communications
VHF channels have been given for each harbour and marina so that you can contact the appropriate authority to arrange a berth, or if you have an emergency on board. As the choice of channel can be a cause of confusion, the following explanation may help. Channel M (which may appear on older sets as 37) should be used only in UK waters. Abroad it is an international duplex channel for ship-to-shore communication. If you try to use it you will not hear the other party and may be interfering with another conversation. The RYA recommends that in UK waters you use channel 80 in the first instance and use M as a back-up. Harbourmasters in the Netherlands, Belgium and France use a variety of channels and not all English harbours have started using channel 80 yet, so we give channel numbers for all harbours using VHF.

## Price categories

We give an indication of the daily charge for visitors at each of the harbours and marinas, based on 1991 high season rates for a 10m boat: £ = under £5, ££ = under £10, £££ = under £15, ££££ = under £20, £££££ = £20 and over. In some cases a free night is offered, sometimes the first, sometimes the third – where this is the case we say so. The first night may be more expensive to cover the price of entering a lock – again, we say where this is the case. Prices usually include water and electricity and often showers too. Launderette charges are always extra, paid for by coins or tokens. Mooring charges are often lower at other times of year.

## Ships' services

We have listed boatyards, engineers and other suppliers who will help when you are in trouble. Many of these firms are Cruising Association boatmen who will give members extra attention. They are mentioned as such in the text. The *Cruising Association Yearbook* contains the names of Honorary Local Representatives – they are usually members of the Cruising Association and are on hand to give other members any information that may be of assistance when cruising and to arbitrate in any disputes between members and boatmen.

## Phone numbers and addresses

We have given addresses of or directions to services which are easy to find, telephone numbers where they are further afield or operate a collection service. Other names, addresses and telephone numbers can often be found on harbourmasters' notice boards.

## Clubhouses

In marinas and on the continent these are usually commercially run and are pleased to see all visitors for the business they bring. They should not be confused with the yacht clubs owned by the members – the sort to which many sailors already belong. Most of the latter have a long-standing tradition of welcoming members of other clubs when on passage. If you wish to avail yourself of their hospitality, make yourself known to the Secretary or Steward, who will probably invite you to use the facilities. Bear in mind that it is not your own club, that it is a privilege to be allowed in as a guest, and behave accordingly.

## Food and drink

Nearly all the restaurants and pubs we have mentioned by name are given as a result of personal recommendations by individual yachting visitors and we hope you will enjoy them. We have also included a selection of restaurants featured in *The Good Food Guide 1992* or *Out to Eat*, a guide to good-value food, both published by Consumers' Association and Hodder & Stoughton. Restaurants which are situated

# OUR TOP TEN
# HARBOURS AND MARINAS

One of the great pleasures of cruising is that every place is different; indeed many change from visit to visit. Choosing a 'top ten' has taken much heart-searching, but we believe this list reflects the best of the many kinds of experience cruising has to offer.

**Fowey**'s lovely landlocked harbour endears one to the West Country – never mind that it is crowded. The village is charming and you will be made welcome, be it in club, pub or shop. A visit here is a taste of the best in cruising on the English side of the Channel. See page 59.

**Newtown** is an unexpected haven just off one of the busiest sea lanes in the world. It is a nature reserve owned by the National Trust for the enjoyment of us all. During the week, in particular, it is an idyllic escape. See page 112.

**Brighton Marina**'s appeal lies very largely in its situation: it provides relief after the long haul along the Sussex coast. Although everything you need can be found in the marina, you won't want to move on without visiting the famous Regency town and the equally attractive countryside of the South Downs. See page 161.

**Southwold** – a creek full of boats of all shapes, sizes and states of preservation – offers the prospect of exploring the coastline and the two attractive little East Anglian towns of Southwold and Walberswick close by. A recently discovered Viking ship in Buss Creek adds to its interest. See page 216.

conveniently close to the moorings, or are indeed the only restaurants in the vicinity, are described briefly.

*Help wanted*
Please let us know if you find information in an entry that is no longer correct. Marinas change hands, harbours expand, or close off some

**Veere** is a picturesque old Dutch town with an air of history. Its fortified harbour mouth, old houses along the quayside and impressive Town Hall are all quite out of scale with its present size. There is always a welcome in the miniature harbour and many interesting old Dutch vessels to admire. See page 225.

**Honfleur**'s inner basin moorings, surrounded by the ancient buildings, transport you to a scene of an older France which entices you ashore to explore. After the long passage up the Seine estuary it is very satisfying to turn sharply to starboard out of the current to be greeted by the opening bridge and lock gate – if you have timed it right! See page 274.

**St Peter Port** gives you the feel of being on holiday abroad, yet there is plenty that is familiar, so it is a good 'port of transition'. The approach down the Little Russel, with rocks and islands on every side and the harbour itself, with its town rising behind it, are all that one can ask of a landfall. See page 309.

**Ile de Bréhat** is as rewarding for a brief visit of a few hours as for a longer stay – it offers quiet anchorages and solitary rambles ashore, or you can join others in the popular places. On a sunny day this colourful island with exotic flowers in a setting of wild rocky shores makes you feel you are far from the windswept seas of northern Europe. See page 352.

**Pontrieux** is inland from the Brittany coast. The peaceful reaches of the Trieux River prepare you for the equally peaceful locked-in basin. The little town up river from the moorings has a flower-bedecked charm which must not be missed. See page 356.

**Morlaix** is sited far up a drying river in the middle of a bustling town dominated by a huge railway viaduct, with plenty to explore, ancient and modern. Top-class shops and restaurants are there to tempt your pocket and your appetite. See page 368.

sections to yachts and open others. If you find a harbour, marina or anchorage in the area covered which you think should be included in the next edition, send details to The Which? Guide to Harbours and Marinas, 2 Marylebone Road, London NW1 4DX. A plan of the area and a brief summary of attractions are needed, as well as the harbourmaster's telephone number.

# Never a barrier

*The Channel is there to be crossed.* **Nigel Calder**, *author of* The English Channel, *and winner of the Best Book of the Sea Award 1987, explains the life and times of this famous stretch of water.*

Patrick O'Brian, my favourite nautical novelist, has his naval captain laughing at his doctor friend's suggestion that the 'ancients' hugged the shore, creeping from promontory to promontory. 'I very much doubt the ancients did anything of the kind,' he says. 'Can you imagine anyone in his wits coming within sight of a lee-shore?'

A reader who perhaps feels timid about sailing cross-Channel may have been brainwashed by landlubberly historians who keep going on, not only about boneheaded ancient mariners who allegedly hugged the shore, but about the English Channel being a great barrier between England and France. Even Shakespeare got it wrong:

> '. . . This precious stone set in a silver sea,
> Which serves it in the office of a wall,
> Or as a moat defensive to a house,
> Against the envy of less happier lands,
> This blessed plot, this earth, this realm, this England.'

To think of the English Channel as a 'moat' is as daft as calling the M25 motorway a tank-trap. All right, the M25 could delay tanks if it were jammed as usual with cars, and even the Channel becomes a watery barrier of sorts if there are plenty of warships around. But Shakespeare really should have known better. Less than 80 years before his birth, in the events celebrated in his own *Richard III*, Henry Tudor sailed from Harfleur in Normandy with a French-speaking army, nipped around Land's End to Milford Haven, and snatched the English crown by killing the king. Indeed Shakespeare did know better, when he had the unlucky Richard rallying his army against 'a scum of Bretons' and 'overweening rags of France'. How did those foreign troops get to Bosworth Field except via the 'silver sea'?

A piece of historical idiocy, widely believed even by sailors, is that the last person to invade and capture England from the sea was William the Conqueror – 1066 and all that. Besides Henry Tudor (1485) there was Henry of Anjou (1153) who brought a French-speaking army into Poole Harbour, and compelled the king to make him heir to the throne; next year, he became Henry II. And in 1688, William of Orange sailed from Holland with a Dutch-speaking army. He evaded the English fleet by using an easterly wind to rush through the Dover Strait and down the Channel. After landing his fierce mercenaries in Tor Bay, he forced the king to flee and made himself William III.

Two Williams the Conqueror, then, and two Henrys the Conqueror: that's not counting any of the attempts to invade England that were prevented only by bad weather or fierce battles, nor any of the invading armies that went the other way, from England to France. If the Channel is a moat, why did the English gentry tremble when Napoleon massed his armies at Boulogne? Why did Churchill vow to 'fight them on the beaches' when Hitler's army was similarly poised? The fact plain to anyone threatened with a cross-Channel invasion is that the water itself is all too easy to cross. And until the last moment one is kept guessing about where, on a long coastline, the troops will scramble ashore.

These excursions into military history may help to cure that purely psychological block about the Channel being a barrier. It never was – at least for the past three thousand years. That is how long the sailors have had well-found boats built with metal implements. Shipwrights in this part of Europe first acquired bronze tools around 1100 BC, more than a thousand years before the Romans came. A cross-Channel trade in scrap bronze flourished at that time, as evidenced by cargoes discovered by divers in the seabed off Dover and Salcombe.

Sadly, archaeologists have to rely on occasional shipwrecks, as in these cases, for most of their evidence about prehistoric voyaging. That does not mean the ancients were particularly accident-prone. Merchants would not have trusted valuable bronze to the open sea unless they had reasonable confidence that it would reach the other side safely. And the cross-Channel seafarers of the Bronze Age were certainly not hugging the shore, or even taking the shortest sea-route. The Dover cargo seems to have come, not from Calais, but from the Seine River 120 nautical miles to the south-west. The shortest open-water passage for the Salcombe cargo would have been some 70 nautical miles, from the Channel Islands.

A thousand years later, ships plied regularly between the Rance estuary near present-day St Malo and Hengistbury Head near present-day Christchurch. They carried Italian wine, for which the chieftains of the Ancient Britons had acquired a keen taste – perhaps too keen, if it weakened their resolve to fight the Roman legions that followed soon after.

Broken wine-jars lay a plain trail for the archaeological detective who wishes to trace the route from the vineyards of Italy to the Celtic hill-forts of southern England. It leads via the Mediterranean sea from Italy to France, and then by river and overland across south-western France. The people of the Bordeaux region watched the fermented grape-juice going by on its way to Britannia and thought to themselves, 'We could make that!' From there, ships took the Italian wine to southern Brittany, where a short overland portage between two rivers brought it to the Rance, for loading again into seagoing ships for the 140-mile voyage to Hengistbury.

The route made good sense. It cut out a tiresomely long sea-passage around Spain (not good for the wine) and it avoided the rocky and pirate-infested waters of western Brittany. Otherwise, the wine-traders took their jars as far as possible by seagoing ships and river barges. Nobody in his right mind would have loaded the wine in carts in Italy and trundled it overland to Calais for the short sea route. Waterborne traffic, then as now, was far cheaper than land transport. And until the invention of the steam train in the nineteenth century it was usually quicker by sea. That is something else often overlooked by historians who persist in thinking of the Channel as a barrier. People living in Portsmouth, say, could reach Cherbourg much more easily than London.

To the Normans, descendants of the Vikings, the Channel was nothing. After the Conquest their domains lay on both sides of the water, and they commuted freely. An exception that proved the rule was the *White Ship*. She was wrecked off Cap Barfleur on a drunken evening in 1120, drowning the heir to the throne. That gave Henry of Anjou the chance for his amphibious coup, 33 years later, and his Angevin empire stretched from the Scottish border to the Spanish border. When knights at Henry's impatient word murdered Archbishop Becket in his cathedral, they had first to cross the Channel from Normandy, to reach Canterbury.

The Channel Islands, together with England itself, are relics of that Channel-straddling empire of medieval times, when kings and dukes struggled like gangsters over the geographical range of their protection rackets. Not until Joan of Arc took up her sword in 1429 did anyone seriously start sorting out who were the French and who the English. They shared a common ancestry and history. When the Roman Empire fell, Celts on both sides of the water were overwhelmed by German pirates. The eponymous Anglo-Saxons and Franks settled in England and France, before coming under attack themselves from the Vikings.

The ex-pirates on both sides of the Channel were obedient to the Catholic Church. The only conspicuous difference was in language. The Franks were more impressed with Roman traditions than the Anglo-Saxons were, and they adopted the Latin-based language that evolved into modern French. English remains a Germanic language with a Norman-French overlay. The King of the Franks started calling himself King of France in 1181. The King of England did not *stop* calling himself King of France until 1801.

For better or worse, the Channel became the laboratory in which modern nationalism evolved, as the French and the English defined their identities. They went on to invent the nation-state for the purposes of chronic warfare and imperial rivalry across the world's oceans. The English counterpart to Joan of Arc was the Protestant pirate from Plymouth, Francis Drake. Abetted by Shakespeare, Drake transformed the self-perception of ale-swigging shepherds and fishermen into that of rum-swigging explorers and empire-builders.

English ships began going down Channel to America, India, China and eventually Australia. So effective was Drake's influence that

Shakespeare's language is now the *lingua franca* of the entire world. The only people who object are the French — but that issue was settled when the weatherbeaten ships that blockaded Brest forced Napoleon to abandon his plan for a cross-Channel invasion.

Mutual friends, the Americans and the Germans for instance, are baffled by the undercurrents of mutual disdain that still mar Anglo-French relationships. Although absurd, and contradicted daily in friendly personal encounters by land or sea, the latent animosity remains strong enough to require a strong explanation. In my opinion, the basic reason for it is that the English Channel is no barrier but a highly convenient highway and bridge, for anyone with a boat.

The fact, combined with very close ethnic ties, made any distinction between the peoples on the two sides entirely artificial. It therefore had to be vehement if it was to take effect. The English defined themselves as the haters of the French, and vice versa. The Channel is a highly conspicuous division, like a line drawn between squabbling groups on a playground – and almost as easy to step over.

Such real differences as there are between the English and the French owe something to geology. In basic respects the rocks are similar on the two sides of the various sections of the English Channel. Thus Brittany, the Channel Islands and the Cherbourg Peninsula on the French side have much in common with the Scilly Isles, Cornwall and Devon. There is an awful lot of granite, unforgiving to the hulls of careless boats. It comes from the roots of mountains, long–since vanished, that were formed in two collisions of continents, around 600 and 300 million years ago. Passages, estuaries and harbours occupy fault-lines that crisscross the old highly stressed rock-masses.

The creation of the Channel itself began with the opening of a rift valley between Brittany and England about 115 million years ago. The Channel was not completed until a dam of chalk running from South Foreland near Dover to Cap Blanc Nez near Calais finally burst, probably sometime during the last Ice Age – perhaps 60,000 years ago. The French and English shores of the eastern Channel also have much in common, geologically, with chalk as a dominant theme.

The chalk was built from the corpses of small marine organisms living in a warm sea in the days of the dinosaurs. Knock-on effects of Italy's collision with Switzerland, which made the Alps, pushed slabs of chalk into the air. Older or younger sandstones and clays feature on many shores of the Channel, but on the whole its margins consist of chalk at one end and granite at the other.

The ethno-geological point is that this is much less of an oversimplification on the French side of the Channel than on the English side. The white cliffs of Dover may be more famous, but the white cliffs of Normandy are far more extensive. They stretch from the Seine to the Somme in a great wall, daunting to mariners. Sailing along the English coast, on the other hand, one finds the geology changing at almost every headland: young shingle at Dungeness, old sandstones and clay at Fairlight, the reappearing chalk at Beachy Head, young boulders at Selsey Bill, and so on. Even the granite masses of the far west are modulated with sandstones, mudstones, the transformed granite of the china clay workings near St Austell, and the bizarre serpentine of the Lizard.

England's geology, in short, is much fussier than France's, with everything on a smaller scale. This reflects the fact that the British Isles have been Europe's bumper in a long succession of continental collisions and splits. The economic result is that the regions of southern England are more self-sufficient than those of northern France, with different kinds of farmland and woodland, and often ores too, within easy reach.

Sussex is the classic example. It was organized in Saxon times into 'rapes' – strips little more than 10 miles wide and running from the shore to some 20–30 miles inland. Each rape was a little England, with its river port for trade and fishing, its grazing on the chalk downs, its arable land on the clay beyond the downs, and its timber supplies and iron mines on the forested sandstone ridge of north Sussex.

For equivalent resources, the French had to look much farther afield, from one great geological province to others. This helped to encourage a nationwide economy and centralised government, which until very recently was a good deal stronger in France than in England. The cross-Channel contrast, apparent immediately to any observant sailor, suggests that the tradition of English county loyalties owes more than a little to the richness of geology. So perhaps do the traits that George Orwell applauded in the English – a scorn for high philosophy, and general bloody-mindedness.

These historical and geological glimpses may persuade the reader that the Channel is a highway replete with interest and welcoming to boats. Prudence requires the usual remark about the sea being a treacherous friend, and the need for boats to be well found and navigated with care, having due regard for the weather. But let me end mischievously by recalling the smugglers, who plied to and fro more frequently and unpredictably than even the most enthusiastic cruising sailor. For them, the ideal weather for a Channel crossing was a gale with rain or fog, on a moonless night. Then the revenue men could never catch them.

# Beyond the tin-opener

*Food is an essential part of any cruise. With 25 years'
experience catering aboard small craft from the Baltic to
the Bay of Biscay,* **Sylvia Parker** *offers ideas to the
ship's cook and introduces us to France's justifiably
famous fresh food.*

## IMAGINATIVE COOKING AFLOAT

I believe that interesting food is second only to safety on board; if the
cook finds cooking a chore it will show in the tasting. Some meals on
board will inevitably be routine tin-opening times, but these can easily
be interspersed by more imaginative feasts. They need not be
extravagant. The aim should be maximum enjoyment from a
reasonably economic use of time, effort and gas. A useful rule of
thumb is 20–25 minutes maximum for the cooking time of any one
item by oven, grill or top burner. Avoid being over-ambitious – after an
energetic day very few cooks are capable of intricate cooking of three
courses in a small galley. If one course involves juggling with cooker
and pans, plan two easy courses to go with it.

Forward planning pays dividends. The more orderly your storage of
food and cooking equipment the less effort you will waste in finding
items. Avoid large storage spaces where small items get lost: break up
the space with small cardboard boxes. Make a record of the basic stores
put on board at the start of a holiday and later mark amounts left of each
item and refer to this for the next cruise. A record of daily main meals
will give you a flying start next time: build on your own successes.

Skipper co-operation is invaluable. A skipper relies heavily on your
help on deck, so insist on knowing estimated times of departure and
arrival. Skippers tend to leave at the *first* possible tidal time, but a
slightly later time may enable a quick errand ashore for fresh food, so
negotiate. Prepare meals early so that you can join the others for a
relaxing aperitif before completing last-minute cooking.

*Some extra items of equipment*
- A pressure cooker – saves water and gas and enables cooking of
  several items at the same time
- A heavy bottomed pan – for reheating pre-cooked food
- A small hand-held grater
- A plastic bottle carrier for safe stowage of wine, cooking oil, etc. –
  also handy at table and when shopping
- A Sodastream dispenser – will pay for itself very quickly.

Before buying any of the newer type of cooking pots or a wok, check
that the fiddle on your cooker gives sufficient space.

*Some basic standbys*

- Large jars of good quality bottled mayonnaise – keep well in a locker not exposed to heat
- Tomato purée
- Rice – some types take less water and cooking than others (e.g. Basmati)
- Pasta – use the energy-saving method: follow packet instructions but boil pasta for only 2 minutes; switch off gas, cover with a tight fitting lid (use a teatowel between pan and lid) and leave for the full cooking time given on packet; drain and serve
- Potatoes – a few tins for emergencies. French supermarkets sell *pommes minute* – vacuum-packed bags of whole, sliced or diced cooked potatoes for boil-in-the-bag, sauté or salads
- Herbs, spices, curry paste/powder, capers, gherkins, olives, bottled lemon juice
- Flour, powdered milk, UHT or longlife yogurt and cream for freshly made sauces – much better than packet sauces; if butter is short, use cooking oil and flavour well to compensate; use arrowroot or cornflour for thickening
- Cooking chocolate – keeps remarkably well in a tin away from heat
- Packets of grated cheese – if stowed sensibly, these keep for a few days out of refrigeration
- Breadcrumbs – UK varieties are not as good as French *chapelure*
- A selection of nuts for salads and desserts
- Luxury items to enliven ordinary fare. French supermarkets are particularly good for: tinned asparagus, artichokes, and heart of palms, bottled *carottes râpées* (grated carrot) and *céleri-rave* (raw celeriac) as bases for crudités and hors d'oeuvre; tinned sardines, tuna and mackerel in various sauces for excellent starters with a salad garnish; top-quality tinned soups and packets of garlic croûtons.

## STARTERS
### Crudités/hors d'oeuvre
For example, raw salad vegetables, including sliced mushroom and courgette; tinned fish; prawns; rollmops; ham; olives and gherkins.
### Egg mayonnaise
Serve with paprika garnish.
### Vegetables
- **Mushrooms** cooked in oil with coriander; add lemon juice, salt and pepper. Serve hot or cold.
- Fresh **haricots verts,** cooked and tossed in butter or oil, garlic and freshly ground pepper.
- **Tomatoes** stuffed with cream cheese and herbs.
### Cheese
- **Crottins** (small goat's cheeses) warmed in the oven, or toasted on bread and served with crisp lettuce.

- **Brie** grilled lightly, then sprinkled with flaked almonds and grilled again.

**Seafood**

Look for local specialities such as Guernsey crabs, Breton sardines, Ostend mussels, St Vaast oysters. Try using fresh lime instead of lemon for a sharper taste.

- **Scallops** – simply wrap each cleaned scallop in a rasher of streaky bacon and grill until bacon is crisp.
- **Prawns** – one or two large langoustines are better than six small prawns. Serve in shell with lemon wedge and mayonnaise. Or gently cook unpeeled prawns in oil with oregano, rosemary, garlic and pepper, then add white wine and cook for 3 minutes.
- **Mussels** – clean thoroughly, remove 'beard', and discard any open or damaged shells. For *moules à la marinière*, combine shallots cooked in butter with dry white wine, parsley, thyme and pepper in a saucepan; add mussels and steam until shells open, discarding unopened ones. For *moules farcies*, steam mussels, discard empty half of each shell, and layer mussels in the other half shell in a grillpan; sprinkle with breadcrumbs, parsley, plenty of garlic, and melted butter; grill.
- Fresh **sardines** and **sprats** – descale former; grill.
- **Crab** – serve legs in shell; or try crabmeat mixed with cream or mayonnaise, mustard, Worcestershire sauce, lemon juice and pepper and grilled for devilled crab.

MEAT

**Ham and mushroom gratin**

Layer medium-cut cooked ham (fresh or tinned) on bottom of grill-proof dish. Cover with a layer of drained chopped mushrooms. Cook onion and garlic in butter, then add a little wine vinegar and reduce by half. Add tomato purée and water or wine to make a thick sauce; season. Pour sauce on to ham and mushrooms. Top with grated cheese and breadcrumbs. Grill 10 minutes before serving until top is bubbling and browned.

**Goulash** (when fresh beef is not available)

Cook onion and garlic in oil. Add tinned tomatoes (drained of liquid) and tomato purée, paprika, salt and fresh or tinned cream. Add high-quality tinned stewed steak and heat carefully to prevent meat disintegrating.

**Chicken**

Boned breasts cook quickly but space is a problem when cooking for more than two. Get round this by using ready-cooked chicken and reheating thoroughly in a sauce – the safest way is to skin and cut the chicken into large bite-size pieces before adding to a sauce. Use any available ingredients for a sauce, such as white wine or sour cream with toasted sesame seeds enlivening a white sauce; or cooked onion, garlic and courgettes in tomato purée and red wine.

## Duck breasts

This is a real haute cuisine recipe that is well suited to a small galley. *Magret de canard* (duck breast) tends to be much larger in France than in the UK, so that each breast could give two servings. Season breasts and sauté in oil, skin-side down, for 8 minutes; turn over and sauté for 6 minutes. Remove from the pan, skin and slice. Use pan juices for a sauce: e.g. deglaze pan with a little vinegar, then add orange juice and water or wine and thicken. Taste and season. Reheat the sauce 5 minutes before serving, add breast slices and simmer for 2 minutes. Serve with fresh orange slices.

## Lasagne

This can be made without an oven by pre-cooking the pasta in boiling water. Use either cooked, diced ham or chicken or tinned minced meat (tinned ratatouille and mushrooms for vegetarians) and add to cooked onion and garlic. Mix in tomato purée and water to make a thick sauce. Layer the pasta and meat sauce alternately in a grill-proof dish. Top with a layer of drained spinach and cover with a thick white sauce flavoured with nutmeg, salt and pepper. Sprinkle with grated cheese and breadcrumbs. Grill just before serving until top is bubbling and brown.

FISH

There is a reluctance to cook fish on board, yet fish is often the freshest ingredient available to sailors. Try to overcome inhibitions or prejudice, such as that fish smells the boat out (curry is much more pervasive), or that it is difficult to prepare without large supplies of running water. Ask the fishmonger to head and tail, gut, clean and fillet the fish and rinse it.

Savour local specialities such as the huge scallops and large local plaice fillets in Fowey, local river salmon and trout in Devon and Cornwall.

Really fresh fish needs the minimum of cooking and is full of flavour. For a simple sauce to accompany it, mix together mayonnaise, lemon juice, capers, diced gherkin, pepper and salt.

## Whole cooked crab

Serve this with mayonnaise and fresh bread. The fishmonger will remove the inedible gills, but ask him to show you how to do this so that you are able to check before serving. In France you can buy special crab tools; nutcrackers are essential.

## Fruits de mer

A feast of crab, prawns, oysters, mussels. Serve with lemon, mayonnaise and fresh bread.

## Grilled fillets (plaice, sole, cod, etc.)

Place fillets in a well-oiled grillpan and sprinkle with lemon juice and oil, then with chopped garlic, grated lemon peel, parsley, thyme and breadcrumbs. Dot with butter and grill until browned.

Alternatively, place fillets in a well-oiled grillpan and smear with a coating of mayonnaise or sprinkle with grated cheese, with or without breadcrumbs; grill.

The same methods can be used with fish cutlets but allow extra grilling time and if the cutlets are thick, turn once and coat again during cooking.

**Whole round fish**

These are sometimes offered by fishermen as a gift. Have a bowl of water and plenty of kitchen paper handy before starting to head and gut, etc. If you have an oven, bake the fish whole or cut in two; brush with oil or butter or with yogurt, put in baking dish with wine, cider or stock, and herbs. Cover with foil. Preheat oven and allow 10 minutes' cooking time for each inch depth of fish (measured at its thickest point) at moderate heat. Alternatively, cut into cutlets and grill, or poach gently in milk, a fish bouillon stock, or a water, wine or cider stock. Warm the liquid, simmer the fish for 2–3 minutes, turn it over and poach for another 2–3 minutes. Use the liquid as the sauce base.

**Prawns provençale with rice**

Defrost frozen peeled prawns and add to a thickish sauce of cooked onion and garlic, tinned tomatoes, tomato purée, pepper and lemon juice. Add salt or sugar after tasting.

Cook rice separately. Reheat prawn mix just before serving and add more chopped garlic with a green herb. Peas are a colourful accompaniment.

**Monkfish** (*lotte* in French)

This fish may seem expensive, but there is very little waste. Remove the transparent membrane and grill, shallow fry, bake, poach, or use for kebabs. If poaching, cut the fish in slices and sauté briefly in butter. Remove fish and use the butter to make a sauce such as the tomato sauce in the recipe above or use double cream, grated peel and juice of lemon or lime, ginger, salt and pepper. Reheat the sauce 5 minutes before serving, add fish and simmer gently. If frying, simply dip 1-inch slices in seasoned flour, fry in oil and butter for 3–4 minutes. Sprinkle with garlic and turn the pieces after 2 minutes. Add lemon or lime juice and parsley.

## DESSERTS

- Fresh fruit is hard to beat.
- A little alcohol added to tinned, dried or fresh fruit does wonders. Try Calvados with stewed apple and Kirsch with fresh pineapple.
- In France the fresh apricots, peaches and nectarines are far superior to UK imports. For a change try gently poaching halved fruit with a syrup of honey or sugar, a little water, wine, cider or spirits. Pour sauce over fruit in individual dishes. Sliced apples or pears can also be used.

- Melt cooking chocolate and a knob of butter very gently in water (add rum or brandy if available). Serve tinned pineapple, pears or apricots in individual dishes on the table and quickly carry the hot chocolate from the galley and pour over the fruit – haste is essential. A bowl of chopped nuts for topping can be passed round.
- Pâtisseries in France are more appropriate as a dessert than a tea-time treat. If you are catering for a boatful, the plate-sized fruit flans look very impressive on the table.
- Fromage frais is delicious flavoured with fruit or just sugar.

## JOURNEY BOX
Always prepare before setting off and stow in a handy position a good amount of food and a flask of a hot drink. In fair weather it leaves more time to enjoy the sail, and in foul it is a life-saver. Pack sandwiches, tomatoes, hardboiled eggs, cheese cubes, slices of cake, biscuits, apples, grapes: this is *the* time for basic, non-rich foods.

*Bon voyage!*

## SHOPPING FOR FOOD IN FRANCE

Indulging in French food is an essential part of the French experience on a cruise. Standing in front of a good charcuterie or pâtisserie, or wandering round a colourful French market should whet even the most conservative appetites. If your command of French is not good, buy a small French/English dictionary and carry it with you.

### Supermarkets and hypermarkets
These are usually a short distance out of town but are economic for wine and spirits. Resist the temptation to buy everything under one roof, thereby missing the quality and fun of using the small specialist shops.

### Markets
It is worth staying in port for a market day in town. Superb quality fruit, vegetables, fish, cheese and meat are to be found in all markets, but those in towns are also very entertaining and a highlight of a French holiday. At first glance there is a bewildering number of stalls selling the same produce. Notice where the locals queue and join them.

Markets offer a marvellous range of types and sizes of very fresh onions, garlic, tomatoes, lettuce, peaches and grapes. Stallholders selling mushrooms will be delighted to tell you how to cook and serve their produce.

Cheese stalls are good value and it is nostalgic to see large slabs of country butter and huge bowls of fresh cream on display. It is also an opportunity to wean your crew away from Camembert and Brie – although those too are at their best in the markets along this coast. Try

Cantal for a tasty hard cheese, Bleu d'Auvergne or Fourme d'Ambert for blue types, Chaource, Boursault or Epoisses for creamy cheeses.

Children will love the pizza vans where you watch the chef baking the bases and filling with a wide choice of ingredients.

BOUCHERIE (butcher)
Small boucheries can be off-putting because little meat is on open display. The French give priority to care for the product so they do not pre-cut; the meat is kept refrigerated, and is stripped of excess fat and gristle before weighing. Also, the French way of processing carcasses into various cuts differs from that in the UK, especially for beef.

**Beef cuts**
*Aiguillette:* top rump or flank (braising)
*Bavette:* lower sirloin
*Bifteck:* fillet steak
*Chateaubriand* steak: centre, thickest part of fillet
*Contrefilet/Faux-filet:* eye of the sirloin. Tender steaks
*Entrecôte:* sirloin or rump. A good 1/2-inch thickness recommended.
*Filet mignon/Tournedos:* slices from the fillet
*Jarret de boeuf:* shin
*Onglet:* breast or lower ribs, similar to skirt steak.

Bifteck hâché makes an economical meal, worlds away from beefburgers: lean steak is sliced off in front of the customer, fed into a mincing machine and then moulded into shape. Freshly made and high-quality, it simply needs grilling/frying.

**Veal**
*Côte/Côtelettes:* cutlets from the ribs.

**Pork**
*Côte/Carré/Echine:* chops
*Pointe de filet:* tenderloin
*Noisettes:* cutlets from loin.

There is a much wider use of escalope cuts in France – not just veal, also turkey (*dindon/dindonneau*) and pork, needing only brief cooking.

**Lamb** is the most expensive meat but do try it in a good restaurant. Fresh **duck** breasts *(magret de canard)* are much bigger than in the UK, so that each breast could give two servings. ***Chevaline*** (horsemeat shops) are clearly named.

CHARCUTERIE (delicatessen)
These are often of a much higher standard than charcuterie counters in supermarkets. They have a wide range of cooked meats, hams, pâtés, terrines and stuffings (*farces*) prepared on the premises. Products are not pre-cut so specify the number of slices (*tranches*) you want. Experiment with the savoury pastries on offer.

A charcuterie offers an excellent learning situation – look carefully at salad mixes, which are expensive to buy but cheaper to copy on board. For example, mushrooms à la grecque are tinned or cooked fresh button mushrooms in tomato purée, seasoning, thyme and coriander.

Good buys are freshly made mayonnaise for a richer accompaniment to shellfish, and *céleri-rave rémoulade* (raw celeriac in mayonnaise).

Caution: the French perform culinary marvels with offal and cheap cuts which are not always to our taste, so learn the appropriate words for liver (*foie*), brains (*cervelles*), etc., and the cheaper products such as *fromage de tête de veau* (from calf's head), *rillettes* (potted meat), *boudin noir* (black pudding), and *ris*, which is sweetbreads not rice (*riz*). *Andouillette/andouille* is intestine filled with strips of chitterlings and stomach: a tripe sausage very popular in France.

TRAITEUR (ready-cooked foods)
On offer here are home-cooked dishes, haute cuisine rather than fast-foods. There is usually a range of three or four dishes per day, from *coq au vin, pintade, magret de canard, paupiettes de veau* and *boeuf bourguignonne* to *paella* and *couscous*, to give just a few examples, or fish on Fridays. Compare the full cost of dining ashore with that of a feast on board using a *traiteur* dish with fresh *haricots verts, pommes de terre Dauphine* (a good buy from *traiteurs*), preceded by, say, fresh prawns and followed by cheeseboard and pâtisserie, with wine costing a fraction of that in a restaurant.

*Traiteur* dishes are ready for mid-day meals though still on sale (cold) all day; you will need a heavy bottomed pan for gentle reheating. You can order *traiteur* dishes a day ahead but check what time they will be ready and always, in shop or restaurant, ask for details before ordering *le plat du jour*.

Freshly grilled/barbecued chickens sold in special foil-lined bags for reheating in the oven are recommended, and on Sundays there is often a spit-roasted joint of beef to buy a portion from.

POISSONNERIE (fishmonger)
Where these exist, mainly in towns, they are usually excellent. In very hot weather they may well have no fish on display, merely a list of fish under refrigeration. Large towns, such as Cherbourg, have a permanent fish market (often mornings only) and fish shops (closed 1200–1500/1600). There is no problem about getting fish filleted or gutted.

**Some fish names**

| | |
|---|---|
| *Aiglefin/Eglefin:* haddock | *Merlan:* whiting |
| *Bar/Loup de mer:* seabass | *Morue:* cod |
| *Barbue:* brill | *Mulet:* grey mullet |
| *Colin:* hake | *Plie:* plaice |
| *Daurade:* seabream | *Raie:* skate |
| *Flétan:* halibut | *Rouget:* red mullet |
| *Grondin:* red gurnard | *St Pierre:* John Dory |
| *Lotte:* monkfish | *Saumon:* salmon |

**Shellfish**

*Calmars:* squid
*Coquille St Jacques:* scallop
*Crevettes:* prawns/shrimps
*Ecrevisse:* crayfish
*Homard:* lobster
*Huître:* oyster

*Langouste:* crawfish
*Langoustine:* Dublin Bay prawn
*Moules:* mussels
*Poulpe:* octopus
*Praires/Palourdes:* small clams

BOULANGERIE (bakery)
Go ashore for fresh croissants and bread early in the morning; most boulangeries open at 0600 hours, with a second baking in the afternoon.

- **Croissants** – ordinary or *au beurre* (richer and better).
- **White bread** – mainly baguette or larger loaves referred to as *grands*. Request *bien cuit* and a well-browned loaf will be specially chosen for you. Bread is undoubtedly better on day of purchase, but is still very good the next day either recrisped in the oven or sliced and toasted.
- **Brown bread** – a variety is available, such as *pain de seigle* (rye), *de six céréales, pain complet* (wholemeal), *de maïs* (maize). These make good sandwiches, better than bread sold for that purpose which tends to be tasteless; get the shop to slice it.
- **Pain de campagne** – as its name suggests, this differs from region to region.
- **Brioche** – cake from yeast dough.

PATISSERIE (confectioner)
These usually do not sell bread, though the two functions are often combined in small communities. Apart from a spectacular selection of cakes and pastries they often sell their own-made ice-cream. In France it is no disgrace to buy from the pâtisserie.

*Sunday shopping*
Mondays tend to be poor shopping days, and for good reason. There is an old French tradition of family Sunday lunch gatherings; consequently the following shops are usually open on Sundays until mid-day. The boucherie enables grand'mère to buy her main-course meat in top condition, whilst her offspring and their families bring the other courses from the charcuterie, poissonnerie, boulangerie and pâtisserie. All this is very convenient for visitors but means that these shops have a compensating closed day (*hebdomadaire*) each week, always listed on the door. There is usually provision for local boulangeries to take this in turn, or in small villages for a bread van to fill in at a fixed time, so make enquiries.

*Bon appétit!*

*French restaurants*

However much you buy fresh food, don't miss out on dining ashore. In France restaurants usually display their menus outside their premises, a helpful custom which is spreading to the UK. Set menus tend to vary in the number of courses rather than in quality, so that paying more will often buy you a larger meal rather than a more exciting one. The exception is when they are called *menu gastronomique* (the price is then often *astronomique*). Table wine (*vin ordinaire*), often provided in a carafe, and draught beer (*à la pression*) are relatively cheap but 'British' beverages such as tea and Scotch whisky and 'British' foods such as bacon and eggs are expensive. It is customary for a service charge to be added automatically to the cost of meals and refreshments bought in restaurants and cafés. The service charge may be included in the price shown, in which case it will be called *prix net*. However, if your receipt bears the words *service non compris* add a tip of approximately 15 per cent to the total sum. Children are much more welcome in restaurants on the continent than in the UK and children's helpings are readily available.

# Cruising with children

*The all-too-short summer cruise may be a delight for adults but young crew members can take an entirely different view of a sailing holiday.*
**Trish and Ray Simpson-Davis** *have sailed the Atlantic with their children, and have written this section with their enjoyment in mind.*

As with all family matters, a little forethought and compromise are vital ingredients for a successful cruise. Passages are an unwelcome addition to a bucket and spade holiday for younger children and you may decide to use the boat as a 'floating caravan' for the first years, making short hops as weather and inclination dictate. Our family once spent a week nosing round the Isle of Wight, discovering delights ashore and afloat we had rushed past for years in 'Ushant or bust' days.

A realistic assessment of your children's capabilities is vital: whilst our kids are OK indefinitely in Force 0–1, in upwind conditions, an hour at Force 4–5 is enough, although they do improve as the holiday goes on. In crossing the Atlantic twice, the eldest one was only ever sick once – between Cowes and Swanage! Tuning everyone up beforehand with a few weekends bouncing at anchor will help considerably, but we abort plans to go to sea when the forecast is doubtful. We were very purist before we had children but now motorsail upwind shamelessly to minimise uncomfortable passages. We use fair tides as much as possible, particularly when working westwards; settled weather will often see us anchored in the lee of a headland or in a bay for a few hours waiting the tide and giving the crew a run ashore.

Children need realistic time estimates. It's worth realising that your child's definition of the passage begins as you leave the marina berth and ends when the dinghy lands on the beach at the other end, whereas for you the passage is psychologically much shorter. Murky blobs on the horizon are definitely not interesting for children although they may be riveting to you as the successful navigator. It's probably best to let sleeping (or happily playing) children lie, and discourage expeditions on deck unless conditions are calm.

Two excellent activities for young children on passage are sleeping and eating. Sleeping is the most important, and with a little careful planning can be used with children until they are old enough to be interested in working the boat. Spend the morning on any physical activities ashore, follow with a picnic lunch underway, and the kids will often be prepared to zizz for a couple of hours whilst the adults enjoy the fair-going tide. The children can then stay up late into the evening as you all sample the delights of the new port.

For the longer haul, it's worth considering an overnight passage when the children can sleep for a good part of the time. For example, at the beginning of a cruise to the West Country we might make short hops on the tide from Southampton to Weymouth. Then, after a full day stopover, we would make a night crossing of Lyme Bay having used the inshore passage within a ship's biscuit toss of Portland Bill as an interesting feature before bedtime. This gives us nine hours or so before the children reappear, when we will be close to Salcombe or Dartmouth.

Use of sleep time may be a way to make distance in otherwise unsuitable weather, but two competent watchkeepers, one on watch, one off, are essential for night passages, to allow a safety margin. With children on board someone will also have to cope the next day – it's better for family harmony if the joys and horrors are shared equitably.

Early starts – say 0300 or 0400 – can be useful if the adults can squeeze in an adequate night's sleep before leaving the anchorage. This may prove to be the only alternative if there is just one watchkeeper on board and/or the boat cannot be worked single-handed. In our experience, adapting for single-handed sailing is essential for serious cruising with tiny children who require constant attention from one parent whilst they're awake.

Food that takes a long time to eat is useful. We carry tiny cheesy biscuits, sultanas, or crisps, and supplies of snack foods such as biscuits, chocolate bars and fruit, for meals underway. We have also discovered a marvellous bonus to not having sweets at home: producing surprise packets of sweets during rough passages transforms the ambience immediately.

What else can children do on passage? With very young children, the inescapable truth is that the next best resource after Sleep and Food is You. Cuddling, singing, reading, story telling, and finger games become second nature. Later, provided that conditions are stable enough for them to remain below, they will probably prefer the cuddly toys, games and activities that are the current favourites at home, so as many of these as there is room for should be packed. Add to these a selection of pencils, felt tips, papers, colouring books, etc. In general, choose activities that are at the child's level or below, and if you will be reading to them, go for pictures with lots to talk about or a familiar text that you can read with your eyes closed (you may need to!). Story-telling tapes are excellent: apart from the commercial ones available, we had Grandma reading chapters from a favourite book, a reassuringly familiar voice in a North Atlantic gale!

Reference books on sea birds, seashore life, wild flowers and the next port are worth carrying aboard for older children. Although cards and commercial games are good for an evening session at anchor, they often need a stable platform so are useful only for calm days, but *Guess Who, Connect 4* and travelling sets can be played in a rolling seaway. We also had hours of fun from mini table tennis set up on the saloon table.

If becalmed in hot weather set up a paddling pool in the cockpit (a baby bath is a versatile piece of kit to carry). Any toys – bucket, watering can, plastic tea set – can be fun, and add ad hoc toys from the galley. Encourage older children to get involved in imaginative games, using props from the ship's stores. For example, Coastguards was a wow for a whole summer, using a portable tape recorder as the radio telephone, with frequent weather forecasts broadcast through the main hatch. Another game involved rock climbing up the saloon (we were close hauled at the time). Essentially, though, our children have tended to play the same games that are currently popular at home – doctors, shops, schools, and so on, which you can predict and provision for.

As the children grow they will become more interested in working the ship, and less dependent on adults for entertainment on passage. Cruising with young children is hard work, but if it's enjoyable enough for them, you will all have a great deal of fun and with luck your children will grow into enthusiastic sailors who will still want to cruise with the old salts.

# SOUTH-WEST ENGLAND

# Isles of Scilly – St Mary's

Sailing in the Scillies demands a meticulous standard of seamanship. Visiting yachts must be well found and the inexperienced should not come here. That said, the local people are welcoming and generous with help. The islands are run efficiently and services are very well established for visitors, but all supplies are brought in by sea or air, so not everything is readily available.

The Scillies archipelago was formed by the sea encroaching upon a large area of granite and most of the islands are little more than outcrops of rock. Of the larger ones, five are inhabited. St Mary's, the largest of all, has a coastline of nine miles and the only harbour in the Scillies, Hugh Town. However, there are many anchorages among the islands to enjoy in settled weather.

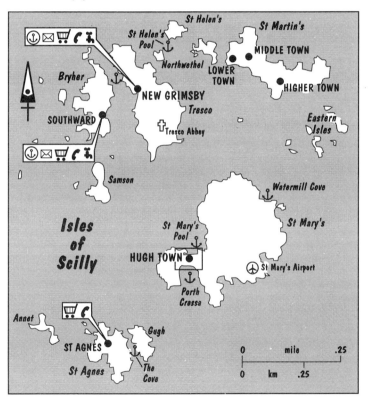

## SHORE LEAVE

### Food and drink

There are several pubs; opening hours are 1100–2300. Tregarthens Hotel in Hugh Town has excellent food and splendid sea views. Other hotels and restaurants are listed in the local guides and all give good value for money. Star Castle is a hotel converted from an Elizabethan castle with inspiring views from the ramparts.

### Entertainment

Events and entertainments are advertised outside the Town Hall. Dances, discos, concerts and plays are held there regularly, and so are slide shows on various aspects of the Scillies. Racing of traditional six-oar gigs takes place on Wednesday and Friday evenings in summer and at the end of August a carnival is held.

### What to see

The museum in Church Street has a display of the islands' history, geology, geography and a fully rigged gig; the **Longstone Heritage Centre** exhibits local and maritime history. There are artists' studios to visit, a glass-blowing works at Porthmellon, potteries near the airport and at the Garrison and an aquarium at Porthcressa Beach.

### Excursions

A well-organised boat system runs to many of the islands from St Mary's from March to October. You can land at **Tresco, St Agnes, St Martin's, Bryher** and **Samson**, see the puffins at **Annet**'s bird sanctuary, the seals on the **Western Rocks** and chat to the keeper of the **Bishop Rock Lighthouse.**

### Exercise

There are many walks of great beauty and interest. A leaflet from the Tourist Information Centre at Porthcressa Beach describes the one-hour circular **Garrison Walk**, the two-hour walk to **Peninnis Headland** and the three-hour **Telegraph Walk** to the highest point on the islands. Guided history and flower walks start from the quay on weekdays. Clubs and trolleys can be hired at the golf club. There is organised diving in clear water, and all the islands have safe, clean beaches with plenty of room, although the water is cold. Porthmellon Beach has a Windsurfing Centre.

### TRANSPORT AND TRAVEL

**Buses** On St Mary's
**Planes** Helicopters fly to Penzance every day except Sundays. The Skybus flies regularly to Land's End in summer, with a car service to Penzance railway station
**Ferries** Daily to Penzance from Monday to Saturday and on about six summer Sundays

**Taxis** St Mary's Taxi Service
☎ (0720) 22555
**Car and bicycle hire** Buccabu Hire
☎ (0720) 22289
**Travel agent** Isles of Scilly Steamship Co
☎ (0720) 22357

**Further information** from Tourist Information Centre at Porthcressa Bank – look for the flag. Open 0830–1700, 0900–1700 Saturdays. Closed Sundays.

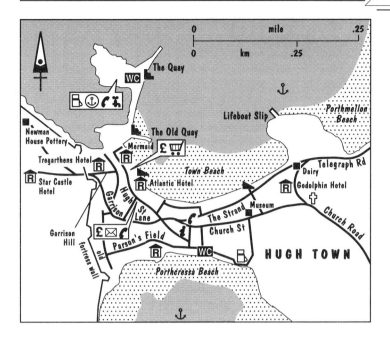

# Hugh Town Harbour

| | |
|---|---|
| **Harbourmaster** ☎ (0720) 22768 | **VHF Channels** 16 (working 14) |
| **Callsign** St Mary's Harbour | **Daily charge** ££ |

Hugh Town is not an enclosed harbour. There is no marina here and very little alongside berthing, so anchorages are the general rule. Changes in weather may require a shift of berth, as anchors can drag in strong westerlies. A crew of two cannot explore ashore and look after the boat unless the weather is settled. Although the weather can be heavy, and it is not advisable to leave a boat here except in an emergency, security is good.

## STEP ASHORE

**Nearest payphone** At the rear of the quay buildings
**Toilets, showers** On the quay
**Launderette** At Porthcressa (open 0900–1750)
**Clubhouse** Isles of Scilly Yacht Club on the quay
**Shopping** Hugh Town, St Mary's main commercial centre, is little more than a village by mainland standards. There are about 20 shops, including a chemist, post office, and Lloyds and Barclays banks (with cash dispensers), which will buy foreign currency notes. Some shops stay open late in summer. Early closing Wednesdays in winter

### SHIPS' SERVICES

**Water** on the quay, but respect the island's short supply: do not waste it. Water is charged at 2p a gallon, the cost price

**Fuel** (diesel and petrol) At the rear of the quay buildings; prices are expensive compared with those in mainland England and France because of shipping costs. You should make arrangements with the harbourmaster before taking on fuel or water because of the needs of commercial shipping

**Gas** (Camping and Calor) From H K Solomon and **Chandler** Scillonian Marine. The Isles of Scilly Steamship Co also sells chandlery

**Boat repairs** Tom Chudleigh
☎ (0720) 22505

**Engineer** D Parr, Unit IBS Porthmellon Industrial Estate; Isles of Scilly Steamship Co

**Sailmaker** K Buchanan
☎ (0720) 22037

# Tresco

Tresco is the second largest island in the Scillies. It is renowned for its gardens, which were started by Augustus Smith in 1834, with plants not seen in other parts of the British Isles.

Also in the grounds is Valhalla, a figurehead collection from ships wrecked around the islands. Yachts may anchor between the quay and Cromwell's Castle but must leave access to the quay clear for local craft.

Tresco is a private island and there is a landing charge. The Island Hotel is in *The Good Food Guide 1992*, recommended particularly for its local fish.

# Penzance

Once the major centre for the fishing and tin trades, Penzance has declined in importance as a port, but it remains a busy market town with plenty of charm, popular with tourists. It offers much of historical interest, notably Chapel Street at the top end of town, which has contrasting styles of architecture from the seventeenth and eighteenth centuries and the ornate Egyptian House. You may wish to hire a car to explore the coast or take a bus to Land's End to enjoy the magnificent scenery, but if you want to keep all your illusions about Land's End intact, don't go: it has recently been commercialised with a theme park.

The Minack Theatre is in a spectacular open-air setting on the cliffs at Porthcurno, three miles from Land's End. Remember to take a cushion for sitting on the stone seats; take a picnic too.

Penzance is a good springboard for reconnaissance by ferry or helicopter of the Isles of Scilly for a future sailing trip, or just to get away from it all. Be warned, though, that overnight accommodation there may well be difficult to find, even impossible, in the holiday season.

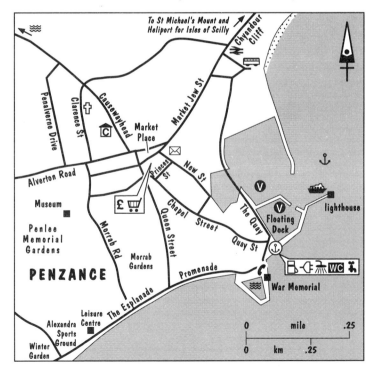

# SHORE LEAVE

### Food and drink
Penzance has a good selection of take-aways, bistros, pubs and restaurants. The Ganges in Old Bakehouse Lane serves excellent Indian food: it is both a restaurant and a take-away. The Admiral Benbow Inn in Chapel Street is good value for bar food. The Turk's Head Inn has a separate restaurant, but may be crowded, particularly during the tourist season.

### Entertainment
There is one cinema, the Savoy in Causewayhead ☎ (0736) 63330. The open-air **Minack Theatre** is at Porthcurno, nine miles away ☎ (0736) 810694. Buses and coaches run there.

### What to see
For a rainy day the museums and art galleries are a good resort. The **Nautical Museum** in Chapel Street displays hundreds of articles salvaged from wrecks. **Penlee House** in the Penlee Memorial Gardens has a permanent collection of the Newlyn Painting School. The **Egyptian House**, so called for its flamboyant Egyptian façade, was built about 1830 as a geological museum and, after years of neglect, restored by the Landmark Trust in 1973. It is now run by the National Trust and the Landmark Trust.

### Excursions
Day trips can be made to the **Isles of Scilly** by helicopter or by sea in the *Scillonian III*. **St Michael's Mount**, a twelfth-century Benedictine Priory and fourteenth-century castle, 275 feet above sea level, with harbour and hamlet at its foot, is accessible at low water across the causeway from Marazion. The harbour dries out so it may be easier to visit by land from Penzance than to sail there. Fishing trips and coastal cruises are on offer, if you can't keep away from the sea.

### Exercise
You can swim from the beach half a mile east of Penzance opposite the heliport, or enjoy the seawater swimming pool.

## TRANSPORT AND TRAVEL

**Buses** From the harbour (Station Road)
**Trains** To Plymouth and London with easy connections for many major cities
**Planes** British International Helicopters fly daily to St Mary's, Isles of Scilly, from Penzance; in summer the Skybus service is in operation from Land's End with a car service from Penzance railway station

**Ferries** From Penzance Monday to Saturday, and some summer Sundays, to St Mary's, Isles of Scilly
**Taxis** Harveys Taxis ☎ (0736) 66666
**Car hire** Vospers, Coinage Hall Street ☎ (0736) 69169
**Bicycle hire** Bike About, 1 Mount Street (about 100 yards from railway station) ☎ (0736) 50345

**Further information** from Tourist Information Office by the railway station, Alverton Street and The Guildhall, Street-an-Pol.

# Penzance Harbour

| | |
|---|---|
| **Harbourmaster** ☎ (0736) 66113 | **VHF Channels** 16, 12, 9 |
| **Callsign** Penzance Harbour | **Daily charge** ££; third night free |

There is no marina here, but a wet dock where visitors can berth. The berthing master will tell you where to lie. The outer drying harbour is full of local boats but you can anchor there (contact the harbourmaster first). The dock is secure in any weather and boats can be left unattended without concern for a few days, which makes it a good base to explore west Cornwall and the Land's End peninsula. That said, in strong southerly or south-easterly winds the lock gates cannot be opened and then it is probably wiser to keep away from Mount's Bay altogether. The dock is not the most attractive place to berth but that is more than compensated for by the warm and helpful welcome from the dock staff and the harbourmaster.

### STEP ASHORE

**Nearest payphone** On promenade opposite bathing pool or the harbour office in an emergency
**Toilets, showers** On the quay; get a key from the berthing master
**Shopping** Two minutes along Quay Street there are plenty of shops. Some close on Wednesday afternoons, but the main high-street shops stay open. Only newsagents open on Sundays. All the usual banks, building societies, bureaux de change, and a post office

### SHIPS' SERVICES

**Water and electricity** See berthing master
**Fuel** Diesel by arrangement with berthing master; petrol from local garage
**Gas** (Camping and Calor) From Bennetts, close to the railway station
**Chandler** Two good chandlers in Newlyn, a limited selection of chandlery at R Curnow on Albert Pier and Penzance Chandlers

**Boatyard** Facilities are limited. Drying out on Albert Pier by arrangement with harbourmaster in emergency
**Engineer** Albert Pier Engineering
☎ (0736) 63566
**Sailmaker** Matthews, New Street
☎ (0736) 64004

# Newlyn

| | |
|---|---|
| **Harbourmaster** ☎ (0736) 62523 | **Daily charge** ££; third night free |

Newlyn is a large fishing port but has limited moorings and facilities for visiting yachts. It is a sheltered port accessible at all stages of the tide. Water, petrol and diesel are available and there is the usual range of high-street shops. Newlyn is the home of the Newlyn School of artists which first developed around the turn of the century. Their works, which mostly make use of the harbours, sea, boats, landscape and sky of the area, and those of later painters, can be seen in the Newlyn Art Gallery.

# Mousehole

**Harbourmaster** ☎ (0736) 731511                 **Daily charge £**

The harbour is very small and dries out, but in good weather a visit to this picturesque village provides a worthwhile diversion. Yachts can anchor outside the harbour but should contact the harbourmaster on arrival. Water, petrol and diesel are available.

# Helford River

Here is a superb unspoiled river, a must for a visit on a west country cruise. Deep-sided wooded valleys and creeks wind in among quays and waterside houses. If you can take the ground you can go right up the river to Gweek on the tide.

Cars are banished to a car park at the top of the hill from Helford Village during the summer, fortunately for the residents, since the picturesque streets are narrow and draw tourists.

Helford Passage is the most commercialised part of the Helford River, centred round the Ferry Boat Inn.

## SHORE LEAVE

### Food and drink
There are restaurants and pubs serving food in Helford Village, Helford Passage and Gweek. Meals are also available at Porth Navas Yacht Club. The Shipwrights Arms in Helford is a charming thatched pub recommended in *Out to Eat*. Mellanoweth in Gweek serves good-value crêpes for summer lunches, full restaurant meals at other times, and is in both *Out to Eat* and *The Good Food Guide 1992*. Riverside in Helford offers more expensive evening meals and is featured in *The Good Food Guide 1992*.

### What to see
Historic boats on loan from the Exeter Maritime Museum can be seen on the river. The **Seal Sanctuary** at Gweek is especially popular with children. **Frenchman's Creek**, scene of Daphne du Maurier's book of the same name, draws intrigued readers. **Trebah Gardens** on the north bank of the river offers a pleasant day ashore, with acres of rare trees, shrubs and ferns and a wooded ravine leading to a private beach. You can leave your dinghy there and climb up to the gardens to pay. Put ashore on the public beach at Durgan for neighbouring **Glendurgan Garden**, owned by the National Trust, which is equally delightful.

### Exercise
There are plenty of walks with magnificent scenery; a good walk from Helford Passage crosses fields to Durgan with lovely views of the estuary. See also the *Holiday Which? Town and Country Walks Guide*, walk 14. You can swim from the beach at Helford Passage, and windsurf at Helford Point.

## TRANSPORT AND TRAVEL
The Helford River is easy to reach by road from Falmouth. See Falmouth (page 51) entry for more information.

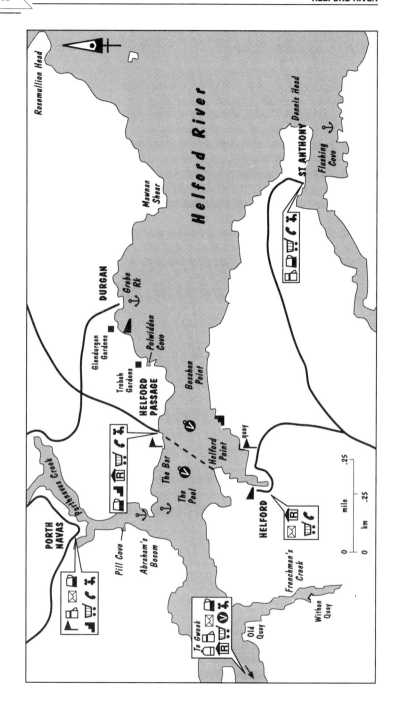

# Helford River Moorings

| | |
|---|---|
| **Moorings Officer** ☎ (0326) 280422 | **VHF Channel** M (occasionally) |
| **Callsign** Moorings Officer | **Daily charge** £ |

There are limited facilities but Falmouth is close if problems arise. The Helford River Sailing Club is very hospitable. The mooring officer is helpful and always ready to assist, particularly with information on local facilities. There is no water taxi but the passenger ferry from Helford Passage to Helford Point will pick up yachtsmen if hailed. There are dinghy landings at Helford Boatyard jetty where there is a small charge, or you can beach a dinghy at Helford Passage or Helford Village, and at Porth Navas on the tide.

## STEP ASHORE

**Nearest payphones** Durgan, St Anthony, Helford Village, Helford Passage, Porth Navas and Gweek
**Toilets and showers** Helford River Sailing Club when bar is open. Ferry Boat Inn,

Helford Passage, open 24 hours
**Clubhouse** Helford River Sailing Club
**Shopping** Most basics can be found at Helford Village, Helford Passage, Porth Navas and Gweek. Early closing Wednesdays

### SHIPS' SERVICES

*Fuel (diesel and petrol) Can be obtained alongside Porth Navas Yacht Club at high water. Diesel available at Gweek Quay*
*Gas (Camping and Calor) From Gweek Quay Boatyard*

*Chandler, boatyard, engineer Gweek Quay Boatyard; Sailaway, St Anthony*
*Sailmaker Spargo, King and Bennett Ltd, Penryn ☎ (0326) 72107; South West Sails, Penryn ☎ (0326) 75291*

---

*Alternative moorings*
**Gweek Quay** has drying moorings alongside which there is water and electricity, a chandler, café and pub and a general store, all useful for a short visit. **Flushing Cove** (St Anthony's Village) just south of the entrance to Helford River is also worth a visit. Here you must anchor and row ashore.

# Falmouth

Falmouth was once the main reporting point for sailing ships, homeward or outward bound, which might wait for days or weeks in the Roads for a fair wind. The fine natural harbour is on the estuary of seven rivers and has plenty to interest sailors both ashore and afloat. The main features are Falmouth Docks, Pendennis Castle and ocean-going shipping berths in Carrick Roads and beyond up the River Fal to King Harry Ferry. Look out for Peter de Savary's port development at Falmouth Docks. Gaffers racing in the Roads make a fine spectacle.

Falmouth is a good centre for exploring the creeks and rivers of the Fal Estuary, such as St Mawes, St Just-in-Roseland (with its exceptionally beautiful church by the water's edge), Mylor and Restronguet. Don't miss a cream tea at Smugglers Cottage, Tolverne Point.

As well as two marinas, there are Harbour Authority moorings and some moorings off the Royal Cornwall Yacht Club.

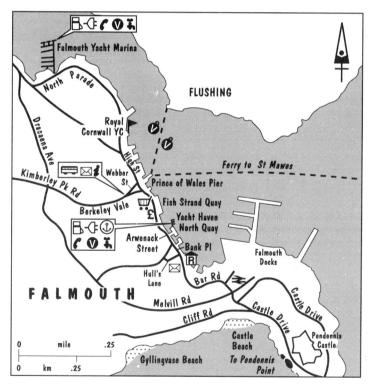

# SHORE LEAVE

*Food and drink*

Falmouth boasts plenty of pubs. Secrets is a very good bistro, as are The Pipe and Bonton Roulet; the Bamboo House Chinese Take-away is recommended and so is the Chainlocker for bar snacks. *Out to Eat* recommends DeWynne's Coffee House, 55 Church Street, for freshly made cakes and light lunches. Cornish Kitchen, 28 Arwenack Street, is a seafood bistro featured in *The Good Food Guide 1992*.

*Entertainment*

The **Arts Theatre** presents a wide variety of plays, as does the **Princess Pavilion**, which also stages concerts and variety shows. The nearest cinema is the Plaza in Truro ☎ (0872) 72894.

*What to see*

**Falmouth Art Gallery** and **Falmouth Maritime Museum** are interesting at any time and useful resorts in bad weather, but Falmouth is an outdoors town, with sights such as the 1929 Steam Tug *St Denys* used in the television series *The Onedin Line* – it now belongs to Falmouth Maritime Museum and lies at Custom House Quay. **Pendennis** and **St Mawes Castles** were built by Henry VIII in 1543 to protect Falmouth Harbour; both are open to the public. To visit St Mawes Castle, take the ferry from Falmouth at Prince of Wales Pier.

*Excursions*

Falmouth Harbour cruises last two hours, or you can take a trip up the Fal and Truro Rivers to **Truro**, visiting various creeks on the way; this is probably the best way to visit Truro as moorings and facilities are very limited there. If you do go up river, visit the National Trust **Trelissick Gardens**, which are only 100 yards from the ferry landing at King Harry Passage on the west bank of the Fal. These large gardens, planted with magnolias, camellias and rhododendrons as well as many rare shrubs, have commanding views over the Fal Estuary and Falmouth Harbour as well as riverside walks through the woods. There is also an exhibition gallery and an open-air theatre.

*Exercise*

There are cliff walks to **Swanpool Point** and **Maen Porth**. The good swimming beaches at Swanpool and Gyllingvase (some distance from the town) offer plenty of activities, too: windsurf, jetski and waterski at Gyllingvase and parascend at Swanpool, which also has a leisure centre and a swimming pool. Falmouth Regatta Week is the second week in August, when Falmouth Harbour is full but fun.

## TRANSPORT AND TRAVEL

**Buses** Coach services from The Moor, Falmouth

**Trains** Local to Truro, then fast to London

**Ferries** Local ferries to St Mawes and Truro

**Taxis** A1 Cabs ☎ (0326) 312404

**Car hire** Godfrey Davis Europcar Ltd ☎ (0326) 311093

*Further information* from Tourist Information Office at 28 Killigrew Street, off The Moor (Town Centre).

# Visitors' Yacht Haven, North Quay

| | |
|---|---|
| **Harbourmaster** ☎ (0326) 312285 | **VHF Channels** 16, 11 (working 12) |
| **Callsign** Falmouth Harbour Radio | **Daily charge** on pontoons ££, on trots £ |

This marina, open from April to October, is the first one on the port side on entering Falmouth Harbour. It is the best for shopping and useful for a short stay. Falmouth Harbour Commissioners run the marina and also provide two trots of bookable visitors' moorings between Greenbank Quay and Prince of Wales Pier, marked K1 to K6 and T1 to T5.

### STEP ASHORE

**Nearest payphone** In entrance to Chainlocker pub
**Toilets, showers** On Custom House Quay

**Shopping** Full selection of high-street shops, banks, building societies, bureaux de change and a post office in town centre nearby

### SHIPS' SERVICES

**Water and electricity** On pontoons
**Fuel** (diesel and petrol) From barge on visitors' pontoon, 0900–1800
**Gas** (Camping and Calor) From West Country Chandlers, Falmouth Yacht Marina

**Chandler** West Country Chandlers and Bosun's Locker, both in Falmouth Yacht Marina
**Boatyard** Falmouth Boat Construction Ltd (Cruising Association Boatman), Falmouth Yacht Marina
**Engineer** Marine-Trak, Falmouth Yacht Marina
**Sailmaker** Spargo, King and Bennett Ltd, Penryn ☎ (0326) 72107

# Falmouth Yacht Marina, North Parade

| | |
|---|---|
| **Harbourmaster** ☎ (0326) 316620 | **VHF Channels** 80, M |
| **Callsign** Falmouth Yacht Marina | **Daily charge** £££ |

This large modern marina is still expanding. It has good facilities and is open all year.

### STEP ASHORE

**Nearest payphone, toilets, showers** In marina
**Laundry** A collection service returns it the same day
**Shopping** Nearest shop is North Parade Stores opposite the marina entrance. Full

selection of high-street shops, banks, building societies, bureaux de change and a post office in the centre of Falmouth, about 15 minutes' walk away. Buses run there from the marina every 20 minutes

## SHIPS' SERVICES

**Water and electricity** *On the pontoons*
**Fuel** *(diesel and petrol) and* **gas** *(Camping and Calor) Available in the marina*

**Chandler, boatyard, engineer** *In the marina*
**Sailmaker** *Spargo, King and Bennett Ltd, Penryn* ☎ *(0326) 72107*

# Mylor Yacht Harbour

| | |
|---|---|
| **Harbourmaster** ☎ (0326) 72121 | **VHF Channels** 80, M |
| **Callsign** Mylor Yacht Harbour | **Daily charge** ££ |

This marina at the entrance to Mylor Creek has four pontoon berths for visitors and 12 moorings. It is well equipped with the usual marina facilities, such as telephone, toilets and showers, water and electricity on the pontoons, a fuelling berth, a chandlery and an engineer.

Mylor Yacht Harbour Ltd is the Cruising Association Boatman. Mylor was once the site of Britain's smallest Royal Dockyard but is now a popular yachting centre. The church merits a visit.

---

*Alternative moorings*
A little way up the Percuil river, round Polworth Point, is the **St Mawes Sailing Club Quay**. There are a few visitors' moorings, but it is necessary to book. The Club welcomes visitors, serves light lunches and suppers and will let you use the showers.

---

# Truro

It is an interesting sail through wooded valleys from Falmouth up the Truro River and Truro is well worth a visit, but one night is probably enough. The main attraction of this fine Georgian city is the cathedral. Holidaymakers come from all over Cornwall for shopping and sightseeing and Truro is to be avoided on a wet day when trippers are not on the beach.

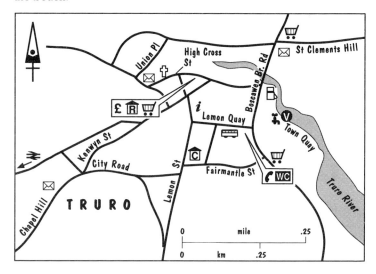

## SHORE LEAVE

### Food and drink
The Wig and Pen in Frances Street is good value; the William IV pub in Kenwyn Street offers both cold and hot food with friendly service; the Heron Inn (Malpas) is in a good position with a lovely view though the atmosphere is disappointing; bar food ranges from sandwiches and pies to quite elaborate dishes in the evenings. The Bustopher Jones wine bar, 62 Lemon Street, is good value and has a choice of vegetarian dishes and a welcoming atmosphere; it is featured in *Out to Eat*. Alverton Manor is a converted convent that is now as luxurious a restaurant as Truro has to offer and is recommended in *The Good Food Guide 1992*.

### Entertainment
The Plaza cinema is in Lemon Street.

### What to see
The **County Museum** in River Street is full of Cornish history and folklore; the **Museum of Entertainment** in Old Bridge Street focuses on the background to films, music hall, circus, radio and TV and has a puppet collection. **Truro Cathedral** is a fine late nineteenth-century building in early-English style. The Georgian houses in Lemon Quay, the main architectural feature of Truro, are the best west of Bath.

*Excursions*

There are coach trips to **Falmouth**, **St Mawes** and **Newquay**, and buses to **Trelissick Gardens**, where there are exhibitions and an open-air theatre in the grounds.

*Exercise*

From **Victoria Garden** to **Boscawen Park** and **Swan Pool** makes a pleasant circular walk. There are swimming pools at the Hydro Leisure Centre, Carricle Recreational Centre and at St George's Road. Cornwall Windsurfing Centre is at 63 Fairmantle Street ☎ (0872) 75342.

## TRANSPORT AND TRAVEL

**Buses** Cornwall Bus and Coachways, Lemon Quay to all parts of Cornwall
**Trains** Fast trains from Station Road to London

**Taxis** City Taxis ☎ (0872) 73053/73479
**Car hire** Europcar ☎ (0872) 76825; Vospers ☎ (0872) 73933

*Further information* from Tourist Information Centre, Boscawen Street.

# Truro Harbour

| | |
|---|---|
| **Harbourmaster** ☎ (0872) 72130 | **VHF Channel** 12 |
| **Callsign** Carrick 1 | **Daily charge** £ |

Truro is only accessible three hours either side of high water. You can berth at the eastern arm of the town quay.

## STEP ASHORE

**Nearest payphone** Lemon Quay
**Toilets** Lemon Quay
**Shopping** Shell garage at the bottom of Tregolls Road open till 0100. Truro has a full selection of high-street shops with

banks, building societies and a post office. Tesco superstore is adjacent to the town quay and is open until 2000 on Thursdays and Fridays

### SHIPS' SERVICES

*Water* Available on town quay
*Fuel* (diesel and petrol) From Reg Langdon, New Bridge Street, adjacent to town quay

*Engineer, sailmaker* Penrose Outdoors on town quay

# Mevagissey

| | |
|---|---|
| **Harbourmaster** ☎ (0726) 843305 | **Daily charge** £ |

This charming old Cornish fishing village has a few moorings for visiting yachts in the outer harbour, but it is advisable to contact the harbourmaster in advance to find out whether there will be room for you.

Situated to the west of Fowey, across St Austell Bay, it is very sheltered except from the east and south-east. Water, petrol, diesel, Calor and Camping gas are all available here and there are shops, including a chemist, a post office and several banks. There are pubs and restaurants, too: Mevagissey is popular with visitors. The **Model Railway Exhibition** in Meadow Street is of special interest. Mr Bistro on East Quay is a fish restaurant recommended in *Out to Eat*.

## Charlestown

This is a commercial port in St Austell Bay with lock gates where coasters load china clay for shipment through the canals of Europe. It is a picturesque place with sandy beaches on either side of the little harbour. Although not a pleasure port, there have been reports of yachts being well received and the crews finding it an interesting place.

Scenes from *The Onedin Line*, *Voyage of the Beagle* and other films have been shot here. The Charlestown Visitor Centre has very good displays of shipwrecks, around the Cornish coast in particular, including many artefacts brought up from the sea bed.

# Fowey

Fowey is an exceptionally attractive little town in a wooded valley on the estuary of the Fowey River. Houses from every period of its long history line the steep streets that climb the hillside. Because it has deep water and easy access, Fowey developed as a port in the twelfth century when Lostwithiel silted up, although the river is still navigable to Lostwithiel on a good tide. In the Middle Ages a large proportion of England's fleet was anchored in the river.

The town becomes very crowded at the height of the holiday season and cars are restricted, but it still retains its charm. The harbour is packed for the Fowey Royal Regatta and Carnival in August, when gaff-rigged working boats and Troys, 18-foot three-quarter-decked sloops dating from 1929, come to race.

Polruan, the fishing village across the harbour, intrigues with its little cottages and gardens clinging to an even steeper hillside. Its picturesque beauty, particularly when lit by the evening sun, tempts one to visit and explore. Polruan is easy to reach, either by the passenger ferry from Whitehouse Slip in Fowey or in your own dinghy.

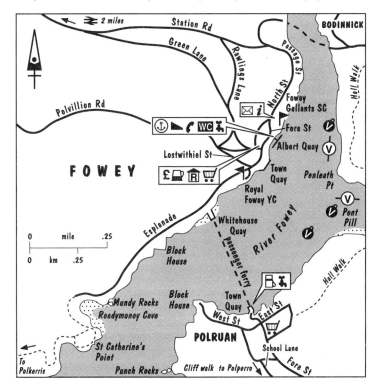

## SHORE LEAVE

*Food and drink*
The town has a very good selection ranging from fish and chips to bistro to restaurants. Try the Old Ferry Inn, Bodinnick, 400 years old, which overlooks Bodinnick Ferry; or the Ship Inn, Fowey, close to the town quay; the Galleon Inn welcomes children on the riverside patio. Food for Thought on the quay is recommended in *The Good Food Guide 1992*; it serves meat dishes which match the quality of the local fish.

*Entertainment*
The nearest cinema is at the Film Centre, St Austell ☎ (0726) 73750.

*What to see*
Blockhouses with a protective chain to seal the harbour against invading ships were built about 1380 and their ruins can still be seen. The **Polruan blockhouse** is accessible but not the one on the Fowey side of the harbour. The **Fowey Museum** is below the Town Hall (the entrance is in Trafalgar Square); it is very small, so there is not much space to display the wealth of evidence of Fowey's past, such as artefacts found during building excavation, items of clothing and old photographs. You can't miss the **aquarium** if you come ashore at Town Quay – it is in the bottom part of the Town Hall, in the same building as the museum. It specialises in local fish. **The Haven**, home of Sir Arthur Quiller-Couch, is on the Esplanade by the Whitehouse passenger ferry slip.

*Excursions*
Walk to **St Catherine's Point** at the harbour entrance and see the chapel where a light was kept burning as a lighthouse in medieval times. Below is a fort built by Henry VIII. Explore the upper reaches of the Fowey River in a dinghy. Look out for Par Docks, the principal outlet for china clay, used in porcelain and paper-making and shipped worldwide. It is the main industry for the St Austell area. Wheal Martyn on the Bugle Road out of St Austell is now the **China Clay Museum** and well worth a visit if you hire a car.

*Exercise*
There are many scenic and historically interesting walks round Fowey. The most famous is **Hall Walk**, sometimes called King's Walk as it was from here that Charles I was fired upon by the Roundheads. Start from Bodinnick, taking the ferry from Caffa Mill, and walk through the village to where the walk proper is signposted. Alternatively, take the passenger ferry to Polruan and climb up through the village to the headland to walk along the cliff path to **Polperro**. For views of the sea and ships in St Austell Bay, walk from **Readymoney Cove** to **Polridmouth Cove**, then on to **Polkerris**. A long-distance ramble (26 miles) would take you along the **Saints' Way** to Padstow. A free leaflet describing several walks is available from the Tourist Information Centre.

There is safe bathing from the sandy beaches of Readymoney Cove and Whitehouse Beach at Fowey, from Carne Beach opposite Town Quay and from Polruan Quay Beach; also from Lantic Bay, Lantivet Bay, West Coombe Cove and Polridmouth Cove east of the estuary.

## TRANSPORT AND TRAVEL

**Buses** Local buses run to Truro
**Trains** The nearest main line railway station is at Par
**Ferries** Local passenger and cycle ferry from Whitehouse Quay to Polruan, car and passenger ferry from Caffa Mill to Bodinnick
**Car hire** David Shand at St Austell

☎ (0726) 851816 – delivery and collection service available
**Taxis** Tony Baseley ☎ (0726) 833385
**Water taxi** A good service runs from Albert Quay 0800–2330 seven days a week; VHF Channel 16 or 6 ☎ (0726) 832450

*Further information* from Tourist Information Centre, 4 Custom House Hill (in the post office).

# Fowey Moorings

| | |
|---|---|
| **Harbourmaster** ☎ (0726) 832471 | **VHF Channels** 16 (working 12) |
| **Callsign** Fowey Harbour Radio | **Daily charge** £ |

Fowey is virtually equidistant from Plymouth and Falmouth, which makes it a convenient place to put into. There is no marina and the main area for visitors' moorings, opposite the Royal Fowey Yacht Club, can be uncomfortable in south-westerly blows. Off Polruan it can be quite rough when there is wind against the tide. Communications by land are poor and changing crews will need to travel via St Austell.

## STEP ASHORE

**Nearest payphone** Near town quay or Royal Fowey Yacht Club
**Toilets** Town quay or Royal Fowey Yacht Club
**Showers** Royal Fowey Yacht Club
**Launderette** Dhobi Room in Passage Street by Fowey Boatyard 0800–2000 (1200 Sundays)
**Clubhouse** Royal Fowey Yacht Club, Whitford Yard, has excellent facilities for visitors, including a good bar and meals by arrangement. The Fowey Gallants

Sailing Club, upstream of Albert Quay, also welcomes visitors; the bar is open during the week and food is served at weekends
**Shopping** A small selection of high-street shops meets all general requirements. There are three banks and a main and sub-post office. VG Foodstore opens Sunday mornings. Cottage Stores, 19 West Street, Polruan is open seven days a week. Early closing Wednesdays and Saturdays except during high summer

### SHIPS' SERVICES

*Water On Albert Quay pontoon – free mooring for up to two hours at Albert Quay pontoon, which is dredged and accessible at all states of the tide*
*Fuel (petrol and diesel) From floating barge, Fowey Refueller (VHF Channel 16) and from Winkle Picker Chandlery at Polruan Quay*
*Gas (Camping and Calor) Troy Chandlery,*

*Lostwithiel Street, and Upper Deck Marine on Albert Quay*
*Chandler Troy Chandlery, Winkle Picker Chandlery, Upper Deck Marine and Fowey Marine at Caffa Mill*
*Boatyard Fowey Boatyard, Passage Street*
*Engineer C Toms and Sons (Cruising Association Boatman) in Polruan*
☎ *(072687) 252*
*Sailmaker Mitchell Sails, North Street*

# Polperro

The harbour dries and has little room for yachts and no facilities for them. It is safe to anchor in the outer harbour in settled weather. This old fishing village is attractive and colourful although commercialised and overcrowded in the season; the pubs and restaurants are usually full. There are small shops, a post office and two banks in the village. The Kitchen in The Coombes is a small, popular restaurant recommended in *The Good Food Guide 1992*. *Out to Eat* features the Sun Lounge, which serves meals all day.

# Looe

This small port dries and has little room for yachts. It is on a useful branch-line railway leading to the main line and to Plymouth. Looe has an active fishing fleet: don't lie alongside fishing boats. The *Holiday Which? Good Walks Guide* walk 9 describes a route around both these villages.

# Plymouth Sound

Plymouth is a delightful mixture of old and new – despite severe destruction during the Second World War and subsequent rebuilding, there are still many old buildings, such as Foulton's Oddfellows Hall, the eighteenth-century houses in St Aubyns Street and the Merchant's House in St Andrews Street. The district round Sutton Harbour, known as the Barbican, has kept its character as an old port, with cobbled streets and a fish market on the quay. The Naval Dockyards have many eighteenth-century buildings. This major naval port has witnessed the departure of ships and seafarers of all descriptions, from pirates, Elizabethan sea-captains and the Pilgrim Fathers to the great battleships of recent times and Sir Francis Chichester on his circumnavigation of the world.

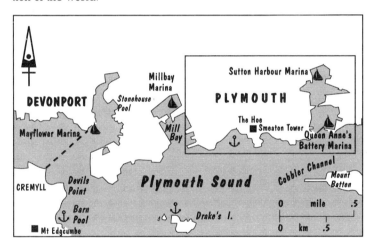

## SHORE LEAVE

*Food and drink*

Finding somewhere to eat in Plymouth is never a problem: there is a wide choice, particularly in the Barbican where restaurants, bistros, wine bars and pubs are all around. Two recommended restaurants are Hosteria Romana, 96 Embankment Road and Piermasters in Southside Street. *Out to Eat* suggests Clouds, a simple restaurant at 102 Tavistock Street, the Training Restaurant at the College of Further Education in Kings Road, Devonport, and Yang Cheng, an old-style Chinese restaurant at 30A Western Approach. *The Good Food Guide 1992* also recommends the last of these and adds Barretts of Princes Street, Chez Nous, an expensive bistro at 13 Frankfort Gate and Trattoria Pescatore, 30 Admiralty Street – an authentic Italian restaurant with a cheerful ambience.

*Entertainment*

The **Theatre Royal** in Royal Parade is the largest theatre, where there are often pre-West End shows; the **Barbican Theatre** in Castle Street is very small and

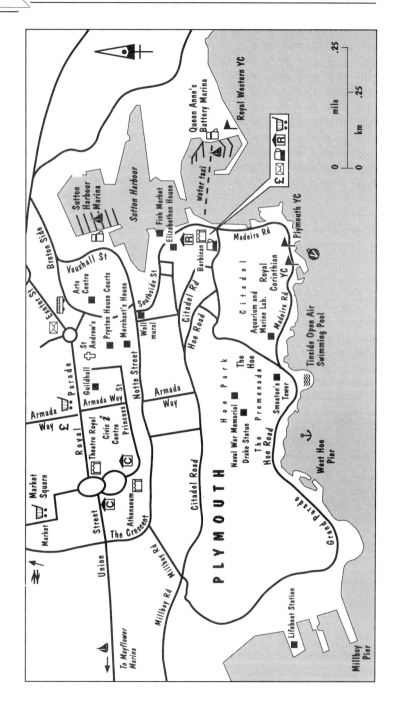

productions usually use local talent. Amateur operatics are performed at the **Athenaeum** in Derrys Cross where you will also find the Drake-Odeon and Cannon cinemas.

*What to see*

The **Plymouth Arts Centre** in Looe Street shows films and specialises in visual arts exhibitions – the vegetarian restaurant there is worth knowing about. The **Elizabethan House** in New Street contains sixteenth and seventeenth-century furniture. The **City Museum and Art Gallery** at Drake's Circus displays the natural history of Plymouth, Cornish minerals, Plymouth porcelain and fine paintings – new art exhibitions are held every month. Fifteenth-century **Prysten House** has Mayflower exhibits and in the **Plymouth Dome** on the Hoe audio-visual displays of local history include an Elizabethan Street complete with sounds and smells. Also on the Hoe are a large aquarium with marine research laboratories and the old **Eddystone Lighthouse**, built in 1759 by Smeaton and moved to the Hoe as a memorial when it was replaced. You may enjoy simply exploring and absorbing the atmosphere of the **Barbican**, with its cobbled streets and alleyways, or taking a trip up the River Tamar or round the harbour to get a feel for the whole area.

*Excursions*

A short trip across the Tamar by the Cremyll Ferry will take you to **Mount Edgcumbe Park**, stretching along 10 miles of spectacular coastline, with views of Plymouth Sound from the beautiful eighteenth-century landscaped parkland. See the *Holiday Which? Town and Country Walks Guide* walk 16. From **Whitesand Bay** you can walk to **Sharrow Point** for its cliff views and to **Sharrow Grot** to see the rock chamber. There is a **Wildlife Park** near Sparkwell. All of south Devon and Cornwall is yours to explore by car or bus – most parts of both counties can be reached on a day trip.

*Exercise*

The beaches at Cawsand, Whitesand and Bovisand are sandy and safe for swimming; alternatively, try the open-air salt water swimming pool on the rocks below the Hoe. Plymouth Pavilions at the west end of Citadel Road is a leisure centre with an indoor swimming pool. Windsurfing is popular at Queen Anne's Battery Marina.

## TRANSPORT AND TRAVEL

**Buses** From Breton Side

**Trains** Frequent service to London from Saltash Road

**Planes** From Plymouth Airport four miles from the city centre, to Heathrow, Gatwick, Jersey, Guernsey, Cork, Morlaix and Brest

**Ferries** Brittany Ferries operate from Millbay Docks to Roscoff and Santander

*Further information* from Tourist Information Offices in the Barbican and in Civic Centre, Royal Parade; there is also a Tourist Information kiosk in Mayflower International Marina.

# Sutton Harbour Marina

| | |
|---|---|
| **Harbourmaster** ☎ (0752) 664186 | **VHF Channels** 80, M |
| **Callsign** Sutton Harbour Radio | **Daily charge** ££££ |

This is a working commercial harbour with the marina at the inshore end. The marina is well managed and the facilities are good, but the management fight a losing battle against debris. The immediate surrounds are commercial dockland and fish wharves. Because of the location, security needs to be – and is – excellent, and boats can be left unattended quite safely. It is surprisingly quiet at night. Sutton Harbour does not have much room for visitors and is not recommended for an extended visit, but it has the unique advantage of easy access on foot to all the amenities of Plymouth.

## STEP ASHORE

**Nearest payphone** In marina watch-office
**Toilets, showers, launderette** In building within marina complex
**Shopping** Within three minutes' walk a late-night shop open till 2000, take-aways, pubs and restaurants.

Full selection of high-street shops, banks and building societies, a post office and a bureau de change in the Barbican
**Taxis, car and bicycle hire** Arrange through marina watch-office

### SHIPS' SERVICES

**Water and electricity** On pontoons
**Fuel** (diesel and petrol) In the marina from 0700 till dusk
**Gas** (Camping and Calor) From garage five minutes' walk from marina

**Chandler** In marina
**Boatyard, engineer, diver and sailmaker** Outside marina, but within Sutton Harbour, about five minutes' walk away

# Queen Anne's Battery Marina

| | |
|---|---|
| **Harbourmaster** ☎ (0752) 671142 | **VHF Channels** 80, M |
| **Callsign** Queen Anne's Battery Marina | **Daily charge** ££££ |

This is an attractive, well-appointed, secure and very up-to-date marina with all water sports available. The marina frequently hosts special races and gatherings during the summer. If you like your sailing full of jolly fellow-sailors and the aura of money, this is the place for you. It is very handy for Plymouth city centre, via a water-taxi run by the marina. The marina is surrounded on the land side by its own buildings, a car-park, and a boat-park. Visiting boats are usually moored inside the marina's protecting wall, so don't expect sea views.

STEP ASHORE

**Nearest payphone** By the marina watch-office
**Toilets, showers, launderette** In the marina
**Clubhouse** The Royal Western Yacht Club in the marina welcomes visitors and has showers and a comfortable bar and restaurant
**Shopping, food and drink** A late-night shop, a restaurant and a bar within the marina; take-aways, pubs and restaurants in the Barbican 200 yards away by water-taxi followed by a two-minute walk. Main shopping area is a further short walk away, where there are all the major stores as well as local shops, banks, building societies, a post office and a bureau de change
**Taxis, car and bicycle hire** Arrange through marina watch-office

*SHIPS' SERVICES*

*Water and electricity* On pontoons
*Fuel* (diesel and petrol), *gas* (Camping and Calor), *chandler, boatyard,* *engineer, diver and sailmaker* All available in the marina

# Mayflower International Marina

| | |
|---|---|
| **Harbourmaster** ☎ (0752) 556633 | **VHF Channels** 80, M |
| **Callsign** Mayflower International Marina | **Daily charge** ££££ |

This is the marina most often used by sailors visiting Plymouth. It is friendly, clean and quiet and bound to enhance any cruise. In heavy southerly weather visitors' berths can be slightly uncomfortable but are safe. Boats can be left confidently at any time. The marina is backed by a modern block of flats, though visitors look out over the Tamar River to Cremyll at interesting passing traffic. Don't choose this marina if you wish to spend your time shopping – you need buses or taxis to get into the city. Further information is available from the Tourist Information kiosk in the marina.

STEP ASHORE

**Nearest payphone** By landing point from pontoons
**Toilets, showers, launderette** In building within marina complex
**Shopping** Late-night shop one-and-a-half miles away in city centre; take-away, pub and restaurant and an excellent bistro all in the marina. Main shopping is in the city centre one mile to the east – there is a coach service in and out of the city three or four times daily from the lane by the exit from the marina
**Taxis, car and bicycle hire** Arrange through marina watch-office

*SHIPS' SERVICES*

*Water and electricity* On pontoons
*Fuel* (diesel and petrol) and *gas* (Camping and Calor) From fuel pontoon in the marina *Chandler, engineer and diver* In marina; *Boatyard* 200 yards away and *sailmaker* 100 yards away

---

*Alternative moorings*
There are moorings at the **Millbay Marina** and the **Royal Plymouth Corinthian Yacht Club** welcomes visitors at the club moorings.

# River Yealm – Newton Ferrers

A visit to Newton Ferrers is a must. The picturesque scenery as you enter the River Yealm is breathtakingly beautiful, with high hills and woods surrounding the villages of Newton Ferrers and Noss Mayo. Up river the woods come down to the river edge, encouraging an abundance of bird life. The villages themselves are a picturesque reminder of their links to the fishing trade at the turn of the century. Although much of the land adjoining the river is private property, there are walks around the River Yealm and further afield to the coast and west to Plymouth Sound, and these are particularly recommended, as indeed are those inland.

## SHORE LEAVE

### Food and drink
The pubs are very much part of village life: excellent local food can be obtained at a reasonable price both at lunchtime and in the evening – or eat in the Yealm Yacht Club (see Step Ashore).

### What to see
It is worth being in the area for the Yealm Regatta at the end of August and beginning of September when there are sailing races, barbecues and fireworks.

### Exercise
Details of **Heritage Coast** walks are described in Coast Path Guide leaflets which are obtainable at the local post offices. The South Devon Heritage Coast covers 58 miles from Sharkham Point to Wembury Beach. There are public footpaths from the landings at Wide Slip or Parish Steps round Yealm Head returning through Noss Mayo; from Yealm Steps north through Court and Newton Woods; and from Warren Point west to Wembury. The tide runs very hard in the Yealm River and it is not suitable for swimming, but there is a small beach, Clitters Beach, on the west bank of the Yealm River, half a mile north of Warren Point.

## TRANSPORT AND TRAVEL

**Buses** Service to Plymouth via Yealmpton and Brixton stops at the Village Hall in Noss Mayo, below the Yealm Hotel and at the top of Newton Hill

**Ferries** From Warren Point to Yealm Steps and from Yealm Steps to Wide Slip
**Taxis** ☎ (0752) 872682

# River Yealm Moorings

Harbourmaster ☎ (0752) 872533        **Daily charge** £

The harbourmaster is usually in the Harbour Office on the Yealm Hotel driveway 1000–1200 and 1430–1530; he is afloat in his launch in the early morning and evening.

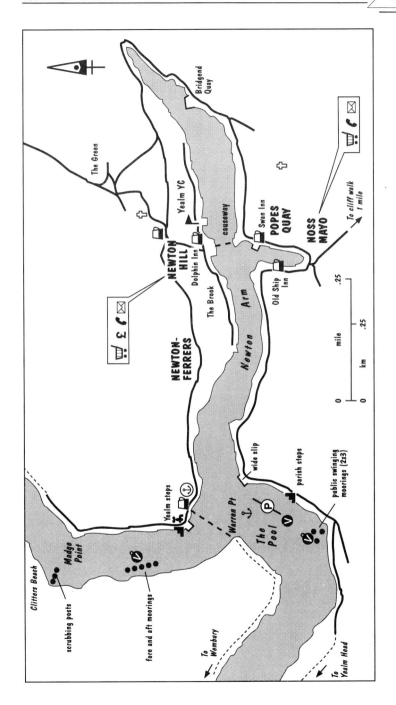

Newton Ferrers and Noss Mayo are easily accessible from one to the other via a causeway at low water. The whole area is extremely sheltered, especially up river.

## STEP ASHORE

**Nearest payphones** Outside post offices in Noss Mayo and Newton Ferrers

**Toilets, showers** Yealm Yacht Club

**Clubhouse** Yealm Yacht Club serves evening meals on Wednesdays, Fridays and Saturdays as well as Sunday lunches. Temporary membership (£6) gives access to the facilities, which include showers

**Shopping** Shop in the village in Newton Ferrers. Go ashore at Yealm Steps and walk half a mile east up Newton Hill to the post office/general store (open Sundays, early closing Wednesdays), Barclays Bank (open Tuesdays and Thursdays) and a chemist. There is also a post office and general store at Popes Quay on the south bank of Newton Creek

### SHIPS' SERVICES

*Water* From the ferry pontoon water point and the Yealm Hotel

*Fuel, gas* Contact harbourmaster

*Rubbish* Visitors are asked to bag their rubbish securely and leave it in the bins provided at Yealm Steps where there is a collection several times a week. There are no other collection points

# Salcombe

Salcombe, Devon's southernmost resort, is completely protected from the sea and delightful to visit. Besides sailing, there is excellent fishing. The upper reaches of the estuary are particularly attractive, with abundant wildlife. The town has quaint, picturesque houses facing the estuary, with old narrow streets lending a rather 'olde worlde' atmosphere. A week here in fine weather would not be too long. The numerous beaches are sheltered and safe. There are many walks, both short and long, on shore and through countryside.

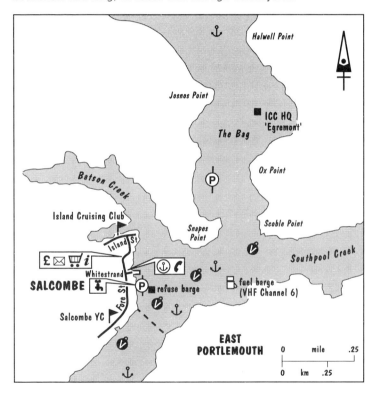

SHORE LEAVE

### Food and drink

Salcombe has an excellent selection of restaurants within a few minutes of the Town Quay. The Marine Hotel, overlooking the harbour, is traditional and very comfortable. The Mariners Pub in the High Street serves very good pub food at a medium price. Crossleigh Restaurant, Fore Street, has excellent seafood but prices are high. The Chivelstone pub is in a delightful setting and popular with sailors: it can be reached at high water by small craft.

*Exercise and excursions*

There are several good picnic places at sheltered beaches, such as South Sand Bay, Mill Bay and East Portlemouth, and plenty of walks: cross the estuary and walk south to the Bar, which is covered by barely three feet of water at low tide and a cause of wrecks as long ago as the Bronze Age. You can continue along the cliffs east of **Start Point** to the disappearing village of **Hallsands** – it was destroyed by a gale in 1917 and the sea continues to encroach on the ruins. Start Point lighthouse is open to the public. The cliff top path is part of the South-West Peninsula Coast Path. A pretty, partly inland walk takes you from East Portlemouth to South Creek and north to Chivelstone. An interesting excursion is to explore the ruin of **Salcombe Castle**, built by Henry VIII and the last fortress in England to hold out for Charles I in the Civil War. You can windsurf upstream from Salcombe, off Halwell Point and north to Kingsbridge. At South Sands a wide choice of water sports ranges from windsurfer and dinghy hire to surf canoes and waterskiing.

### TRANSPORT AND TRAVEL

**Buses** To Kingsbridge every 30 minutes      **Car hire** Quay Garage, Kingsbridge
**Taxis** From several garages in Salcombe      ☎ (0548) 852323

*Further information* from Salcombe Information Centre, High Street and 66 Fore Street.

# Salcombe Harbour

| | |
|---|---|
| **Harbourmaster** ☎ (0548) 843791 | **VHF Channel** 14 |
| **Callsign** Salcombe Harbour | **Daily charge** mooring ££; anchoring in estuary £ |

The safe anchorages and sheltered conditions of the Salcombe estuary, with its many creeks and inlets, have made Salcombe an active sailing centre, particularly in August. For such a popular harbour, facilities are both basic and primitive, but this adds to its charm: for example, you attract the water boat by hoisting a bucket. You can sail to Kingsbridge at high tide.

### STEP ASHORE

**Nearest payphone, toilet** Adjacent to Harbour Office

**Clubhouses** Salcombe Yacht Club and the Island Cruising Club both welcome visitors. The Yacht Club is worth visiting both for advice on local attractions and for its facilities: there is a bar and hot food is available; visitors may use the showers and toilets

**Shopping** The usual range of high-street shops, banks and a post office (early closing Wednesdays)

## SHIPS' SERVICES

**Water** There is a water point on the town pontoon; hoist a bucket to call the water boat

**Fuel** (petrol and diesel) From floating barge downstream from Town Quay; VHF Channel 6

**Gas** (Calor) From Winters Marine or Water Barge; Camping from Winters Marine and Hardware Store in Fore Street (this is a small shop but well stocked with basic tools)

**Chandler** Winters Marine Ltd, Island Street a quarter of a mile from main quay

**Engineer** Starey Marine Services, Cottles Quay, Thorning Street (Volvo Penta agents); B D Carter, Island Street

**Sailmaker** John McKillop & Co, Ebrington Street, Kingsbridge, is particularly recommended and will collect from Salcombe ☎ (0548) 852343

**Rubbish** All refuse should be put in the floating refuse barge near Whitestrand

# River Dart

The entrance to this very sheltered river lies between steep wooded hills rising to about 500 feet, which have made it easy to defend British fleets anchored here through the centuries. Dartmouth, on the west bank of the Dart, has always been an important naval port and is the home of the Britannia Royal Naval College. Although a working port, it is a very attractive town with medieval houses in small winding streets that lead to the old quays. As a consequence it is popular with tourists, particularly in July and August. The pontoons off the Dartmouth Yacht Club, and the anchorage and visitors' buoys in Dartmouth Harbour are as crowded as the town. If you are lucky enough to find a vacancy, you will probably have to move from time to time. However, there are several choices of berth in the river. Above the higher car ferry on the west bank lies the Dart Marina and on the east bank of the river is Darthaven Marina, at Kingswear. A mile up stream, off Dittisham, you will find further visitors' moorings.

## SHORE LEAVE

### Food and drink
Dartmouth is hospitable, with plenty of good pubs and restaurants. The Carved Angel, 2 South Embankment, is one of the most renowned restaurants in England and is recommended in *The Good Food Guide 1992*, along with the bistro Billy Budd's, 7 Foss Street, and Ford House, 44 Victoria Road. Fingal's at Old Coombe Manor, Dittisham is also suggested. *Out to Eat* picks out the Cherub, 11 Higher Street, a timber-framed pub offering sound, inexpensive food.

### Entertainment
The Royalty Cinema in Mayor's Avenue is popular.

### What to see
The town itself is old and fascinating, particularly the wool merchant's house built in 1380. The **Henley Museum**, in Anzac Street, is a small private museum housing items of local interest. There is a **Maritime Museum** in **The Butterwalk** – an attraction in its own right – and an original beam engine in working order in the **Newcomen Engine House** in Mayor's Avenue.

### Excursions
Take a **Dart Valley Light Railway** steam train from Kingswear to Paignton along the Dart Estuary and Torbay coast. Visit **Dartmouth Castle**, built in 1481, where the Dart joins the sea; a chain once stretched across the river to **Godmerock Castle**, Kingswear (also open to the public) to prevent enemy ships entering the port. South of the lower ferry on the west bank is Baynards Cove, where there are many attractive old houses and castle ruins.

### Exercise
Walk from Dartmouth Castle to Compass Cove for interesting views of Dartmouth Harbour. See the *Holiday Which? Good Walks Guide* walk 13. There are also plenty of short easy walks along the grassy banks of the River Dart. One of the best beaches for swimming is at Goodrington (take the steam railway from

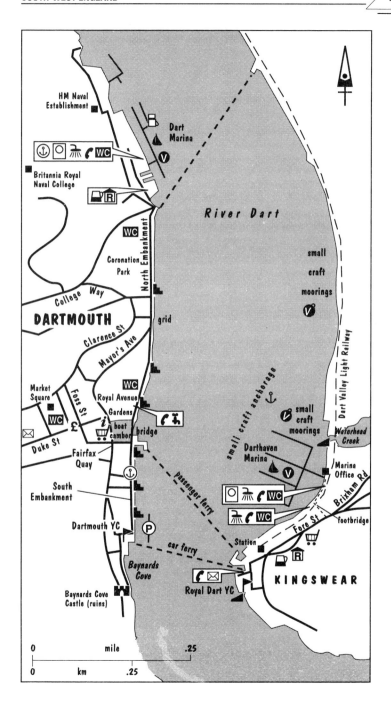

Kingswear); another is at Blackpool Sands, which has a car-park, shop and restaurant; windsurfing is popular there as well as at the river mouth. In Dartmouth itself the heated outdoor swimming pool is convenient if you want a swim without the effort of going to a beach.

### TRANSPORT AND TRAVEL

**Buses** Several times a day from Kingswear to Paignton

**Trains** Several steam trains every day from Kingswear to Paignton (trains run from Paignton to Bristol and London)

See also **Darthaven Marina.**

*Further information* from Tourist Information Office in The Butterwalk.

# Dart Harbour and Dittisham

| Dart Harbour and Navigation Authority ☎ (0804) 832337 | VHF Channel 11 |
| --- | --- |
| **Callsign** Dartnav | **Daily charge** ££ |

As well as the moorings and pontoons in Dartmouth Harbour, there is an anchorage below Dittisham, south of the Anchor Stone. The moorings at Dittisham are crowded. It is possible to go right up to Totnes with the tide, but consult the River Officer before proceeding above Dittisham.

### STEP ASHORE

**In Dartmouth:**
**Payphone, toilet** By bandstand
**Clubhouse** Dartmouth Yacht Club welcomes visitors
**Shopping** Selection of usual shops, banks, building societies and a post office; some food shops stay open late. See also Dart Marina, below

**In Dittisham:**
**Shopping** A pub, and a general store

### SHIPS' SERVICES

*Water* By bandstand in Dartmouth and on quay in Dittisham

*Other services* See Dart Marina and Darthaven Marina, below

# Dart Marina

| Harbourmaster ☎ (0804) 833351 | VHF Channels 80, M |
| --- | --- |
| **Callsign** Dart Marina Two | **Daily charge** £££ |

This is a safe, well-managed, clean and secure marina, with good views across the river and within easy walking distance of Dartmouth. It is attractive and has the added advantage of a hotel on-site, but being small the marina is often full. Push in here if you can: you will probably be asked to move to a berth belonging to a temporarily absent owner.

STEP ASHORE

**Nearest payphone** In Dart Marina Hotel
**Toilets, showers, launderette** In building
within marina complex
**Shopping** In Dartmouth, seven minutes'
walk to the south along the quay, where
there is a full selection of high-street
shops, banks, building societies, post
office and bureau de change. Early closing
Wednesdays. No late-shopping night
although some food shops stay open late.
Take-away, pub and restaurant in Dart
Marina Hotel
**Taxi, car and bicycle hire** Arrange through
marina office

SHIPS' SERVICES

*Water, electricity* On pontoons
*Fuel* (diesel and petrol), *gas* (Camping
and Calor) In marina
*Chandler, boatyard, engineer* Available
on-site
*Sailmaker* Dart Sails, 26 Foss Street

# Darthaven Marina, Kingswear

| Harbourmaster ☎ (0804) 25545 | VHF Channels 80, M |
|---|---|
| Callsign Darthaven Control | Daily charge ££££ |

This is another very crowded marina and you will be lucky to find a
vacancy here; if you do, you may have to move from time to time.
Because boats are tightly packed, there is not much in the way of views
from your berth. However, the marina is pleasantly situated, quiet,
clean and secure. Kingswear is a rather run-down small village but it is
very easy to ferry over to Dartmouth. The scenic round trip, run by the
Dart Valley Light Railway, starts from the station just behind the marina
but creates no undue noise.

STEP ASHORE

**Nearest payphone** At entrance to marina
**Toilets, showers, launderette** In marina
**Shopping** Five minutes' walk away there is
a late-night shop in Kingswear, where you
will also find a pub, restaurant and take-
away. There is a full selection of
shops, banks, building societies and a
post office. Early closing Wednesdays. No
late-shopping night. The main shopping
centre is across the river in Dartmouth,
but the ferry service is frequent

SHIPS' SERVICES

*Water, electricity* On pontoons
*Fuel* (diesel and petrol) From barge in
the river
*Gas* (Camping and Calor) Available in
marina
*Chandler, boatyard, engineer* In marina
*Sailmaker* Dart Sails, 26 Foss Street,
Dartmouth

TRANSPORT AND TRAVEL

**Buses** Several buses run from Kingswear
to Paignton every day
**Trains** Several steam trains every day
from Kingswear to Paignton
**Taxi, car and bicycle hire** Arrange through
marina office

# Brixham

Brixham is a working port for the fishing industry, which adds the interest and hazards of a commercial area. This may make it less welcoming to many, although the recently established marina, protected by the east breakwater, gives a new dimension of convenience and cleanliness.

Brixham falls into two parts: the old village on the hill and the fishing village half a mile below. Much of Brixham slopes steeply, so the harbour is overlooked on the south-west and south-east sides. The narrow streets with their hairpin bends are connected by pedestrian ways with long flights of steps. There is the usual range of shopping facilities, but if you take the ferry to Torquay you will find access to most other requirements.

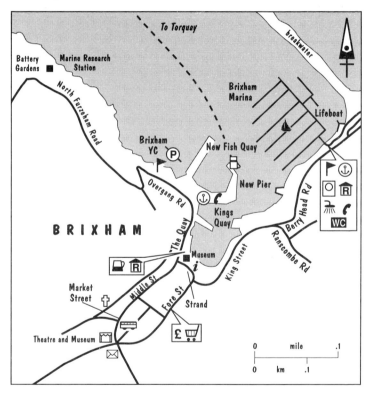

## SHORE LEAVE

*Food and drink*
Berry Head Hotel on edge of town in Berry Head Country Park has a pleasant restaurant. Of numerous pubs the Blue Anchor, the Maritime and the Crown have been recommended by visitors.

*What to see*
The **Brixham Coastguard Museum**, the **Maritime Museum** and even the **Fisheries Museum** appeal to yachting visitors. Other marine attractions include the **Perils of the Deep** exhibition, which simulates the excitements of the undersea world, and a harbourside aquarium. You can admire a full-sized replica of Drake's *Golden Hind* on Brixham Quay.

*Excursions*
A visit to **Berry Head Country Park**, with its Castle and Fort, nature trail and reserve, makes a pleasant day ashore; or take the **Dart Valley Light Railway** round trip from Paignton.

*Exercise*
Three walks start from **Broadsands** car-park and one from **Sharkham Point** car-park; all are described in a leaflet available from the Tourist Information Office. You can swim in Churston Cove and from Shoalstone Beach, Breakwater Beach and Fishcombe Beach – they are all mostly pebble beaches. At Ranscombe Road there is a heated indoor pool or if you prefer there is an unheated outdoor saltwater pool at Shoalstone. Windsurf in Paignton Harbour.

### TRANSPORT AND TRAVEL

**Buses** Several buses every day to Paignton
**Ferry** Western Lady Ferry Service to Torquay from New Pier

**Taxis** ☎ (0803) 882090/882100
**Car hire** (from Torquay) Hertz ☎ (0803) 294786

*Further information* from Tourist Information Office, The Old Market House, The Quay.

# Brixham Marina

| Harbourmaster ☎ (0803) 882929 | VHF Channels 80, M |
|---|---|
| Callsign Brixham Marina | Daily charge £££ |

The marina complex is new and security is good: visitors must obtain a pass from the marina office (open 24 hours a day) in order to be able to enter and leave the shoreside part of the marina.

## STEP ASHORE

**Payphone, toilets, showers, launderette** In a utility block across the walkway from the marina office
**Clubhouse** Marina clubhouse/restaurant
**Shopping** General store in the marina. Full selection of high-street shops, banks and building societies, a post office and a bureau de change in town. Early closing Wednesdays

## SHIPS' SERVICES

**Water and electricity** *On pontoons*
**Fuel** *Fuel berth may be operational by 1992, meanwhile fuel (diesel only) has to be obtained on New Pier*

**Gas** *(Camping and Calor) From Brixham Chandler adjacent to marina*
**Boatyard, engineer, sailmaker** *Marina office keeps list of phone numbers and will make recommendations*

---

*Alternative moorings*

Outside the marina the **Brixham Yacht Club** has two offshore pontoons available to visitors using the club facilities. Fuel has to be obtained on New Pier and is diesel only. Access is rendered hazardous by trawlers which may be alongside. Other possible hazards include an occasional tanker delivering fuel to a terminal at the north end of the breakwater and the existence of a lifeboat fairway between the breakwater and the marina. Despite these things, and given the pleasantness of the Brixham Yacht Club building, a visit can be worthwhile, be it for a drink and sandwich or a longer stay. The Yacht Club has a bar and a restaurant.

# Torquay

Situated on the English Riviera, Torquay is a large holiday resort and shopping centre, with most of the associated pros and cons. In July, August and September the town is very crowded. There are two large covered shopping precincts within a stone's throw of the harbour area with amenities for tourists and sailors alike, including gift shops, coffee bars and a chandlery. The Princess Theatre backs on to the marina in the western part of the harbour and there is a selection of amusement arcades and eating and drinking places within walking distance.

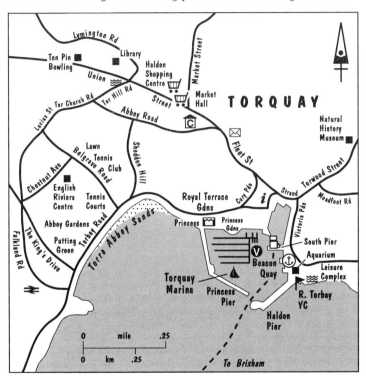

## SHORE LEAVE

### Food and drink

Torquay has a great variety of restaurants and several have been recommended, such as the Ganges in Tor Hill Road and the Pizza Hut in Fleet Street, this with the comment 'good but expensive'. The Old Vienna in Lisburn Square has a good atmosphere and excellent wine but is expensive. La Table du Capitaine in Fore Street is very good and medium-priced but the most strongly recommended is another French restaurant, The Vaults at 23 Victoria Parade. A short stay at the Osborne Hotel, Hesketh Crescent, whether from need of a little luxury or just to eat at Raffles bar, is enjoyable. *The Good Food Guide 1992* recommends Capers, an unpretentious restaurant at 7 Lisburn Square, as well as The Vaults and the Mulberry Room, 1 Scarborough Road, a café also featured in *Out to Eat*.

### Entertainment
The Odeon Cinema is in Abbey Road and the Princess Theatre in Torbay Road.

### What to see
**Torquay Natural History Museum** in Torwood Street is well worth a visit and **Aqualand**, at Beacon Quay, claims to be the largest aquarium in the West of England.

### Excursions
The **Exeter Maritime Museum**, the world's finest collection of boats from every continent, will interest every sailor. **Marlden Stately Home**, **Berry Pomeroy**, the haunted castle, **Kents Cavern** (caves), the **Model Village** at Babbacombe and **Paignton Zoo** are all within easy reach of Torquay.

### Exercise
Walks to the headland and cliffs give good views across Torbay. You can swim off the beaches at Meadfood Abbey Sands and Corbyn Sands or undercover at the English Riviera Leisure Centre in Chestnut Avenue and at Swim Torquay at Plainmoor. Other attractions are the dry ski slope – ☎ (0803) 313350 – and waterskiing, parascending and speedboats from Ski Torquay, Beacon Quay ☎ (0803) 295445.

## TRANSPORT AND TRAVEL

**Buses** From the Strand to Teignmouth and Exeter

**Trains** From Torre and Torquay stations to London, change at Newton Abbott

**Planes** From Exeter Airport to the Continent and the Channel Islands

**Ferries** Torbay Steamways to Channel Islands ☎ (0803) 214397; *Western Lady* plies between Torquay and Brixham

**Taxis** Rank outside Royal Torbay Yacht Club; also Torbay Taxi Services ☎ (0803) 211611

**Car hire** Hertz ☎ (0803) 294786

**Bicycle hire** Colin Lewis, 15 East Street

**Further information** from Tourist Information Office, Vaughan Parade, on western side of Old Harbour.

# Torquay Marina

| | | |
|---|---|---|
| **Harbourmaster** ☎ (0803) 214624 | **VHF Channels** 80, M |
| **Callsign** Torquay Marina | **Daily charge** £££ |

As a harbour, Torquay benefits from the protection afforded by Torbay and the high and rocky north peninsula.

## STEP ASHORE

**Nearest payphone, showers, toilets, launderette** In marina
**Clubhouse** Royal Torbay Yacht Club gives a warm welcome to visitors and any advice they may need. The Club caters for lunch and evening meals, parties by arrangement. **Showers** and **toilets** in the

Club open 0900–2300
**Shopping** Numerous take-aways, pubs and restaurants along the east side of harbour; main shops are also adjacent to harbour. Branches of most major banks on the Strand, also building societies, a post office and a bureau de change

### SHIPS' SERVICES

**Water, electricity** In marina
**Fuel** (diesel and petrol), **gas** (Camping and Calor), **engineer** At Queen Anne Marine, Beacon Quay

**Chandler** At Queen Anne Marine, Beacon Quay and Torquay Chandlers, The Pavilion
☎ (0803) 211854

# Lyme Regis

Lyme Regis is a charming little town where anything you are likely to need on holiday can be obtained. It is popular in the summer with a friendly and hospitable atmosphere wherever you go. Much of the surrounding country belongs to the National Trust. There are exciting cliff walks, fascinating beaches and the intriguing fossil remains for which Lyme is famous. Rock pools are a delight at low water, for the children especially. The bay is a great favourite with windsurfers. Among the many items of historical interest, the thirteenth-century harbour is famous for the landing of the Duke of Monmouth in 1685 at the start of his ill-fated rebellion.

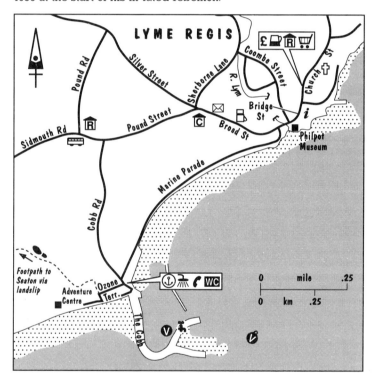

## SHORE LEAVE

### Food and drink

Lyme Regis has plenty of places to eat and drink. Drake's take-away, Broad Street is useful. The Beachcomber Restaurant, 47 Combe Street is recommended and The Cobb Arms by the quay is refreshing and full of character.

### Entertainment

There is a cinema in Broad Street, and the Marine Theatre in Bridge Street.

*What to see*

Visit the **Philpot Museum** in Bridge Street for excellent examples of local fossils, and look for fossils yourself, especially in the rocks to the east and west and along the beaches. There is an aquarium on the Cobb. Explore the town with its Norman church and Victorian sea-front and thatched cottages. On Tuesdays a historical tour is guided by the Town Crier.

*Excursions*

Go to **Chideock** for its charming thatched cottages or **Chard** to see **Forde Abbey**, a Cistercian monastery founded in 1140, set in 30 acres of gardens and lakes.

*Exercise*

The Tourist Office provides a leaflet which suggests three day-long walks: to **Pinhay Bay**, to **Charmouth** and to **Seaton**, all of which are interesting geologically as well as scenically. Swimming and windsurfing are safe and popular from the beaches.

### TRANSPORT AND TRAVEL

**Buses** From the coach station at the junction of Pound Street and Pound Road, go to Axminster, Salisbury, Exeter and Sherborne

**Trains** Main line from Axminster to London and the West Country; there is a bus link from Lyme Regis to Axminster

**Planes** From Exeter
**Ferries** From Weymouth
**Taxis** Lyme Regis Taxi Hire
☎ (02974) 3181
**Car hire** Escort Travel, 28 Talbot Road
☎ (02974) 2185

*Further information* from Tourist Office, The Guildhall, Bridge Street.

# Lyme Regis Harbour

| | |
|---|---|
| **Harbourmaster** ☎ (02974) 2137 | **VHF Channel** 16 |
| **Callsign** Lyme Regis harbour | **Daily charge** alongside pier ££; on visitors' buoys outside harbour £ |

It is a long haul across Lyme Bay in a small boat and Lyme Regis can be regarded as a very pleasant break in the passage or a useful bolthole should the weather forecast be pessimistic. The harbour is small and most of it dries out. A nasty swell develops in a south-easterly, and in strong onshore winds the approach is rough. Once inside it is sheltered from the north-west and south-west. The harbour is mainly used by fishermen and sees only the occasional visiting yacht. It is not a place to leave a boat unattended for long, but a delightful stopover in settled conditions and very welcoming. The harbourmaster is particularly helpful – see him if the boat has to be left. The harbour is well kept and efficiently run.

## STEP ASHORE

**Nearest payphone** By Cobb Arms in Cobb Square, at the 'root' of Victoria Pier
**Toilets** Public WCs in Cobb Square
**Showers** In the sailing club boat store – ask harbourmaster for key
**Clubhouse** Lyme Regis Sailing Club is upstairs in a building on Victoria Pier
**Shopping** A 10-minute walk to the east along Marine Parade leads to the main shopping centre with a good selection of shops, banks, building societies and a post office

### SHIPS' SERVICES

**Water** *Taps on Victoria Pier*
**Fuel** *(diesel and petrol) Available in cans from garages*
**Gas** *(Camping and Calor) From P L Turners & Co, Uplyme Road*
**Engineer** *R J Perry Marine, The Cobb*

# Weymouth

At the southern tip of Dorset, Weymouth is in one of the most beautiful parts of England. The rolling Dorset hills run back from the English Channel in a great loop of chalk downland. The Dorset Coast Path extends round Portland Bill, very impressive in windy weather, and along Chesil Beach, a storm beach of stones. To the west is Abbotsbury, a swannery set behind the Chesil Bank overlooked by the monument to Captain Hardy, who commanded *Victory* at the Battle of Trafalgar. To the north are Dorchester, Sherborne and Shaftesbury (Thomas Hardy country). To the east are the chalk cliffs of Ringshead and Lulworth. But note that the roads out of Weymouth are poor.

Weymouth itself is an old-fashioned English seaside resort, with candy-floss stalls and donkeys on the beach, cheap gift shops and a live theatre with popular summer shows. Weymouth is always an interesting place to visit, with shore amenities, shops, museums and chandlers all very close to the harbour. Another, historical, aspect to the harbour can be seen in the Cove with its old warehouses on Custom House Quay, many of which are now pubs, restaurants and museums. The most attractive parts of Weymouth are the streets round the old harbour.

## SHORE LEAVE

*Food and drink*
Sea Cow on Custom House Quay is an excellent and informal restaurant with a wide variety of unusual dishes in the English and continental vein, recommended in *Out to Eat*. Mallams at the Quay, Trinity Road, is more formal. Casual Restaurant, Hope Square serves good fish dishes. *The Good Food Guide 1992* suggests Hamilton's, 5 Brunswick Terrace.

*Entertainment*
Cannon cinema is in Gloucester Street and the Pavilion Theatre on the Quay.

*What to see*
**Tudor Museum**, Brewers Quay, is worth a visit and so is **Nothe Fort**, on the south side of the harbour entrance, built in 1860 as part of the defences for Portland Harbour and full of Victorian cannon, uniforms and military equipment.

*Excursions*
Visit **Athelhampton**, near Dorchester, a fifteenth-century house set in a walled garden; **Sherborne Castle** in north Dorset, built by Sir Walter Raleigh in 1594; the hill fort, **Maiden Castle**, scene of a battle between Celts and invading Romans; Dorchester county town (Casterbridge of Hardy's novels) with the excellent **Dorset County Museum**; or **Thomas Hardy's Cottage** near Dorchester. All are within easy reach by public transport. You could go to the village of **Abbotsbury** with its unspoilt sixteenth and seventeenth-century thatched cottages, fourteenth-century tithe barn and eleventh-century abbey. **Abbotsbury Swannery** was originally established by Benedictine monks as a source of birds for their table.

*Exercise*
Walk to **Chesil Beach**, a stretch of pebbles extending west from Portland Bill for

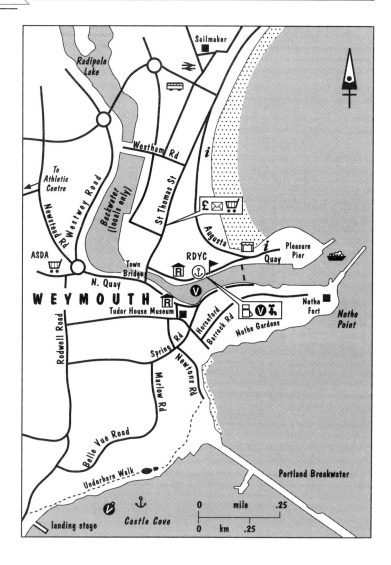

16 miles to West Bay near Bridport. The size of the pebbles gradually changes from coarse sand to large stones weighing as much as 12lb. Swift currents make bathing dangerous. See the *Holiday Which? Town and Country Walks Guide* walk 38. The **Dorset Coastal Path** turns inland at Abbotsbury and joins other walks with some of the most spectacular scenery in England. Try walking to **Portland Bill lighthouse** – especially impressive in stormy weather, though take care.

George III came to Weymouth for sea bathing – notice his statue on the sea front – Weymouth Beach is still good for swimming and there is windsurfing in Weymouth Bay. The athletics centre and swimming pool at Knightsdale Road has a sauna, solarium, weights room and two pools.

## TRANSPORT AND TRAVEL

**Trains** To London via Dorchester, Poole and Bournemouth every hour
**Ferries** Condor catamarans and hydrofoils to Channel Islands
**Taxis** Fleetline ☎ (0305) 781025/748252

**Car hire** Avis ☎ (0305) 760078
**Bicycle hire** Westham Cycles, 128 Abbotsbury Road; Weymouth Cycles, King Street (near station)

*Further information* from Tourist Information Office, Royal Terrace, The Esplanade.

# Weymouth and Portland Harbours

| | |
|---|---|
| **Harbourmaster** ☎ (0305) 206421 | **VHF Channel** 16 (working 12) |
| **Callsign** Weymouth Harbour Radio | **Daily charge** ££ |

Facilities for yachts are sparse. There are visitors' yacht moorings on the north side of the harbour by the Royal Dorset Yacht Club and on Brewers Quay on the south side. You can cross the harbour by the Town Bridge (a lifting bridge) or, lower down, by cross-harbour ferry. It is also possible to anchor in Portland Harbour, in Castle Cove, a less crowded and often cooler alternative to Weymouth. You can row ashore and walk across the hill into the town, which takes about 20 minutes by road, longer by the Underbara Walk.

## STEP ASHORE

**Nearest payphones** On the north side of the harbour by the Town Bridge; on the south side of the harbour in Hope Square close to the Cove
**Toilets, showers** 13 Custom House Quay on north side of harbour open during harbour office hours; on south side, close to Cove, open 24 hours

**Clubhouse** Royal Dorset Yacht Club, 11 Custom House Quay, on the north side of harbour, welcomes visitors
**Shopping** Plenty of fast-food outlets in town on the north side of the harbour. For main shopping there is a full selection of high-street shops. Early closing Wednesdays

### *SHIPS' SERVICES*

*Water* Taps on north and south quays
*Fuel* Raybar Fuels for marine diesel; a mobile tanker usually moors at Custom House Quay at weekends and west side of Town Bridge during week; VHF Ch 6 ☎ (0305) 771351/783677, mobile ☎ (0860) 589571/564105
*Gas* (Camping and Calor) From Small Boat Company, Commercial Road, on east side of inner harbour

*Chandler* Weymouth Chandlers on north side of harbour; Small Boat Co, Commercial Road and W L Bussell, Hope Street south of Cove
*Boatyard* W L Bussell (Cruising Association Boatman) will repair afloat
*Engineer* Small Boat Co, Commercial Road
*Sailmaker* Buglers, rear of 2 Chelmsford Street, near station

# Lulworth

Lulworth is an anchorage which must be visited by all yachtsmen and women at least once in their sailing careers, if only to see the unique pool formed by the sea breaking through limestone and washing out softer rocks behind. Once you are inside, the striations of the rock are marvellous to observe. A little to the west is Stair Hole with its contorted rock strata. The geology of the whole area is spectacular, with chalk cliffs, contrasting rock layers, fossils and petrified forests.

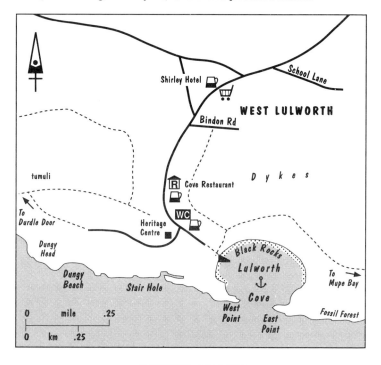

SHORE LEAVE

If you follow the road which forks to the west from the beach you will come to the **Heritage Centre**. Walks are limited by the Ministry of Defence tank training area. If the area is open, **Tyneham Village**, north of Worbarrow Bay, which is being restored, is worth a visit. Just north of Wool (a small town north of Lulworth) is the **Bovington Tank Museum**, one of the world's largest collections of armoured fighting vehicles. The **Dorset Coastal Path** is steep but the scenery is dramatic. You can walk to **Durdle Door**, a chalk area, and on to Weymouth and to West Swanage via **St Alban's Head**, **Worbarrow** and **Kimmeridge** in the east. The coast path is closed during the week, except in late July and August, because of firing on the Lulworth firing ranges. See also the *Holiday Which? Good Walks Guide* walk 27. Lulworth Cove, Durdle Door and Mupe Bay all have shingle beaches. Windsurfing is popular in Lulworth Cove. The Castle in West

Lulworth is recommended in *Out to Eat*, especially for its casseroles. The Weld Arms in East Lulworth has a nautical theme and is in *The Good Food Guide 1992*.

## TRANSPORT AND TRAVEL

**Bus** Daily to Wool by Little Red Bus

**Taxis** Garrison Cars
☎ (0929) 462467/463395

# Lulworth Cove

Visit Lulworth in settled weather because, due to the nature of the anchorage, a swell can build up. The shoreside facilities are virtually non-existent for the yachtsman and are uninspiring for the landlubber. If the anchorage gets very crowded, an alternative is Mupe Bay about a mile to the east.

## STEP ASHORE

**Nearest payphone** Outside Cove Restaurant

**Toilets** 100 yards along the road running north from the beach

**Shopping** Cove Restaurant stays open until about 2000 in summer. Further along the road are village shops. The Pastry Shop sells local bread and pastries and a limited range of groceries. There is also a butcher, a post office/general store and a wine shop which offers a selection of more than 100 varieties, including English wines and fruit wines. The Lulworth Cove Hotel provides a reasonable evening meal; last orders 2100

## SHIPS' SERVICES

**Water** *Taps in both the ladies' and gents' toilets can be used to fill containers*

# Swanage

Swanage is a pleasant, old-style, English seaside resort which time seems to have passed by. The town is at the eastern end of the Isle of Purbeck with landward access via Corfe Castle or across the chain ferry at Sandbanks. The harbour, part of the seafront of Swanage Bay, is open to the east. Swanage is a good place to wait out a south-westerly or westerly gale, or just to enjoy a peaceful anchorage, providing high-life is not expected. You can take pleasant walks along the Dorset Coastal Path to Old Harry in the north, Durlston Head in the south and the stone quarries at Worth Matravers in the west.

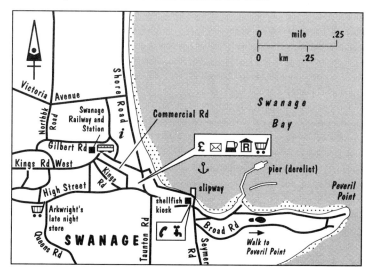

SHORE LEAVE

The **Town Museum** is in Church Hill and the **Mowlem Institute** in Shore Road has both a cinema and theatre. The **Swanage Railway** runs hourly in the high season from Swanage station to Harmans Cross village, stopping at Herston Halt, and back again. The **Dorset Coastal Path** will take you to **Anvil Point lighthouse** (open to the public), **St Alban's Head** and **Chapman Pool**. You can either walk or bus to **Durlston Head Castle** where there is a restaurant, pub and **Great Globe**, a map of the world carved out of a 40-ton stone sphere.

Buses also run to **Corfe Castle**, a medieval ruin and scene of the murder of King Edward in 978, which gives its name to the village at the foot of the hill on which it stands. In West Street there is a model of the old village and the castle before its destruction in the Civil War.

Take a bus to **Blue Pool**, between Swanage and Wareham. This is a deep, vivid blue pool set in peaceful woods but you cannot swim there. Swimming is safe in Swanage Bay, which is also popular with windsurfers. There is a children's play park above Shore Road.

The Galley restaurant, 9 High Street, is recommended in *The Good Food Guide 1992*.

### TRANSPORT AND TRAVEL

**Buses** From Swanage railway station forecourt to Wareham, Poole and Bournemouth

**Taxis** Swanage Associated Taxis
☎ (0929) 422788/425350
**Bicycle hire** From Purbeck Pedal Power
☎ (0929) 426631

*Further information* from Tourist Information Office in Shore Road opposite beach.

# Swanage Harbour

Very few facilities exist for yachts, which are not really encouraged. A proposed marina to revive the derelict pier was turned down in 1989. Dinghies are needed to go ashore from the anchorage to the slipway but they are not allowed along the Blue Flag bathing beach.

## STEP ASHORE

**Nearest payphone** In the High Street, close to the slipway
**Toilets** Near slipway
**Shopping** Late-night shop (Arkwrights) on the corner of the High Street and Queens Road, 0800–2200 Mondays to Saturdays. The main shopping area is along the High Street, Institute Road and Station Road, with the usual high-street shops, banks, building societies and a post office. Early closing Thursdays. There are take-aways (pizzas and burgers) in the High Street half a mile west of town centre (0930–1430 and 1800–2200) and many small restaurants in the centre of Swanage

### SHIPS' SERVICES

**Water** *Difficult to obtain but can be taken from a tap behind the shellfish kiosk near the slipway*
**Fuel** *(petrol),* **gas** *(Camping) From Brook* *Garage, near the station forecourt*
**Chandler** *In the High Street; Swanage Angling near the slipway also stock some chandlery*

# Studland

Studland Bay is a restful place for two or three days' quiet mooring with walks and pleasant relaxation, providing one avoids July and August weekends when it is very crowded, both on and offshore. The whole of the Studland area is administered by the National Trust.

Studland is the anchorage for enjoying the Purbeck Hills with their beautiful walks and the view of Poole, Bournemouth and along the coast to Lymington. On clear days St Catherine's Point can be seen. Studland is a mooring for the visitor who does not want the high life.

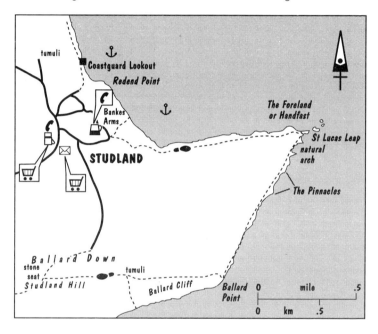

SHORE LEAVE

### Food and drink
The Bankes Arms is a very pleasant pub, popular with sailors – it is open all day and serves cream teas and pub meals; families are accommodated in a room to the side of the bar. Occasional entertainment by folk and jazz groups gives this pub a lively reputation for a small country village. The Manor House Hotel serves morning coffee, lunches and afternoon teas but children are not made welcome.

### What to see
Studland village is south of the **Studland Heath Nature Reserve** where a number of rare species of birds and animals including the Dartford warbler, adders and, occasionally, a smoothsnake can be seen.

*Exercise*

A breezy cliff walk leads to fascinating views of **Old Harry Rocks** from above, where you can see how the crumbling stacks are being eroded by wind and water. A pleasant extension to the walk continues along Ballard Down, part of the Dorset Coastal Path; from **Studland Hill** you have a fine view to the west of Swanage and Swanage Bay, where King Alfred defeated the Danes in 877. Beyond the bay Portland Bill can be seen in the distance. To the north and east the view includes Poole Harbour, Brownsea Island, Bournemouth and the Isle of Wight. See the *Holiday Which? Good Walks Guide* walk 26.

The golden sands of Studland Bay form one of the safest bathing beaches in Dorset. Windsurfers can be hired on Studland Beach and north of Redend rocks.

# Studland Bay

The anchorage can be spoilt by water and jetskiers who power through the anchorage at maximum speed despite the buoys indicating a five-knot speed limit and the presence of Police Launch Alarm.

Mooring facilities are not suitable for a long stay or for leaving your boat.

To reach Studland village from the beach, take the well-marked path to the main road, about a quarter of a mile away; turn left for the village, which is another half-mile, or right into the main road where you will find the Bankes Arms about 100 yards away on your left.

## STEP ASHORE

**Nearest payphone** Bankes Arms Studland Village

**Toilets** On your left if you turn left at the main road. If you anchor north of Redend rocks at Redend Point, you will find another path on the shore that leads to

**Shopping** Studland Stores/post office sells food (early closing Saturdays, closed Sundays). The garage in the village also sells food and is open until 1900

## SHIPS' SERVICES

*Fuel* (petrol) from garage

# Poole Harbour

Poole is a great place to sail to, with its extensive harbour and beautiful surroundings: the Purbecks, Brownsea Island, Furzey Island (which is private) and Green Island. Poole Harbour is the first, second or third largest natural harbour in the world, Europe or UK, depending on whom you listen to. Except for the main channels it is very shallow and is best explored in a shallow draught boat, bilge keeler or multihull, or by dinghy. A boat cannot be left unmanned on the Town Quay for any period of time. If it is to be left, then a berth at Cobbs Quay, Salterns Marina, Poole Yacht Club or the Royal Motor Yacht Club at Sandbanks should be found. Poole is an excellent base for venturing out into Dorset by car, bicycle, bus or train; you can even charter planes from Bournemouth Airport. The surrounding towns of Wareham (a Roman town), Wimborne Minster, Bournemouth, Christchurch, and, further afield, Salisbury, Sherborne and Shaftesbury are all easily reached and worth visiting.

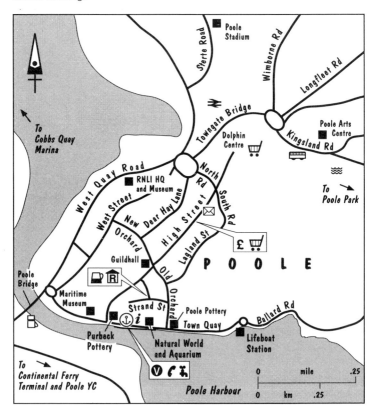

Poole Harbour

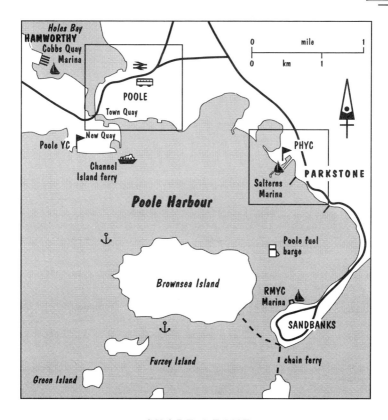

## SHORE LEAVE

### Food and drink
Corkers restaurant and wine bar on the Quay is worth a visit. La Lupa, an Italian restaurant particularly recommended, is informal and suitable for crews still in yachting gear. For a pleasant formal meal (not in yachting gear) choose Barfood in the High Street: Edwardian meals at reasonable, but not Edwardian, prices.

### Entertainment
There is a 10-cinema complex at Tower Park, four miles from the centre of Poole. **Poole Arts Centre**, Kingsland Road, houses the Ashley cinema and a theatre and is home of the Bournemouth Symphony Orchestra.

### What to see
Poole is the headquarters of the Royal National Lifeboat Institution and its museum is particularly interesting for all sailors. The **Maritime Museum** in a medieval building on the Quay has displays of Poole's seafaring history. **Natural World**, also on the Quay, includes an aquarium and a serpentarium. Poole pottery can be seen in the making at **The Pottery** on the Quay, which also offers glass-blowing demonstrations and has a museum.

### Excursions
**Brownsea Island** is a nature reserve with red squirrels, peacocks and deer and

a bird reserve with a hide on the north side. You can get there by ferry from Poole Quay or moor off Pottery Pier on the west side or Blood Alley Lake on the south side. There are no landings on the east or north sides. Places of interest within easy reach of Poole include **Upton Country Park**, an estate four miles north of Poole with formal gardens and an early nineteenth-century house. **Kingston Lacy**, near Wimborne, is a seventeenth-century house with formal gardens, owned by the National Trust.

*Exercise*

A good local walk, easily reached by water, is round the **Arne bird sanctuary**; you can moor off Shipstal Point. There are safe, sandy beaches where you can swim at Studland, Sandbanks and Brownsea Island. If it's too cold to swim in the sea, try the Dolphin Swimming Pool near Poole Park which has three indoor pools, plus sauna, solarium and gym. Windsurfing is popular at Sandbanks, Canford Cliffs and the seaward side of Sandbanks Beach, or learn to windsurf on Poole Park Lake. Waterski in and around the Wareham Channel, north-west of the Arne Peninsula. The leisure centre at the Dolphin Centre offers a variety of sports.

## TRANSPORT AND TRAVEL

**Trains** From Poole to London via Bournemouth and Southampton
**Planes** From Hurn Airport, about nine miles from the marina – to the Channel Islands, Dinard and Paris during the summer
**Ferries** To Cherbourg in the summer and to Channel Islands all year round

**Taxis** ☎ (0202) 672251
**Car hire** Brian Whiteside at quay ☎ (0202) 679980
**Mopeds** Mr Moped ☎ (0202) 716774
**Bicycle hire** None close to the quay; Bikes at Branksome ☎ (0202) 769202; Poole Windsurfer Centre for mountain bikes ☎ (0202) 741744

*Further information* from Tourist Information Office on Town Quay.

# Poole Town Quay

| | |
|---|---|
| **Harbourmaster** ☎ (0202) 685261 | **VHF Channel** 14 |
| **Callsign** Poole Harbour Control | **Daily charge** ££ |

The greatest disappointment is the very limited range of facilities at the quay itself. There are only piles to moor against and in summer rafts of boats cause difficulties for all. But once you have stepped ashore, Poole is alive and kicking.

## STEP ASHORE

**Nearest payphone** On Quay
**Toilets** On Quay by Poole Bridge
**Showers** Lord Nelson Inn on Quay and in gym in Bennets Alley, off Quay, after 1600
**Clubhouse** Poole Yacht Club ☎ (0202) 674706 on the south side of New Quay, over the Poole Bridge, is the nearest
**Shopping** General stores for late-night food shopping near the Quay. If you need fast food there are many burger bars and fish and chip shops as well as pubs and restaurants on the Quay. The main shopping areas are in the High Street and the Dolphin Shopping Centre with all major stores and shops as well as local shops, banks and building societies with cash dispensers, a post office and a bureau de change
**Water taxi** VHF Ch 6 ☎ (0836) 537485

## SHIPS' SERVICES

**Water** *Available on the Quay*

**Fuel** *(diesel and petrol) From Poole Bay Fuels. Fuel barge near Aunt Betty buoy; VHF Ch 37*

**Gas** *(Camping and Calor) From GasLink Ltd, 3 Willis Way and all boatyards in harbour*

**Chandler** *Piplers on Quay and several others*

**Boatyard, Engineer** *Ridge Wharf at Wareham is recommended ☎ (0929) 556288. Several more up river*

**Sailmaker** *Several, but Quay Sails, 20 Lagland Street is recommended*

# Salterns Marina

| | |
|---|---|
| **Harbourmaster** ☎ (0202) 709971 | **VHF Channel** 80, M |
| **Callsign** Salterns Marina | **Daily charge** ££££ |

Salterns, on the east bank of Poole Harbour, is about one-and-a-half miles from Poole Quay by water and about four miles by road. The marina itself is very pleasant with all facilities, helpful staff and a yacht club (although this is a proprietary rather than a members' club). Salterns is situated in a residential area with a parade of shops. With the poor facilities for mooring at the Quay, this is a good place to leave a boat in safety.

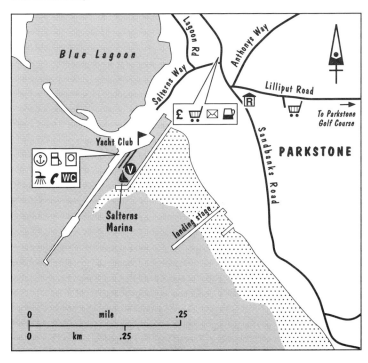

## STEP ASHORE

**Nearest payphone** By marina office
**Toilets, showers, launderette** (with drying room) In marina building
**Clubhouse** Poole Harbour Yacht Club
**Shopping** Late-night shop on Sandbanks Road – turn left at the end of Salterns Way leading from marina. There is a post office/general store and a bank in Sandbanks Road. Main shopping centre in Poole or Bournemouth, both about four miles by road. Tower Park has a large Tesco and entertainment park

### SHIPS' SERVICES

*Water and electricity* On pontoons
*Fuel* (diesel and petrol), *gas* (Camping and Calor), *boatyard, engineer* All available in marina

## SHORE LEAVE

*Food and drink*
The restaurant in Salterns Hotel is good but expensive. The Beehive pub is excellent for meals and snacks. Barrie – Le Pêcheur (known locally as Barrie the Fish) has an excellent seafood restaurant on Sandbanks Road. Allan's, 8 Bournemouth Road, Lower Parkstone is an unpretentious seafood restaurant recommended in *The Good Food Guide 1992*.

*Excursions*
**Compton Acres Gardens** are famous private gardens with rock and water gardens, a woodland walk, a heather dell and Japanese garden. They are about a 15-minute walk away, or a short bus ride.

*Exercise*
Salterns is situated on the harbour in a residential area but you can take a bus to Sandbanks and then a ferry for a walk on Studland Heath, or walk to Constitution Hill and win a marvellous view of Poole Harbour and the Purbecks to the south. Parkstone Golf Club is close by. There are beaches where you can swim at Sandbanks, both in the harbour and seaward to the east.

# Cobb's Quay

| **Mooring Master/Harbourmaster** ☎ (0202) 674299 | **VHF Channels** 80, M |
|---|---|
| **Callsign** CQ Base | **Daily charge** £££ |

Cobb's Quay is west of the Town Quay and is approached via a lifting bridge, which is only raised every two hours to a schedule. In high summer and at weekends there is an unholy scramble to get through the bridge particularly in the morning and evening.

At the other side of the bridge, the channel passes through an industrial area and then opens out into Holes Bay. The channel is not very deep, especially towards Cobbs Quay Marina. One of the problems with Holes Bay is that it is gradually silting up. Although the marina claims to be accessible at all states of the tide, the depth is often less than three feet at low water spring tides on a generally mud bottom.

The marina is about one-and-a-half miles from Poole Quay by water and two-and-a-half miles by road. The land entrance is in the middle of a residential housing area with no immediately accessible shops. Access for a visitor without land transport is inconvenient. The great plus for Cobb's Quay is that it provides all facilities for yachts and, apart from Salterns Marina, is the only safe place to leave – for more than a few hours – a visiting, unmanned yacht in Poole Harbour.

## STEP ASHORE

**Payphone, toilets, showers** All within marina complex
**Clubhouse** Cobb's Quay Yacht Club

(proprietary)
**Taxis, car and bicycle hire** Can be arranged through marina office

### SHIPS' SERVICES

**Water and electricity** *Available on pontoons*
**Fuel** *(petrol and diesel) Available in marina*

**Gas** *(Camping and Calor) From chandler in marina*
**Boatyard, engineer, sailmaker** *All available in marina*

## SHORE LEAVE

There is a licensed restaurant in the marina.

Two miles from Cobb's Quay, at the northern end of Holes Bay, is **Upton House** and **Upton Country Park**, easily visited on foot. Parts of the elegant early nineteenth-century house are open to the public on Sunday afternoons. The landscaped gardens lead into areas of farmland, woodland and saltmarsh with three nature trails from which to observe wildlife.

---

*Alternative moorings*
Other berths can be found at **Royal Motor Yacht Club** and **Poole Yacht Club** although both are busy and have only limited visitors' facilities.

---

# SOLENT
## and
# ISLE OF WIGHT

# Yarmouth

Yarmouth is a pocket-sized town – one of the oldest on the Isle of Wight –
with an attractive square and a castle. In the Domesday Book Yarmouth
is called Ermud, later Eremue. It was the main port on the Isle of Wight
in the twelfth century, when it received a royal charter, and remained a
borough till 1891. Yarmouth Castle, built as a fortification by Henry VIII,
put an end to the trouble the town had endured at the hands of the
French, who twice ransacked and burned it to the ground.

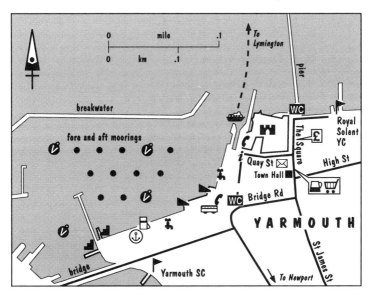

## SHORE LEAVE

### Food and drink
Yarmouth caters well for sailors on the eating front, with plenty of pubs serving
meals of various types. The Bugle Hotel has a barbecue in a small courtyard.
There are children's rooms at the Bugle, King's Head and Wheatsheaf.

### What to see
Yarmouth has an old church and an unusual Town Hall rebuilt in 1763. **Yarmouth
Castle** was built as part of Henry VIII's very necessary coastal defences; in 1597
the Governor's House, which later became the George Hotel, was added to it –
look out for the original oak staircase. **Fort Victoria Country Park** is about a 10-
minute walk from Yarmouth – the fort is one of three built to defend the Solent at
its narrowest point. The park includes a nature trail through 50 acres of
woodlands, wetlands and seashore, with spectacular views of the Western
Solent, and an aquarium. **Golden Hill Fort** is a little further away (about a mile),
but is more ambitious, with a military museum, craft centre, antiques and gift
shop; and it has fine views over Christchurch Bay towards the Purbeck Hills.

*Excursions*

Coaches run from the ferry terminal to **Alum Bay**, which has a bathing beach, although its main attractions are its coloured sand cliffs and breathtaking scenery. The climb down is steep, but you can use the chairlift. A rather unexpected find at Alum Bay is the **Museum of Clocks**, the only one of its kind in the south of England. There is also a pottery and a glass blower.

A bus runs to the Needles from Yarmouth: the National Trust own the **Needles Old Battery**, a former Palmerstonian Fort built in 1862. It is 250 feet above sea level with a 200-foot tunnel leading to spectacular views of the Needles rocks and lighthouse. In the parade ground there is an exhibition of the history of the headland, a children's exhibition and an original gun barrel mounted on its carriage.

**Carisbrooke Castle**, where Charles I was imprisoned, is on the bus route to Newport. Coach tours of the island, which take five hours, leave Yarmouth Ferry Terminal at 1140 every day.

*Exercise*

The beaches to the west of Yarmouth are the best for swimming. If you are energetic, walk to **Cliff End** or even to **Alum Bay**. A good walk is along High Down Ridge towards Tennyson's Monument and over Tennyson Down. See the *Holiday Which? Good Walks Guide* walk 41. If you want to take part in an organised walk, details can be found in the sports pages of the *County Press*. There is plenty of organised sport on the island.

## TRANSPORT AND TRAVEL

**Buses** Hourly to Newport
**Ferries** To Lymington every 30 minutes
**Taxis** Cab rank by ferry on pier
**Car hire** Panda Hire, The Square

**Bicycle hire** Nearest is Vectis Products, The Broadway, Totland
☎ (0983) 752455

*Further information* from Tourist Office on the quay by the ferry terminal.

# Yarmouth Harbour

| Harbourmaster ☎ (0983) 760300 | VHF Channel 80 |
|---|---|
| Callsign Yarmouth Harbour | Daily charge ££ |

In spite of its popularity as a yacht harbour, which in the summer months means queueing at the entrance and waiting to be shepherded to your mooring by a flotilla of harbourmaster's assistants armed with radios, Yarmouth remains enjoyable to visit. The rows of piles, which make up most of the visitors' berths, can call for some slick boathandling. The inconvenience of being on piles is compensated for by the Sandhard ferry which runs a service to the quay until midnight, costing 50p.

In the height of summer, when the harbour is full, and therefore closed, you may have to anchor or pick up a buoy outside.

## STEP ASHORE

**Nearest payphone** At south-east corner of the harbour
**Toilets** Also at south-east corner
**Showers, toilets** At Royal Solent Yacht Club
**Clubhouses** Royal Solent Yacht Club, The Square; Yarmouth Sailing Club, Bridge Road

**Shopping** In The Square, five minutes' walk from the harbour. There are several food shops, a bank, a post office and a bookshop which sells charts. Try taking your dinghy up the Yar to Puffins Fisheries at Saltern Wood Quay where you can buy freshly-cooked local shellfish

### SHIPS' SERVICES

**Water** On the quay
**Fuel** (diesel and petrol) On quay
**Gas** (Camping and Calor) From Harold Hayles Boatyard across the bridge and chandler

**Chandler** Harwood's Ltd, The Square
**Boatyard, engineer** Harold Hayles Boatyard
**Sailmaker** Saltern Sail Company, Saltern Wood Quay

# Lymington

Set at the edge of the New Forest and just inside the Solent, Lymington has a long history as a seaport. It was favoured by the Romans who had a large camp at Bucklands Ring, the iron age fort, itself dating back to 500 BC. Like Yarmouth, on the other side of the Solent, it was sacked several times by the French in the fourteenth and fifteenth centuries. Jack-in-the-Basket, the beacon at the entrance, appears on a seventeenth-century chart. The narrow fairway is lined with moorings right up to the Town Quay, and the sight of the huge ferry bearing down on you can be daunting. However, once you have tied up you will find the town delightful, with its many old streets lined with Georgian houses.

There are two crowded marinas, both expensive; the Town Quay, with public lavatories alongside, is one-third the price.

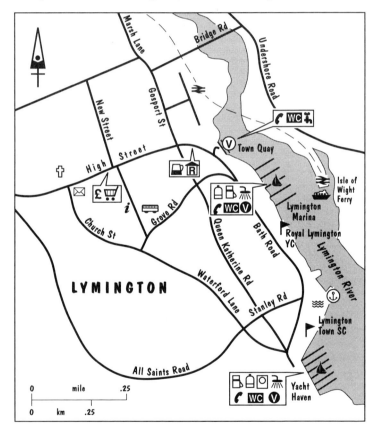

## SHORE LEAVE

### Food and drink

A wide selection exists for all tastes and pockets, from tea-shops to wine bars. Many of the hotels in the High Street were old coaching stations; many of the pubs were used by smugglers. Eating ashore around the Town Quay can be expensive. The Tollhouse, an old inn at the top of the town in Southampton Road, is a friendly place and is recommended for its home-cooked vegetables and Sunday lunches. Provence in Gordleton Mill Hotel, Silver Street, Hordle, is an excellent restaurant, recently refurbished, which is featured in *The Good Food Guide 1992*.

### Shopping

There is a full range of high-street shops, banks with bureau de change facilities and outside cash dispensers, building societies and a post office. Early closing is on Wednesdays. There is a market on Saturdays.

### Entertainment

Lymington Community Centre in Cannon Street has a small cinema, but is closed in August.

### What to see

The **Buckland Heritage Centre** in the **Tollhouse Cottage** tells the story of the iron age rings which may be seen 'live' nearby. **Lymington Vineyard** at Pennington welcomes visitors.

### Excursions

**Hurst Castle** at Keyhaven, one of Henry VIII's many defences, out on its shingle spit, is a good place for a swim and a picnic. At **Brockenhurst**, four miles north of Lymington, the Rhinefield rhododendron drive, Bolderwood arboretum and deer sanctuary offer a pleasant outing away from the sea.

### Exercise

There is an indoor swimming pool at Lymington Recreation Centre in North Street, Pennington and an open-air pool near the harbourmaster's office. Guided walks around Lymington start from the Parish Church on Sunday afternoons and Wednesday evenings during the summer.

### TRANSPORT AND TRAVEL

**Buses** Every hour from the bus stop half-way up the High Street to Southampton and Bournemouth

**Trains** Every 30 minutes to Brockenhurst where they connect with trains for Poole, Southampton and London

**Planes** From Southampton–Eastleigh airport

**Ferries** To Yarmouth every 30 minutes

**Taxis** Lymington Taxis ☎ (0590) 672842

**Car hire** ☎ (0590) 673227

*Further information* from Tourist Office in the car park behind Waitrose in the High Street.

# Lymington Yacht Haven

| | |
|---|---|
| **Harbourmaster** ☎ (0590) 677071 | **VHF Channel** 80 |
| **Callsign** Lymington Yacht Haven | **Daily charge** ££££ |

This is the first marina on the west bank on entering the river. It is about a mile from the centre of Lymington.

## STEP ASHORE

**Nearest payphone** By harbour office
**Toilets, showers, launderette** All in harbour office block
**Clubhouse** Berth holders are welcome at the Lymington Town Sailing Club near the marina
**Shopping** Waterford Stores and post office are near the marina, the Riverside Stores with off licence in Bath Road.

Otherwise it is a 15-minute walk into town to the main shops
**Food and drink** Bar and restaurant at Lymington Town Sailing Club; five minutes' walk away is an old pub, The Fisherman's Rest in All Saints Road, which is personally recommended for its varied and good-value menu

### SHIPS' SERVICES

*Water and electricity* On pontoons
*Fuel* (diesel and petrol) From the fuel berth

*Gas* (Camping and Calor) *chandler, boatyard, engineer, sailmaker* All in the marina or nearby

# Lymington Marina

| | |
|---|---|
| **Harbourmaster** ☎ (0590) 673312 | **VHF Channel** M |
| **Callsign** Lymington Marina | **Daily charge** £££££ |

This marina, known as Berthons to those who remember the old firm of boatbuilders, is further up river and closer to the town.

## STEP ASHORE

**Nearest payphone** By dockmaster's office
**Toilets, showers** Behind dockmaster's office, on first floor
**Clubhouse** Lymington Town Sailing Club
**Shopping** Waterford Stores and post office near Yacht Haven and Riverside

Stores with off licence in Bath Road are the nearest shops. Otherwise it is a 10-minute walk into town to the main shops
**Food and drink** Bar and restaurant at Lymington Town Sailing Club

### SHIPS' SERVICES

*Water and electricity* On pontoons
*Fuel* (diesel and petrol) From fuel pontoon
*Gas* (Camping and Calor) *chandler,*

*boatyard, engineer, sailmaker* All in the marina or nearby

# Town Quay

**Harbourmaster** ☎ (0590) 672014          **Daily charge** ££

The Town Quay is more convenient for shore-based activities than either of the marinas but there are few facilities and no security.

## STEP ASHORE

**Nearest payphone** On Town Quay
**Toilets** On Town Quay
**Launderette** 11 New Street

**Shopping** Main shops within five minutes' walk

## SHIPS' SERVICES

**Water and electricity** Available on Town Quay
**Gas** (Camping and Calor) From chandler

**Chandler** Yachtmail Co Ltd, Admiral's Court, The Quay

# Newtown River

Newtown River once served as a harbour for Newtown, a busy port with flourishing salt works and oyster beds. It is now a wildlife reserve frequented by migrating birds and protected by the National Trust. The river is a rare haven where nature takes precedence, and it is a delight to explore by water or land – there are lots of creeks and shore-side walks. The moorings get very crowded at summer weekends, so, if you can, time your visit for midweek when space will be found to anchor or tie up to one of the visitors' buoys and enjoy the wildlife and walks.

Newtown River is old-fashioned yachting: its main attraction is peace and quiet – somewhere to recharge your personal batteries at the height of a balmy summer. There used to be mussel beds at low water, some of which can still be found, and if you feel brave and know how to prepare them, there is great satisfaction in being self-sufficient at dinner. In season some superb blackberries can be picked.

## SHORE LEAVE

### Food and drink
The only pub within walking distance of Newtown River moorings is the New Inn at Shalfleet (mentioned in the Domesday Book) – it has an imaginative menu and serves good seafood. You will need to book in summer to avoid disappointment ☎ (0983) 78314. Local morris dancers occasionally perform outside the New Inn.

### Excursions
Landing on the east side of the River, at Newtown Quay, will lead you after about a mile to **Newtown** itself. In spite of its name, Newtown was the old capital of the Isle of Wight, sacked by the Romans and later burned by the French. It once returned two members to Parliament. This ancient borough is now reduced to a small village, although the outlines of the thirteenth-century town are clearly defined. As well as a few old houses there is the very fine brick and stone seventeenth-century **Old Town Hall**, later used as a school and a meeting house. It is now owned by the National Trust. It is still used for parish council meetings and the rooms, including the council chamber, the robing room and the mayor's parlour, can sometimes be visited. Copies of ancient documents of the borough and a facsimile of the mace are available at the Hall. There is a church in the village but no shops or post office.

**Clamerkin Farm Park** has a working farm, with many small hand-reared farm animals, on the Newtown estuary overlooking **Clamerkin Lake**. Many species of water birds can be seen from hides placed behind an old sea wall. There is good walking here, along banks purple with sea lavender and with lovely seascapes.

On the west side of the river you can land at Shalfleet Quay and walk the two miles to the main road and picturesque **Shalfleet Village**. On the way along the riverside you will pass the old mill with its millstream, footbridges and an exceptionally luxuriant garden. It is possible to take a dinghy up **Shalfleet Lake** almost to Shalfleet, but because the creek dries you can't delay at Shalfleet, so

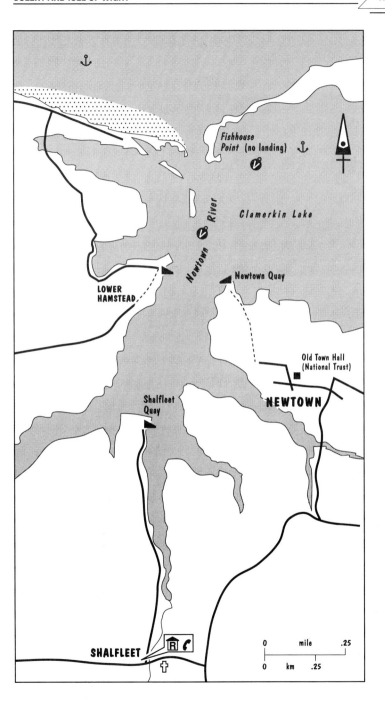

Fishhouse Point (no landing)

Clamerkin Lake

Newtown River

Newtown Quay

LOWER HAMSTEAD

Old Town Hall (National Trust)

Shalfleet Quay

**NEWTOWN**

**SHALFLEET**

| 0 | mile | .25 |
| 0 | km | .25 |

it's best to stretch your legs by walking. The post office at Shalfleet, which sells some groceries, is also a mini craft centre with a 'farmyard zoo'. The village has an attractive old church.

### TRANSPORT AND TRAVEL

**Buses** The Newport–Freshwater bus, which passes Yarmouth Ferry Terminal, stops at Barton's corner, a mile from the Newtown Old Town Hall

# Newtown River Moorings

**Berthing Master** ☎ (0983) 78424

**Daily charge** visitor's buoy ££; own anchor £

Anchoring is restricted to marked channels in order to preserve the delicate oyster beds – these are signposted with white on green boards – and to avoid foul ground. The National Trust Berthing Master collects harbour dues. You will need a dinghy to get ashore.

### STEP ASHORE

**Nearest payphone** Newtown village
**Shopping** Post office at Shalfleet, two miles from Shalfleet Quay. Many cottages sell fresh fruit and vegetables at their gates

# Beaulieu River – Buckler's Hard

Two hundred years ago Buckler's Hard, a couple of miles up the Beaulieu River, was a busy shipyard building frigates for Nelson's fleet with timber from the New Forest. So many trees were needed that the forest was permanently changed. Now Buckler's Hard is a sleepy village street, except for the tourists, set in beautiful countryside.

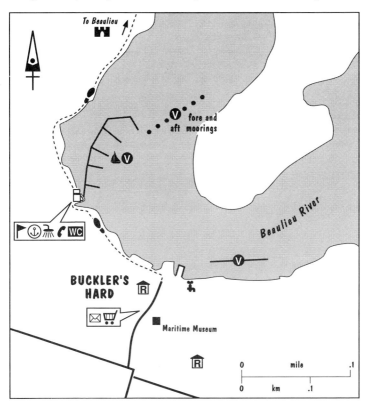

SHORE LEAVE

*Food and drink*
The Mainsail Cafeteria near the Maritime Museum is good for light snacks. The Master Builder's Hotel serves both pub food and restaurant meals.

*What to see*
Several residential cottages have been restored and furnished according to their use and period. Henry Adams (the Master Builder) can be seen through the window of his house, poring over plans, attended by his foreman. The **Maritime Museum** reflects the history of the village, with an evocative model of the old shipyard in full production.

*Excursions*
Go to **Beaulieu** to see the **Motor Museum**, the **Palace House** and gardens and the ruins of **Beaulieu Abbey**.

*Exercise*
The two-and-a-half mile riverside walk, through woodlands, to **Beaulieu** is very pleasant. The trail begins by the pier – a guide leaflet is available from the Information Centre. The harbourmaster suggests walking there and returning by taxi. A New Forest guidebook, available from the Information Centre, includes information on walking in the Forest.

## TRANSPORT AND TRAVEL

**Buses** From Beaulieu to Southampton

**Taxis** From Beaulieu: Maurice Badland ☎ (0590) 612267

***Further information*** from the Harbour Office and from the Buckler's Hard Information Centre in the Maritime Museum.

# Beaulieu River and Buckler's Hard Moorings

**Harbourmaster** ☎ (0590) 616200

**Daily charge** own anchor £; on piles ££; marina ££££

You can anchor in the peace of the lower reaches of Beaulieu River, alongside Gull Island nature reserve, go on up to Buckler's Hard to moor to piles, or go into the marina. The river and marina are owned by Lord Montagu, chairman of British Heritage, and superbly maintained. The marina is very well run and welcoming but only simple facilities are available.

## STEP ASHORE

**Nearest payphone** By harbour office at the landing stage
**Toilets, showers, launderette** In purpose-built block by harbour office

**Shopping** There is a well-stocked village shop a quarter of a mile away at the top of the village street, reached by the footpath along the river bank

### SHIPS' SERVICES

***Water and electricity*** *On the pontoons*
***Fuel*** *(diesel and petrol),* ***gas*** *(Calor and Camping) At landing stage*

***Chandler, boatyard, engineer, sailmaker***
*All available in the marina*

# Cowes and the Medina River

Cowes is famous for racing but also welcomes cruising yachts and provides excellent facilities for enjoyment or repairs. Families are welcome everywhere but the town is often too crowded for very young children, especially during Cowes Week, which runs from the first Saturday in August. If you are there at that time, don't miss the fireworks on the last Friday. The harbour is always busy and yachts should beware of ferries, large trading vessels and hydrofoils.

The banks of the Medina River are interesting and busy places, from the wharves in East and West Cowes to Osborne and Whippingham, with their memories of Queen Victoria, to the more tranquil shores of the west bank till finally at Newport the boatyards reappear. The Medina River is administered by the Cowes Harbour Commissioners up to the Folly Inn, upstream of which it is under the jurisdiction of the Newport harbourmaster.

## SHORE LEAVE

*Food and drink*
Cowes has numerous restaurants, pubs and take-aways – hungry crews are well catered for. An old favourite is Murrays Seafood Restaurant, 106 High Street.

*Entertainment*
Amateur plays can be seen at Trinity Theatre, off Bath Road.

*What to see*
The **Maritime Museum**, in the same building as Cowes Library in Beckford Road, contains, among other items, a fine series of ship models, mostly of vessels built by the Cowes shipbuilding company J Samuel White, Ltd. The **Sir Max Aitken Museum** in the High Street features maritime artefacts of sailing vessels from Nelson's day to modern times.

*Excursions*
You could visit **Arreton Manor**, where barns and farm buildings have been converted into workshops and studios, and jewellery, pottery, furniture and other goods are made and sold. The **Seaview Flamingo Park**, in a lake set in spacious grounds overlooking the Solent, has a large colony of breeding flamingos, and many other birds.

*Exercise*
There are various beaches where you can swim, but watch out for strong currents. The coastal walk towards **Gurnard Point** is excellent; otherwise take a bus to **Freshwater**, the **Needles** or **Alum Bay** and walk from there.

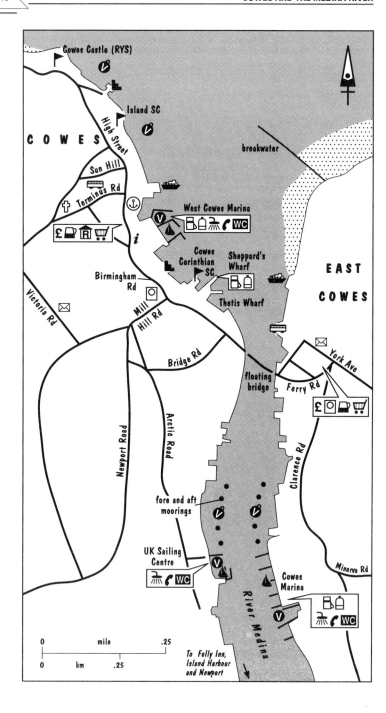

## TRANSPORT AND TRAVEL

**Buses** From Carrel Lane, off the High Street, to the rest of the Isle of Wight, in most cases via Newport
**Trains** From Southampton
**Planes** From Southampton-Eastleigh airport
**Ferries** Red Funnel Ferry and hydrofoil to Southampton. Local chain ferry runs almost continuously from West to East Cowes and back
**Taxis** There are ranks at Fountains Yard and at the Bus station
**Car hire** Solent Self Drive
☎ (0983) 822247
**Bicycle hire** Cowes Cycle Centre, High Street

*Further information* from Tourist Office on Fountain Quay.

# Cowes Harbour Commission

| | |
|---|---|
| **Harbourmaster** ☎ (0983) 293952 | **VHF Channel** 69 |
| **Callsign** Cowes Harbour Radio | **Daily charge** ££; short stays up to 4 hours £ |

The harbourmaster has a number of moorings for those who do not want to use the many private facilities in the river. The four buoys just past the Royal Yacht Squadron on the starboard hand are usually far too restless for a long stay. North of Thetis Wharf is a public pontoon landing for a short stay or overnight. South of the floating bridge there are pile moorings on both sides. The many landing places can be recognised by the dinghies tied to them. The harbourmaster and his staff are always in evidence on the water in their launches and will be pleased to give help and advice.

## STEP ASHORE

**Nearest payphone** This varies according to where you land: try pubs and yacht clubs, also several phone kiosks in Cowes High Street
**Toilets** Pubs and yacht clubs, or public WCs
**Showers** Yacht clubs
**Launderette** Washeteria, Mill Hill Road
**Clubhouses** There are six yacht clubs in Cowes; the Island Sailing Club and Cowes Corinthian specifically welcome visitors
**Shopping** Cowes High Street has a good range of shops, banks and a post office. Hewitt & Son is open for provisions seven days a week. Limited bureau de change service available at Cowes Tourist Information Centre at 4 Marine Walk as well as at banks

### SHIPS' SERVICES

*Water* Old Town Quay; Whitegates public pontoon; Watch House slipway; Thetis Pontoon
*Fuel* (diesel and petrol) Available from West Cowes Marina (open 24 hours) and Souters Yard
*Gas* West Cowes Marina, Hurst Ironmongers, High Street
*Chandler, boatyard, engineer, sailmaker* All can be found in abundance in Cowes, and they are often willing to work late or at weekends

# West Cowes Marina

| | |
|---|---|
| **Harbourmaster** ☎ (0983) 295754 | **VHF Channels** 80 |
| **Callsign** West Cowes Marina | **Daily charge** ££££ |

This is the first marina you come to on entering the river, but it is also the most restless berth because of the permanent swell which enters the harbour. It is, however – when not crowded with racing yachts – the most convenient place for getting ashore to enjoy the many pleasures and amenities which Cowes has to offer.

## STEP ASHORE

**Nearest payphone** Under the harbourmaster's office
**Toilets, showers** In building at back of marina, behind Fastnet Restaurant

**Shopping** Just outside the gates
**Food and drink** Fastnet Restaurant in marina

### SHIPS' SERVICES

*Water and electricity* On pontoons
*Fuel* (diesel and petrol), *gas* (Camping and Calor), *chandler, boatyard, engineer, sailmaker* All in marina or nearby

# UK Sailing Centre

| | |
|---|---|
| **Harbourmaster** ☎ (0983) 294941 | **Daily charge** £££ |

The UK Sailing Centre is on the starboard hand of the Medina River, a quarter of a mile above the floating bridge. It is a residential sailing school but is happy to welcome visitors if there is room on the pontoons. It is cheaper and quieter than downstream, but is a long walk from the town.

## STEP ASHORE

**Nearest payphone** In entrance lobby to main block
**Toilets and showers** In building behind the main block

**Clubhouse** Bar on the first floor
**Shopping** Small grocery in Arctic Road; turn right outside the gate

### SHIPS' SERVICES

*Water and electricity* On pontoons

# Cowes Marina

| Harbourmaster ☎ (0983) 293983 | VHF Channel 80 |
|---|---|
| Callsign Cowes Marina | Daily charge £££ |

This marina is on the east bank, opposite the UK Sailing Club. There are plenty of grassed areas where you are invited to have a barbecue. The marina has a programme of improvements for its shore facilities in progress.

### STEP ASHORE

**Nearest payphone** By harbour office
**Toilets and showers** In marina
**Launderette** In East Cowes shopping area, half a mile from the marina
**Clubhouse** The Barge, a floating vessel with restaurant and bar
**Shopping** Essentials are available from the café by the harbour office; otherwise go to East or West Cowes

### SHIPS' SERVICES

*Water and electricity* On pontoons
*Fuel* (petrol and diesel), *gas* (Camping and Calor), *chandler, boatyard, engineer* All in marina

### SHORE LEAVE

This is a good place from which to visit **Osborne House** as it is only a half-mile walk away. Most of Osborne House, which overlooks the Solent, was built between 1845 and 1851 under the supervision of Prince Albert. Queen Victoria died at Osborne in 1901 and her apartments have been preserved largely unchanged since then. There are more than four hundred works of art, pictures and pieces of furniture. The Royal Nursery on the second floor has been restored and is also open to the public.

# The Folly Inn

| Harbourmaster ☎ (0983) 295722 | VHF Channel 16 |
|---|---|
| Callsign Folly Launch | Daily charge ££ |

Mooring here is to Harbour Commission piles. The main attraction is the peace of the river, away from Cowes, and the Inn itself. The original building was once a barge called La Folie – perhaps French. It was abandoned on the beach some two hundred years ago but was quickly taken over by a local and turned into a pub; some parts of the hull remain in the building. The Folly is long-established as a weekend rendezvous for Solent sailors, so, if you want a quiet time, go there midweek.

## STEP ASHORE

**Nearest payphone** At Folly Inn
**Toilets, showers, launderette** All available at Folly Inn
**Shopping** Medina Park Stores in Folly Lane, a quarter of a mile away, open Sundays
**Food and drink** Folly Inn serves pub food and has a restaurant

### SHIPS' SERVICES

*Water* On landing pontoon

## SHORE LEAVE

The unusual **Whippingham Church** in the village was built to the order of Prince Albert and used regularly by Queen Victoria and the Royal Family when they were in residence at Osborne. Well-signposted footpaths lead to **Newport**.

# Island Harbour

| | |
|---|---|
| **Harbourmaster** ☎ (0983) 526020 | **VHF Channels** 80, M |
| **Callsign** Island Harbour | **Daily charge** ££ |

This is a really rustic marina, sited in a dredged basin with a lock useable above half tide. There is little here but a fine harbour control building, a toilet block and a few sheds: it is a pleasant spot, rather like mooring on the edge of a meadow. The harbourmaster will lend you barbecue equipment. The old paddle steamer, *Queen of Ryde*, sits in the mud alongside – it was used as a restaurant, but old age overtook it, leaving a sad and rusty sight. Planning permission has been sought to develop the marina.

## STEP ASHORE

**Nearest payphone** In the harbour office
**Toilets, showers** In the blue building at the back of the site

### SHIPS' SERVICES

*Water and electricity* On pontoons
*Fuel* (diesel and petrol) From berth by lock

## SHORE LEAVE

To make your way back to civilisation, follow the well-marked footpaths to the **Folly Inn** and to **Newport**.

# Newport Harbour

| Harbourmaster ☎ (0983) 525994 | VHF Channel 69 |
| --- | --- |
| Callsign Newport Harbour | Daily charge ££ |

This harbour is at the head of the river and it dries right out. The old commercial quay has been attractively developed and there are pontoons for yachts. The centre of Newport is a few minutes' walk away. Newport is the capital of the Isle of Wight, as well as being a port and a market town.

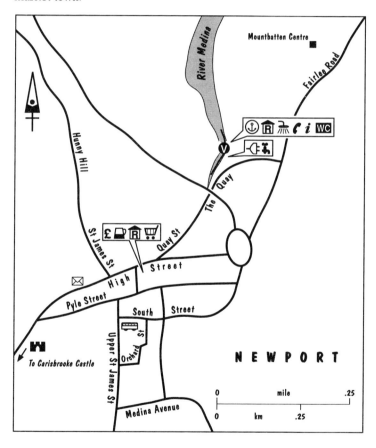

STEP ASHORE

**Nearest payphone** In Riverside Restaurant
**Toilets, showers** Below the harbour office
**Launderette** The Castle Launderette, in Carisbrooke

**Shopping** The main shopping area, with all facilities, is five minutes' walk from the harbour; market on Tuesdays

### SHIPS' SERVICES

**Water and electricity** *On pontoons and quayside*
**Fuel** *(petrol and diesel),* **gas** *(Camping* and Calor)*, **chandler, boatyard, engineer, sailmaker** *All available but more easily obtained down river*

## SHORE LEAVE

### Food and drink

Newport has restaurants of every kind, including a McDonald's. Personally recommended are Valentinos, 93 High Street, Carisbrooke (closed on Sundays), and Tamarisk – which incorporates a tea-shop, the Bakers Oven – at 73 High Street.

### Entertainment

The Studio 1 cinema is in the High Street, Newport. The **Mountbatten Centre** in Newport houses the Medina Theatre, as well as being an exhibition and leisure centre.

### What to see

The **Quay Arts Centre**, just upstream of the harbour, is a restored eighteenth-century warehouse in which there are two art galleries. The **Roman Villa** in Cypress Road has an under-floor heated bath system, tessellated floors and corn-drying kiln.

    **Carisbrooke Castle** is one-and-a-quarter miles south-west of Newport. Part Roman, part Norman and part Elizabethan, it is best known for its connection with Charles I, who was imprisoned there for the ten months before his execution. You enter the moated castle through an impressive gatehouse and find yourself with some seven acres of castle and earthworks to explore. **Carisbrooke**, on the eastern boundary of Newport, is an attractive village.

### Excursions

Virtually everywhere in the Isle of Wight is accessible from Newport. **Godshill**, to the south, is a charming thatched-roofed village. The **Toy Museum** on the ground floor of a Victorian house near the centre of the village is a draw to children of all ages; it has one of the largest displays of post-1945 toys in the country. In the gardens of the Old Vicarage is a large scale **model village**; each house has its own tiny garden with miniature trees and shrubs.

### Exercise

If bad weather stops you enjoying outdoor pursuits, visit the swimming pool at the Medina Recreation Centre in Fairlee Road which has a water slide and learner pool.

### TRANSPORT AND TRAVEL

**Buses** From town centre all over the island
**Taxis** Amar Taxis ☎ (0983) 522968

**Car hire** Wight Drive, 318 Gunville Road, Newport ☎ (0983) 522304

**Further information** from Tourist Office, Quay Store, Town Quay.

# Southampton Water and the Itchen River

Southampton Water, from Calshot Spit to Southampton Docks, is lined on both sides with a mixture of rural and industrial landscapes. Calshot Power Station and Fawley Refinery to port allow glimpses of the New Forest, while Netley Country Park appears to starboard after the oil installations at Hamble Point. At the top of Southampton Water the scenery becomes completely industrial around the dock areas, with the bright new buildings of Ocean Village lending a splash of colour. Many small yards have their quotas of yachts, but for visitors the only suitable places are the marinas: Hythe, Town Quay, Ocean Village and Shamrock Quay.

## SHORE LEAVE

*Food and drink*

Eating and drinking places of every sort can be found in Southampton. La Margherita, an Italian restaurant near the Mayflower Theatre in Commercial Road, is recommended for its varied and reliably good food. *Out to Eat* recommends Hasty Tasty, 48 High Street, for a bumper-sized breakfast, Kohinoor, 2 The Broadway, Fortswood and Kuti's, 70 London Road (also in *The Good Food Guide 1992*) – both for Indian food – and finally Town House, a vegetarian restaurant at 59 Oxford Street.

*Entertainment*

**The Mayflower Theatre**, Commercial Road, stages plays, opera, ballet, musicals and concerts – often before they reach the West End. Concerts are held at the **Guildhall** in West Marlands Road. Both Cannon and Odeon cinemas are in Above Bar Street. There are several night clubs and discos.

*What to see*

The **Civic Art Gallery** in the Civic Centre has an exceptional collection and has quizzes for children. **Tudor House Museum**, St Michael's Square, is in a medieval timber-framed house built for a wealthy merchant – the banqueting hall is furnished in sixteenth-century style and the garden is based on sixteenth-century texts and illustrations. **The Medieval Merchant's House**, 58 French Street, is a recently restored English Heritage property. The **Bargate Museum**, High Street, in a room over what was once the northern gateway to the town, is a local history museum. The **Maritime Museum**, Bugle Street, housed in a fourteenth-century wool warehouse, features the history of the port of Southampton including a model of the docks in the 1930s.

*Excursions*

**Eling Tide Mill**, near Totton, is now restored and working. The New Forest offers plenty of space for walks and picnics. **Broadlands**, on the River Test in Romsey, is an elegant Palladian house, once the home of Lord Palmerston and more recently of Lord Mountbatten of Burma, whose life is depicted in a permanent exhibition in the stables.

*Exercise*

There are swimming baths at Western Esplanade. Walk round what is left of the town walls or take part in a guided walk round old parts of the town.

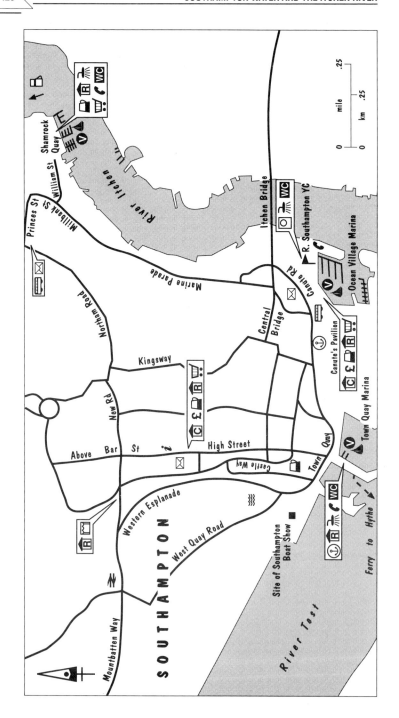

### TRANSPORT AND TRAVEL

**Buses** Comprehensive local services; also to Winchester, Eastleigh and Portsmouth
**Trains** To London, Portsmouth and the West Country
**Planes** From Southampton-Eastleigh airport, trains stop at Eastleigh

**Ferries** To Isle of Wight and Hythe; also to Cherbourg
**Taxis** Fleet Cars ☎ (0703) 466339
**Car hire** Kenning Car Hire ☎ (0703) 639788
**Bicycle hire** Hargroves ☎ (0703) 227179

*Further information* from Tourist Office, Above Bar Precinct.

# Hythe Marina Village

| | |
|---|---|
| **Harbourmaster** ☎ (0703) 207073 | **VHF Channel** 80 |
| **Callsign** Hythe Marina | **Daily charge** £££ |

This is more a property development with a waterside theme than a marina. Access is through a lock, available at most states of the tide, and the welcome for visitors is courteous and efficient, although facilities are few and a long way from where you will be berthed. The main attraction is the view across to Southampton Docks and any large ships which may be in. In the other direction is Hythe, half a mile away. This is a peaceful place to be moored and the New Forest is within easy reach. Alternatively, you can take the ferry across Southampton Water.

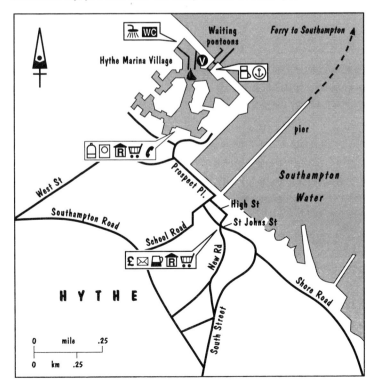

## STEP ASHORE

**Nearest payphone** By marina shops, a quarter of a mile away

**Toilets, showers** In the sanitary block, five minutes' walk away. The key is available, on deposit, from Lock Control

**Launderette** By marina shops

**Shopping** The marina convenience store is a quarter of a mile from the moorings; Hythe village, half a mile away, has a modest range of shops, banks and a post office

### SHIPS' SERVICES

*Water and electricity* On pontoons
*Fuel* (diesel and petrol) From fuel berth
*Gas* (Camping and Calor) From chandler

*Chandler, boatyard, engineer, sailmaker*
*All available on-site*

## SHORE LEAVE

A restaurant and pub sit by the marina shops and Hythe has several pubs and restaurants. The **New Forest**, for walks and picnics, is on the doorstep and **Eling Tide Mill**, near Totton, is within easy reach. Take the ferry from the end of the pier across to Southampton.

### TRANSPORT AND TRAVEL

**Buses** To Fawley and Southampton – it is quicker and cheaper to take the ferry from the end of the pier across to Southampton

**Taxis** Hythe Taxis ☎ (0703) 843390
**Car hire** Jennings Motors, Dibden Purlieu ☎ (0703) 842171

*Further information* from Tourist Office, Above Bar Precinct, Southampton.

# Town Quay Marina

| | |
|---|---|
| **Harbourmaster** ☎ (0703) 234397 | **VHF Channel** 80 |
| **Callsign** Town Quay Marina | **Daily charge** ££ |

The marina at Town Quay was opened in June 1991 and at the time of inspection the pontoons were just being moved into position, so there is no information about what the marina is like in use. All the usual facilities of a modern marina are planned and toilets and showers were ready for use. The adjoining building houses two restaurants; there will be shops in the same building. This marina is very much the nearest to the city centre and the staff are anxious to attract visitors – the comparatively low charges will help them in this. It is also close to the site of the Southampton Boat Show, which may lead to overcrowding in September.

# Ocean Village Marina

| | |
|---|---|
| **Harbourmaster** ☎ (0703) 229385 | **VHF Channel** 80 |
| **Callsign** Ocean Marina | **Daily charge** £££ |

Set in the old Eastern Docks, Ocean Village is backed by an extensive shoreside development. The colourful Canute Pavilion houses a selection of tourist shops, a minimarket and a variety of eating places – a Covent Garden by the sea which lends a holiday atmosphere to the marina.

## STEP ASHORE

**Nearest payphone** At top of ramp leading from pontoons
**Toilets** At top of ramp
**Showers, launderette** Under Yacht Club building
**Clubhouse** Royal Southampton Yacht Club on the edge of the marina welcomes members of affiliated yacht clubs

**Shopping** Minimarket and other shops in the Canute Pavilion
**Food and drink** Pubs and restaurants of various types in or near the Canute Pavilion
**Buses** From outside the marina to the city centre

## SHIPS' SERVICES

*Water and electricity* On pontoons
*Fuel* (petrol and diesel) At weekends from a fuel barge in the river outside the marina or from the Itchen Ferry Boatyard (diesel

only) a mile upstream
*Chandler* Kelvin Hughes near marina entrance

## SHORE LEAVE

Ocean Village has its own five-screen Cannon cinema and street entertainers perform in and around the Pavilion. The **Hall of Aviation**, five minutes' walk from Ocean Village in Albert Road South, presents the story of aviation in the Solent. The prize exhibit is the Sandringham flying boat: go on board and sample travel 1920s style.

# Shamrock Quay Marina

| | |
|---|---|
| **Harbourmaster** ☎ (0703) 229461 | **VHF Channel** 80 |
| **Callsign** Shamrock Quay | **Daily charge** £££ |

This marina is the furthest up the Itchen River in an industrial area, some way from the city centre. Shamrock Quay was once the yard of Camper and Nicholson where many of the huge yachts which raced in the Solent at the start of the century were built. They left when the Itchen Bridge was built downstream and tall-masted yachts could no longer reach them. The old warehouses and workshops have been converted to modern use and form a pleasing backdrop to the marina.

STEP ASHORE

**Nearest payphone** By the buildings at the back of the quay
**Toilets, showers, launderette** All in the building behind harbourmaster's office
**Shopping** Convenience store, Store Four, in the marina

**Food and drink** Taps restaurant and the Waterfront pub, which serves food, are both in the marina
**Buses** From Northam Road to city centre; the bus stop is ten minutes' walk from Shamrock Quay

## SHIPS' SERVICES

*Water and electricity* On pontoons
*Fuel* None in marina; diesel is obtainable at Itchen Marina across the river

*Gas* (Camping and Calor) From chandler
*Chandler* Shamrock Chandlery in marina
*Boatyard, engineer, sailmaker* All on-site

# River Hamble

River Hamble, at the heart of the sheltered water of the Solent and with the benefit of a two-hour stand at high water, has become the victim of its own attractiveness. From the entrance at Warsash right up to the bridge at Bursledon, the lines of moored boats are almost unbroken. With four of the largest marinas in the Channel, several yards and numerous pile moorings, the visitor may wonder where to put in; at weekends it can seem busier than a motorway.

Until the early part of the century Hamble was a fishing port and famous for its oysters, but now the whole village is geared to sailors and sailing. Large wooden ships were built at Warsash until a hundred and fifty years ago. Yachts are still built at Stone Pier Yard and the hard is often used for scrubbing and antifouling.

Of the many places where you might find a berth we have described the four most suited to visitors for their shoreside facilities; Hamble Point Marina, the Harbourmaster's visitors' piles, Port Hamble Marina and Swanwick Marina. As a starting place for trips inland only Swanwick Marina, at the head of the river, is really convenient, with buses at the gate and the railway station nearby.

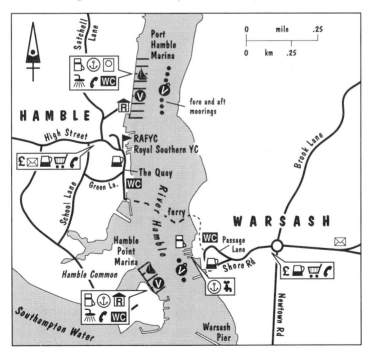

## SHORE LEAVE

**Southampton** and **Portsmouth**, with their many attractions, are within reach but the **Hampshire Farm Museum** and **Upper Hamble Country Park** are close by. A working farm has been recreated to show life as it was 90 years ago, with many breeds of cattle no longer seen on modern farms on show. Walking along the river, which winds through copses in the Country Park, is a delight. The **Royal Victoria Country Park** at **Netley** has views over Southampton Water; the village pub is ideal for a lunch break. A substantial amount remains of **Netley Abbey**, founded in 1239, said to be due to a curse on anyone who tries to remove the stones.

A guided cruise from Bursledon visits all the places on the river featured in the TV series *Howard's Way*.

### TRANSPORT AND TRAVEL

**Buses** From Bursledon, Hamble, Swanwick and Warsash to Fareham, Portsmouth and Southampton
**Trains** From Hamble, Bursledon and Swanwick stations to Southampton and Portsmouth and thence to London
**Planes** From Southampton-Eastleigh airport, trains stop at Eastleigh

**Ferries** A passenger ferry crosses the river at Warsash to Hamble Village; cross-Channel ferries operate from Portsmouth and Southampton
**Taxis** Phipps Radio Taxis ☎ (0703) 452241
**Car hire** Europcar, Hartwells Ltd, The Avenue, Southampton ☎ (0703) 229077

*Further information* from Tourist Offices at Above Bar Precinct, Southampton and Ferneham Hall, Osborn Road, Fareham.

# Hamble Point Marina

| **Harbourmaster** ☎ (0703) 452464 | **VHF Channel** 80 |
|---|---|
| **Callsign** Hamble Point Marina | **Daily charge** ££££ |

This is the first marina on the port hand as you enter the river. It is a long walk from any shoreside facilities and is therefore not really suitable for taking Shore Leave. However, if you wish simply to stop for the night it would be a useful mooring.

## STEP ASHORE

**Nearest payphone** Behind harbour office and toilet block
**Toilets, showers** Beneath harbour office
**Clubhouse** The marina club – The Ketch

Rigger – serves bar meals
**Shopping** In Hamble Village, one mile uphill along a winding country road – no short cuts and no buses

### SHIPS' SERVICES

*Water and electricity* On pontoons
*Fuel* Diesel only at fuel berth
*Gas* (Camping and Calor), *chandlery,*

*boatyard, engineer* In marina
*Sailmaker* J R Williams at Hamble

## TRANSPORT AND TRAVEL

**Buses** The nearest bus stop is in Hamble Village

**Taxi** Phipps ☎ (0703) 452241

# Harbourmaster's Moorings

| | |
|---|---|
| **Harbourmaster** ☎ (0489) 576387 | **VHF Channel** 68 |
| **Callsign** Hamble Harbour Radio | **Daily charge** £ |

Mooring between piles in the good old-fashioned way will give you the lowest prices for miles around. You may also have a more peaceful or interesting time than in a marina, although you will, of course, have to go ashore by dinghy. Piles B1-B4 are opposite Warsash and piles 9-16 are off Port Hamble.

## STEP ASHORE

**At Hamble**
**Nearest payphone** Up the hill in the village
**Toilets** Near the car-park
**Launderette** At the Kings and Queens pub in Hamble Village
**Clubhouses** Royal Southern Yacht Club and Royal Air Force Yacht Club are on the quay

**Shopping** Shops and banks in Hamble High Street
**Food and drink** The Olde Whyte Harte in the High Street has good bar food and is popular with sailors. The Kings and Queens (also called The Pie Pub) in Hamble Village also serves food

**At Warsash**
**Nearest payphone:** In Warsash Village, a five-minute walk
**Toilets** Near car-park at landing
**Shopping** There are rather more shops in

Warsash than in Hamble, and a bank
**Food and drink** The pub on the quay, the Rising Sun, serves food, as does the Jolly Farmer up the hill in the village
**Car hire** Roxby Garage in village

## SHIPS' SERVICES

*At Warsash (none at Hamble)*
*Water At harbourmaster's jetty*
*Fuel (diesel and petrol), gas Camping and Calor), chandlery, boatyard, engineer All available at Stone Pier Yard, next to the*

*harbourmaster's jetty*
*Sailmaker Bruce Banks at Park Gate, towards Locks Heath (signposted at landing)*

# Port Hamble Marina

| | |
|---|---|
| **Harbourmaster** ☎ (0703) 452741 | **VHF Channel** 80 |
| **Callsign** Port Hamble | **Daily charge** ££££ |

This marina is on the west bank of the Hamble River just above Hamble Village.

## STEP ASHORE

**Nearest payphone** Beside harbour office
**Toilets, showers, launderette** All in new block
**Clubhouse** Square Rigger, a slightly run-down proprietary club, serves pub food

**Shopping** Marina shop sells basic necessities. A small selection of shops, banks and a post office in Hamble Village five minutes' walk up the hill

### SHiPS' SERVICES

*Water and electricity* On pontoons
*Fuel* (diesel and petrol) At fuelling berth
*Gas* (Camping and Calor) *chandlery,*

*boatyard, engineer* all on-site
*Sailmaker* J R Williams in Hamble

# Swanwick Marina

| | |
|---|---|
| **Harbourmaster ☎** (0489) 885262 | **VHF Channel** 80 |
| **Callsign** Swanwick Marina | **Daily charge** ££££ |

This marina, near the head of the river, was started by the Moody family; there is still a Moody in the firm and the marina is still referred to colloquially as Moody's.

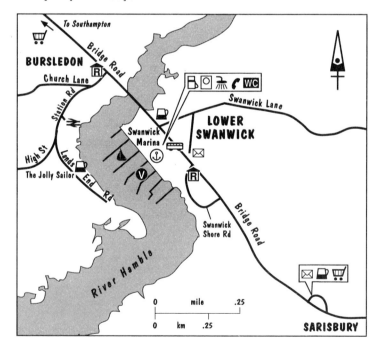

## STEP ASHORE

**Nearest payphone** Behind dockmaster's office
**Toilets, showers, launderette** In marina
**Shopping** Marina shop sells basic necessities; post office in Swanwick Lane opposite the marina; village shops at Sarisbury Green, half a mile up the hill to the east, sell general supplies; bank half a mile further on at Park Gate. Sailors are often seen staggering down the hill with purchases from the large Tesco at Bursledon – there is a bus
**Food and drink** The Spinnaker and Old Ship are both pleasant pubs and both serve food. Across the river at Bursledon is the Jolly Sailor of *Howard's Way* fame

### SHIPS' SERVICES

*Water and electricity* On pontoons
*Fuel* (diesel and petrol) From fuelling berth
*Gas* (Camping and Calor), **chandlery,** *boatyard, engineer* All in the marina
*Sailmaker* Richardson Sails, Elephant Boatyard

### TRANSPORT AND TRAVEL

**Buses** From outside the marina to Portsmouth and Southampton
**Trains** From Bursledon station, across the river from the marina, with a frequent service to Southampton for London trains

# Portsmouth

At first sight Portsmouth Harbour is not a promising place to visit on holiday, but as you join the traffic sailing through the narrow gap in the fortifications, take a look around. Portsmouth has been the home of the Royal Navy for 500 years. The towers and walls to starboard were started in the fifteenth century and were regularly strengthened and extended up to Victorian times. Also to starboard is the menacing black shape of HMS *Warrior* looking just as it did 130 years ago when it made the world's navies obsolete at a stroke with its superior fire power and steam propulsion. Beyond, in the dockyard, you will probably see some ships of the modern fleet, apparently diminished in size but incredibly more powerful, and beyond them the masts of HMS *Victory*, still in commission nearly 200 years after its last battle. In a shed behind the *Victory* is the *Mary Rose*, lost 250 years earlier still, when it was heeled over by a squall when sailing out of Portsmouth harbour with the gunports open.

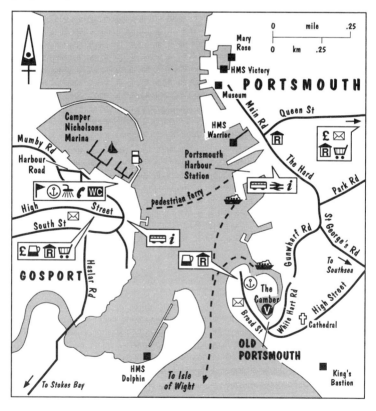

In recent times Portsmouth has seen the start and finish of many round-the-world races and witnessed the triumphant arrival of Tracy Edwards and her all-female crew in *Maiden*.

For access to all Portsmouth has to offer Camper & Nicholsons Marina is the most comfortable berth, with Portsmouth only a five-minute ferry ride away. If the cost of staying there is ruining you, slip across to the Camber, where they welcome visitors – it is oily, rusty and gritty, but who cares? It costs peanuts and is next to the best pubs. Port Solent is comfortable but isolated; Hardway is interesting for the club itself.

## SHORE LEAVE

### Food and drink
Portsmouth and Southsea are never short of places to eat in: our suggestions focus on the area round the harbour. The Bridge serves good pub food and has a restaurant for evening meals. There are other pubs and restaurants nearby, some with a view to watch the comings and goings in the harbour entrance; Still and West's upstairs restaurant has fine views. The Talisman in the High Street serves French food. Keppels Head Carvery and The Mitre in College Street are both near The Hard – conveniently near the Portsmouth–Gosport Ferry terminal. Pizza House, 14 Hilsea Market, London Road, is a lively Italian restaurant recommended in *Out to Eat*.

### Entertainment
Touring productions visit the **King's Theatre** in Southsea and the **New Theatre Royal** in the city centre. The **Guildhall** has a continuous concert programme; musical entertainment is a feature of many Portsmouth pubs, clubs and other nightspots.

### What to see
The Camber is in the heart of what Victorian planners and the Second World War have left of Old Portsmouth. Within a few minutes' walk you will find the **old walls** and the **sally ports** from which Nelson embarked for Trafalgar and the Tolpuddle martyrs for Botany Bay. In the High Street are the old pubs and houses associated with Nelson's navy and the assassination of the Duke of Buckingham. The **Garrison church**, bombed in the last war and now partly restored, was the scene of the marriage of Charles II to Catherine of Braganza on her arrival from Portugal. The twelfth-century parish church, with its unusual square white tower and cupola, became a cathedral earlier this century – a suitably imposing west front is at last being built.

**Southsea Castle**, where Henry VIII witnessed the loss of the *Mary Rose*, contains an exhibition on 'Fortress Portsmouth'. The **D-Day Museum** which features the Overlord Embroidery – larger than the Bayeux Tapestry – is nearby. You can visit **HMS *Warrior*, HMS *Victory*, *Mary Rose*** and the **Royal Navy Museum** in the Docks opposite The Hard. Charles Dickens was born in Old Commercial Road where there is now a museum of life in his times. **Portsmouth Sea Life Centre** at Clarence Esplanade is a modern aquarium.

### Excursions
Go to **Stokes Bay** for picnics and windsurfing, perhaps anchoring off in your own boat, or take a boat trip round Portsmouth harbour with a commentary on the ships in port.

*Exercise*
Swim from the beaches at Southsea or, if the weather is bad, in the indoor pools at the Pyramids on Clarence Esplanade.

## TRANSPORT AND TRAVEL

**Trains** From Portsmouth Harbour and Portsmouth and Southsea stations to London, Southampton, Gatwick, Brighton and the West Country
**Planes** From Southampton-Eastleigh airport and Gatwick
**Ferries** From Portsmouth Continental Ferry Port to Le Havre, Cherbourg, St Malo and Caen. The Portsmouth–Gosport ferry runs every fifteen minutes and takes five minutes, with the last crossing at midnight
**Taxis** From rank at The Hard, Portsmouth Harbour
**Car hire** Europcar, Tricorn Centre, Unit 17 ☎ (0705) 817331

*Further information* from Tourist Offices on Clarence Esplanade, The Hard and by Portsmouth and Southsea station.

# Camper & Nicholsons Marina

| | |
|---|---|
| **Harbourmaster** ☎ (0705) 524811 | **VHF Channels** 80, M |
| **Callsign** Camper Base | **Daily charge** £££££ |

This is an excellent port to be stormbound in, with plenty to occupy the children or crew on a rainy day, if a bit short on scenic walks. It is also a fine place for stocking up before a channel crossing. The facilities are modern, the security excellent and it is only a few minutes' walk to Gosport High Street and next to the Portsmouth–Gosport Ferry which takes five minutes to cross the harbour.

## STEP ASHORE

**Nearest payphones** At head of ramp leading up from pontoons and below marina office, also outside marina to the left of the main gate; several payphones at the bus station
**Toilets, showers** Clean and working, if old-fashioned. You can have a bath (or bath the children) for 10p in the 'ladies' showers'

**Launderette** At marina, open 0800–1900
**Clubhouse** Shores Club
**Shopping** The chandler in the marina has food and off-licence sections. Gosport High Street is five minutes' walk away, where you will find banks and building societies, a post office and a selection of high-street shops. Market on Tuesdays

### SHIPS' SERVICES

*Water and electricity* On pontoons; ask for lead at office
*Fuel* (diesel and petrol) On marina fuel barge
*Gas* (Camping and Calor) In marina
*Chandler* In marina; also Solent Marine

*Services:* turn right outside gate
*Boatyard, engineer* Camper & Nicholsons Repairs Office behind marina club
*Sailmaker* W G Lucas & Son, Broad Street ☎ (0705) 826629

## SHORE LEAVE

### Food and drink

For convenience try the restaurant in Shores Club (last orders 2300) or venture outside the marina, where there is plenty to choose from. Alternatively, take your own boat or the ferry across to Old Portsmouth.

### Entertainment

The Ritz cinema is in Walpole Road.

### What to see

**Gosport Museum**, Walpole Road, tells the story of how the fishing village became a naval establishment. The **Submarine Museum** in Haslar Jetty Road offers a guided tour round a Second World War submarine and tells the story of the underwater navy.

### Exercise

Walk the three miles to **Stokes Bay** via Haslar Bridge, or follow the **Solent Way**: for 12 of its 60 miles this follows the Gosport and Fareham shoreline and much of the path offers magnificent views over the Solent to the Isle of Wight.

A *Gosport Walks* leaflet is available free from the Tourist Office at the bus station. If you prefer to swim, Southsea has beaches and the Cascades indoor pool.

### TRANSPORT AND TRAVEL

**Buses** From Gosport ferry building near the marina to Southampton every hour

**Trains** From Portsmouth Harbour

**Ferries** To Portsmouth run every fifteen minutes and take five minutes; last ferry returns at midnight

**Taxis** Rank at Gosport Bus Station near ferry terminal

**Car hire** Southern Self Drive, Mumby Road: turn right outside marina gate

*Further information* from kiosk in marina and Tourist Office at the bus station on roundabout between Mumby Road and High Street: turn left outside marina gate.

# The Camber

**Berthing master** ☎ (0705) 297395 ext 310      **Daily charge** £

This is a welcoming place and if you want some local colour or to be near to Portsmouth City it is a good place for a short stop. Visiting yachts tie up, perhaps two deep, on the end of the jetty in front of The Bridge pub. The berthing master emphasises that space is limited and berths are made available on a first-come-first-served basis – you find your own space and pay at the berthing master's office which is next to the pilots' office. Fishing boats and the Isle of Wight car ferry cause a surge.

## STEP ASHORE

**Nearest payphone** In Broad Street, 200 yards from the dock
**Shopping** No shops in the immediate vicinity but the morning fish market in the docks is not to be missed if you want something worth eating on board – it is just like the markets the French have had the sense to keep. The nearest supermarket is Sainsbury in Commercial Road

### SHIPS' SERVICES

*Chandler, sailmaker* Lucas in Broad Street

# Port Solent Marina

| **Harbourmaster** ☎ (0705) 210765 | **VHF Channels** 80, M |
|---|---|
| **Callsign** Port Solent | **Daily charge** £££ |

This modern, smart, efficient marina is part of a residential estate with a waterside theme, and many of the berths are occupied by boats belonging to the houseowners. There is a sprinkling of interesting vessels, from Sir Malcolm Campbell's *Bluebird* to a Thames barge, to give a saltwater atmosphere, but the Boardwalk and most of the shops look like refugees from *Howard's Way*. It is a very pleasant place for a one-night stop, especially if you need a launderette or would like a slap-up meal, but traffic noise on the nearby motorway may keep you awake. The marina is an oasis in an industrial dormitory area and it is not an easy place to set out from for any sightseeing or travel. The main pleasure to be gained is from the sights in Portsmouth harbour while sailing in and out.

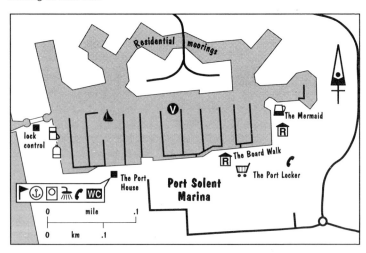

## STEP ASHORE

**Nearest payphone** At the west end of The Port House by the entrance to the pontoons
**Toilets, showers, launderette** All in The Port House
**Clubhouse** The very smart, proprietary

Waterside Club welcomes visitors
**Shopping** Various tourist shops in The Boardwalk (the building at the east end of the basin) with a convenience store out of sight round the back

### SHIPS' SERVICES

*Water and electricity* On pontoons; electric cable available from office on deposit
*Fuel* (diesel and petrol) From berth by lock

*Gas* (Camping and Calor), **chandler, boatyard, engineer, sailmaker**
All available on-site – facilities are comprehensive

## SHORE LEAVE

The Waterside Club and several restaurants and pubs offer meals of all kinds from bar snacks to gourmet standard, Italian, Mexican and Chinese included. A striking architectural contrast to the 1980s marina is **Porchester Castle** on the other side of the entrance channel. The 18-foot high Roman walls still stand after 1600 years and a surprising amount of the Norman castle also remain. Connections with the early Plantagenet kings make it a particularly interesting place to visit. It is easiest to go across by dinghy when your boat is on the holding pontoon outside the lock.

A six-screen cinema is being built for 1992 opening.

### TRANSPORT AND TRAVEL

The nearest public transport is in Portsmouth, so if you are likely to need buses, trains, planes or ferries, it is better to berth at Camper & Nicholsons

Marina in Gosport
**Taxis** ☎ (0705) 386613
**Car hire** Arrange through marina office

# Hardway

**Harbourmaster** ☎ (0705) 581875      **Daily charge** £

Hardway Sailing Club is a 'do-it-yourself' club where everything is in working order and visitors are welcome to use the facilities in a considerate way. It is a good place for a practical scrubbing weekend or a meet on the piles – arrange these with the club secretary first. Be careful if you are moored on the piles in a strong wind: don't leave your boat unattended if there are other boats alongside.

# STEP ASHORE

**Nearest payphone** In clubhouse or near shops in St Thomas Road
**Toilets, showers** In clubhouse
**Launderette** St Thomas Road
**Shopping** In St Thomas Road, a five-minute walk: the Happy Shopper general store, open till 2000 every day, a newsagent and a post box. The nearest post office is in the shopping centre in Elson Road, a 15-minute walk, along with a good butcher and baker, greengrocer, hardware shop and a newsagent. The nearest banks with bureau de change facilities are in Gosport
**Clubhouse** Hardway Sailing Club

## SHIPS' SERVICES

*Water* On landing stage
*Electricity* Clubhouse storeroom
*Fuel* (petrol and diesel), *gas* (Camping and Calor) From Hardway Marine, next to club
*Chandler* Hardway Marine
*Boatyard, engineer* Ask in Hardway Marine

# SHORE LEAVE

The Jolly Roger (last orders 2130) is in Priory Road, a few minutes' walk to the south from the club: the Chinese take-away and the Windsor Castle pub are both in St Thomas Road – all three are recommended. Visit the **Naval Armaments Museum** at Hardway. You could go to **Porchester Castle** by boat and anchor in the creek, or walk to **Fort Brockhurst**, in Gunners Way. This takes half an hour, walking to the north of the club along Elson Road. If you are stuck at Hardway in bad weather you might enjoy the Holbrooke Leisure Centre in Fareham Road where you can swim.

## TRANSPORT AND TRAVEL

**Buses** From the bus stop at the corner of Grove Road and St Thomas Road into Gosport
**Trains** From Portsmouth Harbour or Fareham
**Taxis** ☎ (0705) 511143

# Bembridge

This is still a relatively unspoilt tidal harbour with a good and easily accessible beach and play area for children (plus places to take them if it rains) and lovely walks with superb views.

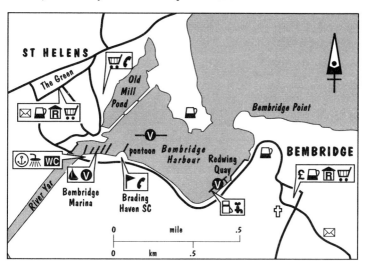

## SHORE LEAVE

### Food and drink
Of the restaurants and pubs in St Helens and Bembridge, St Helens Wine Bar and restaurant, Lower Green Road, is recommended. Bembridge offers tea-shops and fish and chip shops.

### Entertainment
Take a bus to Ryde for the cinema; films are also shown in Bembridge Village Hall occasionally.

### What to see
Visit some of the surprisingly large number of interesting diversions in and around Bembridge. The **Maritime Museum** has a collection of early and modern diving equipment and ship models. **Bembridge Lifeboat Station** is open on Wednesdays, Thursdays, Sundays and Bank Holiday afternoons – it is an operational lifeboat station with a Tyne Class lifeboat. The eighteenth-century **Bembridge windmill**, with much of the original wooden machinery, is worth a visit – it was last used in 1913. In Upper Green Road, St Helens, you will find the **Shell Garden**, where local shells depict 80 Isle of Wight scenes. In nearby Brading is a **Dolls Museum** with antiques dating from as early as 2000BC, a **Wax Museum** with cameos of island history, the figures dressed in authentic costumes. The **Roman Villa** at Brading is an important archaeological find, believed to have been the centre of a rich farming estate. It has fine mosaic floors, painted walls and many luxury articles.

*Excursions*

Buses run from just outside the marina to **Ryde, Sandown, Shanklin** and **Newport**, all of which have their own attractions.

*Exercise*

Fine sandy beaches, ideal for young children, are a 10-minute walk away, or a short trip by dinghy. Windsurfing from the beach is popular. The walk to the windmill via the footpath from the harbour takes 25 minutes. The walk to Brading by the footpath from St Helens takes up to an hour, depending on how long you spend admiring the views.

## TRANSPORT AND TRAVEL

**Buses** From bus stop at Embankment and St Helens to Ryde, Sandown, Shanklin and Newport
**Trains** From Brading to Ryde, Sandown, Lake and Shanklin

**Ferries** From Ryde to Portsmouth
**Taxis** Flint Cars ☎ (0983) 872133
**Car hire** Autorent, 9/11 George Street, Ryde ☎ (0983) 62322
**Bicycle hire** Ask at the marina office

*Further information* from Tourist Office, Western Gardens, Ryde ☎ (0983) 291914.

# Bembridge

| | |
|---|---|
| **Harbourmaster** high water ☎ (0983) 874436; low water ☎ (0983) 873635 | **VHF Channel** 80 |
| **Callsign** Bembridge Marina | **Daily charge** £££ |

The marina is rather cramped for larger boats, especially in high season, so use the free-floating pontoon in the harbour instead; it is only a short row ashore from the fishermen's jetty.

## STEP ASHORE

**Nearest payphone** In marina next to quay office
**Toilets, showers** At marina office – not the Ritz but in working order
**Clubhouse** Brading Haven Yacht Club; visitors are given a friendly welcome

**Shopping** Grocer in the campsite to the north-west of the marina; shops in Bembridge, one-and-a-half miles to the south, include a supermarket, bank, post office and a craft shop; in St Helens, half a mile to the north, is a small general store and a post office

## SHIPS' SERVICES

*Water and electricity* On pontoons
*Fuel* (diesel and petrol) At Redwing Quay (tidal)
*Gas* (Camping and Calor) From St Helens Service Station or try the campsite

*Chandler, boatyard,* Bembridge Boatyard, The Embankment
*Engineer* Bembridge Outboards, Embankment Road
*Sailmaker* Try boatyard

# SOUTH-EAST ENGLAND

# Chichester Harbour

Chichester Harbour is one of the finest natural harbours in England and an area of outstanding natural beauty. With 12 miles of channels and plenty of water from half-tide up, it offers the family sailor an opportunity for pottering and enjoying the surrounding views and the wildlife, including the Brent geese, which are thriving so well under protection that they are becoming a problem. It is best to avoid weekends, when the harbour is crowded with thrusting dinghy sailors and windsurfers who do not allow for yachts' need to keep to the deep water.

## Chichester Harbour Moorings

| | |
|---|---|
| **Harbourmaster** ☎ (0243) 512301 | **VHF Channels** 16, working 14 |
| **Callsign** Chichester (office); Regnum (launch); Ælla (launch) | **Daily charge** £; on visitors' pontoon above Itchenor ££ |

As a whole, Chichester Harbour is not an easy place from which to step ashore right into the centre of things – bus, feet or car are needed. There are no shoreside shops and very limited facilities, so you will have to go into a marina if supplies are needed. But for outstanding scenery and bird life it has plenty to offer. After a cruise, those lucky enough to keep their boats in Chichester Harbour wonder why they bothered to go away. Apart from the marinas there are many rural spots to visit, either for a short stop or an overnight stay.

### Mill Rythe
At the head of this creek is the Hayling Island Yacht Company's yard ☎ (0705) 463592. It can only be reached near the top of the tide, so is not easy to visit for a short stay. However, if you have to leave the boat, it is friendly, secure and well-placed for getting to the mainland by bus or taxi.

### Emsworth Channel
Moor to the piles or try for a berth in **Emsworth Yacht Harbour**. It is convenient for the small town which has all facilities and a selection of pubs and restaurants. Fuel is available from garages in cans. Emsworth Museum, over the fire station in North Street, has much to interest the sailor with its paintings and photographs of Emsworth's maritime past, a model of a sailing gravel barge which once operated in Chichester Harbour and another of *Echo*, the largest sailing fishing vessel ever to have worked out of an English port. *The Good Food Guide 1992* recommends the straightforward Spencers, 36 North Street and the more ornate 36 on the Quay, 47 South Street.

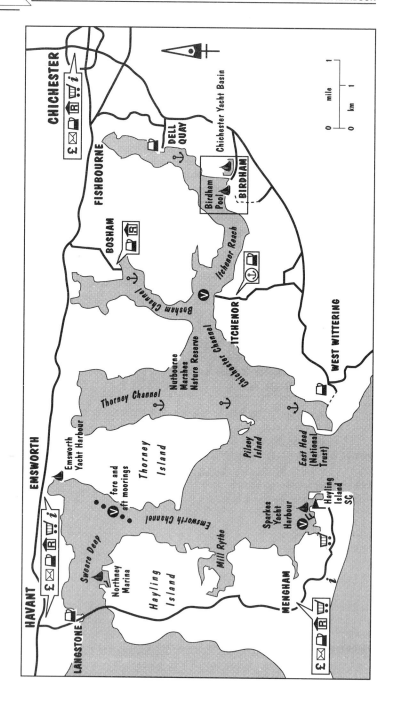

### Thorney Channel

On the east side of Thorney Island this secluded anchorage has no facilities but offers proximity to the bird sanctuary on Pilsey Island. See the *Holiday Which? Town and Country Walks Guide* walk 144 for a route which includes the Nutborne Marshes Nature Reserve.

### Bosham

The harbour dries completely here, but you can tie up to the quay or stand on the hard if you have legs or bilge keels. It is a small and picturesque village with an ancient church where the daughter of King Canute is buried. Bosham Walk is a small covered precinct with attractive little antique and craft shops. For a slap-up meal go to the Millstream Hotel.

### Dell Quay

Right at the top of the harbour, this is as near as the sea now goes to Chichester. In Roman times it went right up to the walls of the Governor's Palace at Fishbourne close by, the excavated remains of which are well worth visiting. The Crown and Anchor at Dell Quay has a good selection of real ales and serves food.

### Itchenor

The Chichester harbourmaster has his office here – you can obtain a harbour guide, booklets on the history of the harbour and leaflets guiding you on walks. A pub is the extent of other shoreside facilities. This is the only place in the harbour with conventional visitors' moorings, which is useful to know if you feel happier on a buoy. Fresh water is available at Itchenor jetty, but waiting time is limited to 15 minutes because of congestion. Fuel is available in cans from the garage.

### East Head

This is a good anchorage beside a large and safe beach and the dunes which protect this corner of the harbour. It is also a nature reserve belonging to the National Trust. There is a danger of the sea breaking through the neck of the spit, which would cause great damage to the harbour and its wildlife, so take great care not to damage the plantings of retaining grasses when you go ashore.

# Sparkes Yacht Harbour (Sandy Point)

| Harbourmaster ☎ (0705) 463572 | VHF Channel M |
|---|---|
| Callsign Sparkes Yacht Harbour | Daily charge £££ |

This is a small, modern and very friendly marina just inside the entrance to Chichester Harbour and thus a useful staging post. The marina is backed by a comprehensive boatyard organisation, so it is a good place to sort out any problems and to leave the boat if necessary.

Sparkes Yacht Harbour is set in the south-east corner of Hayling Island, at the end of a peninsula of residential and holiday development. There is a bus every hour or so to the shops, which you will need because everything except the beach is a long way away. Hayling Island is a simple family holiday resort with good beaches and a fun-fair and is very popular with windsurfers. It is not a good spot for starting inland expeditions.

## STEP ASHORE

**Nearest payphone** In launderette
**Toilets, showers, launderette** At the end of office block
**Clubhouse** Hayling Island Sailing Club, half a mile away, is one of the foremost dinghy racing clubs
**Shopping** One-and-a-half miles to simple shops and three miles to the main shopping centre at Mengham, where

there are banks and building societies. The nearest bank with an outside cash dispenser is at Mengham.
If you are arriving at Hayling Island by car it is easier to park and do your food shopping at the Co-op at Gable Head. There is also a greengrocer, called Penney's, at Gable Head

### SHIPS' SERVICES

**Water and electricity** On pontoons
**Fuel** (diesel and petrol) From end of jetty
**Gas** (Camping and Calor), **chandler,**

**boatyard, engineer, sailmaker** All available in the marina

## SHORE LEAVE

### Food and drink
The Mariners Bistro in the marina serves good simple food. It is also possible to obtain a meal at Hayling Island Sailing Club. Other restaurants on the island are some way away. Ma Baker's in West Town and The Inn On The Beach, at the more westerly end of the beach, are recommended.

### Entertainment
Summer shows are put on at the **Barn Theatre** in Mengham.

### Exercise
You can walk along much of **Hayling Island**'s 16-mile shoreline and from the saltings bordering Chichester Harbour spot the many migrating birds drawn to the area, with the scenic backdrop of the Downs. Swimming is safe along the five miles of beach on the south side of the island, but watch out for strong currents near the entrances to Chichester and Langstone harbours. Windsurfing is permitted off beaches at the western end of the island, where there is also a golf course – one of the finest in the south of England. Seacourt Racquets Club, which offers holiday membership, has one of the few Royal (real) tennis courts in the country.

## TRANSPORT AND TRAVEL

**Buses** Hourly from outside the marina to Mengham and Havant
**Trains** From Havant to London, Portsmouth and Gatwick
**Planes** From Gatwick airport
**Ferries** From Portsmouth to Le Havre,

Caen, Cherbourg, St Malo and the Isle of Wight
**Taxis** Abasmith ☎ (0705) 463022
**Car hire** Beach Road Garage ☎ (0705) 462948
**Bicycle hire** G Team Hire Cycles ☎ (0705) 463886

*Further information* from Tourist Office at Eastoke Corner.

# Northney Marina

| | |
|---|---|
| **Harbourmaster** ☎ (0705) 466321 | **VHF Channel** 80 |
| **Callsign** Northney Marina | **Daily charge** £££ |

Situated at the top of Emsworth Channel, there is little to draw one to this marina in the rural north of Hayling Island, unless you need access to the London to Portsmouth train service from Havant. It is rather isolated and not well served by public transport, but it could be useful for an overnight stop. The general air in the marina is polite but uninterested. Havant and the nearest shops are two miles away.

## STEP ASHORE

**Nearest payphone** In marina office
**Toilets, showers** In marina block
**Clubhouse** Porky's, a café in the marina block, serves lunches at weekends

**Shopping** Havant, two miles away, has the usual range of high-street shops, including Waitrose supermarket (open until 2000 Thursdays and Fridays), banks, and building societies

### SHIPS' SERVICES

*Water and electricity* On pontoons
*Fuel* (diesel and petrol) From fuelling berth

*Boatyard, engineer* Marine Propulsion on-site

## SHORE LEAVE

*Food and drink*
The nearest restaurant is in the Post House Hotel at the entrance to the marina; the nearest pubs are the Ship Inn on the Langstone side of the bridge on to Hayling Island and the Royal Oak in Langstone High Street; both are waterside pubs with outside tables looking over Chichester Harbour.

*What to see*
St Peter's Church in North Hayling Village was built in 1140; its bells, the oldest in England, date from 1350. It is a fine example of a Norman village church and noted for having no foundations but being supported by boulders from the post-glacial period.

Films and plays are put on at **Havant Arts Centre** in East Street; **Havant Museum** next door has five rooms presenting aspects of local history and three rooms housing the nationally important **Vokes Firearms Collection**. The new extension gallery shows a range of temporary art and craft exhibitions. Admission is free.

*Exercise*

The Windsurfing Centre in the marina offers tuition for the beginner on simulators and supplies all equipment – board sailing began in Hayling Island. There are shore walks from the marina, or you can walk along the foreshore from the Royal Oak at Langstone, past the old mill, to **Warblington** to see the ancient church with its tiny timbered spire and fourteenth-century wooden porch made from old ships' timbers. At two corners of the churchyard are grave watchers' huts built at the end of the eighteenth century and said to have been used to hide smugglers' booty. A single turret and part of the gateway are all that remain of sixteenth-century **Warblington Castle**, built on the site of an earlier fortified building.

## TRANSPORT AND TRAVEL

**Buses** Hourly to other parts of Hayling Island and to Havant

**Trains** From Havant to London, Portsmouth and Gatwick

**Planes** From Gatwick airport

**Ferries** From Portsmouth to Le Havre, Caen, Cherbourg, St Malo and the Isle of Wight

**Taxis** Swift Radio Cars ☎ (0705) 471666

**Car hire** Southern Self-Drive, West Street, Havant ☎ (0705) 492266

*Further information* from Tourist Office, Park Street, Havant.

# Chichester Yacht Basin

| | |
|---|---|
| **Harbourmaster** ☎ (0243) 512731 | **VHF Channels** 80, M |
| **Callsign** Chichester Yacht Basin | **Daily charge** £££ |

Chichester Yacht Basin is one of the new variety of marinas: very much upmarket and perhaps offering more ashore than many sailors want. However, the enterprise is welcoming and the basin is well run. Security is good, with video cameras and patrol staff. Boats can be left safely and professional services are capable. To venture inland you will need to take a bus, walk into Chichester or hire a car.

## STEP ASHORE

**Nearest payphone** At basin office and on north side of basin

**Toilets, showers** Two blocks in the basin

**Launderette** On south side of basin

**Clubhouse** Chichester Yacht Club

**Shopping** Marina Stores in the Yacht Basin and a post box outside it; post office and general store in Birdham village, two miles away; otherwise the nearest shops, banks and post office are in Chichester, four miles away. Chichester has no early closing in the summer, the food shops are open late most nights and the department stores on Thursdays

### SHIPS' SERVICES

*Water and electricity* On pontoons

*Fuel* (diesel and petrol), *gas* (Camping and Calor), *chandler, boatyard, engineer, sailmaker* All in Yacht Basin

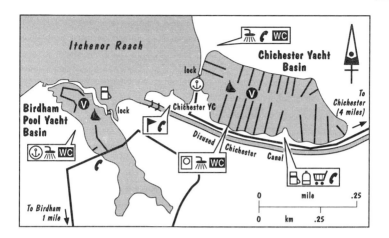

## SHORE LEAVE

### Food and drink
Café Moonshine is the Yacht Basin's restaurant. The Lamb Inn at Birdham, two miles away, is a friendly pub with reasonably priced food and tables in a sheltered garden; the Crown and Anchor at Dell Quay, one-and-a-half-miles away, is a fifteenth-century pub overlooking the harbour with good food – often local fish dishes – but its popularity means it becomes very crowded at summer weekends. Chichester has lots of pubs and restaurants among which Noble Rot, a brasserie and wine bar in 200-year-old wine vaults in Little London, is recommended. Thompsons, 30A Southgate, has a growing reputation as the best restaurant in town and is recommended in *The Good Food Guide 1992*. St Martin's Tea Rooms, 3 St Martin's Street, which is almost exclusively vegetarian, is recommended in both *The Good Food Guide 1992* and *Out to Eat*, where you will also find suggested Pizza Express, 27 South Street, Salad House, 14 Southgate and Shepherds Tea Rooms, 35 Little London.

### Entertainment
**Chichester Festival Theatre** and the new **Minerva Studio Theatre** in Oaklands Park have a summer season of plays. Try the restaurant or picnic in the grounds; whichever you choose, it is a delightful way to spend a summer evening.

### What to see
Chichester's **Market Cross** is in the centre of the city. **Pallant House**, 9 North Pallant, Chichester, built in 1712, displays period furniture and modern paintings. The many beautiful things to see in the **cathedral** include works of art from the Norman period to the present day. Most notable are the well-preserved twelfth-century stone carvings set in the south wall of the quire aisle. The buttery with a walled garden in the tranquil precincts serves coffee and light lunches.

### Excursions
This is a major tourist area and there is a great deal to see and do. **Fishbourne Roman Palace**, just south of Chichester, is the remains of a first-century governor's palace with fine mosaic floors. Four miles from Chichester, at Singleton, is the **Weald and Downland Open Air Museum** set in 40 acres of

grounds, with a collection of historic buildings rescued from demolition and reconstructed as they were when first built. **Goodwood House**, set in beautiful parkland, has rich treasures on show, including Canaletto paintings, Sèvres porcelain and French and English furniture.

*Exercise*
Walk on the **South Downs** and around the harbour or take a guided tour of Chichester. Swimming and windsurfing are popular at West Wittering. Westgate Leisure Centre in Chichester has three swimming pools.

### TRANSPORT AND TRAVEL

**Buses** From outside the marina to South Street, Chichester; from South Street to Portsmouth and Worthing
**Trains** From Chichester station in South Street to Portsmouth, and London via Gatwick or Havant
**Planes** From Gatwick airport; also a private airfield at Goodwood and a helicopter pad in the marina
**Ferries** From Portsmouth to Le Havre, Caen, Cherbourg, St Malo and the Isle of Wight
**Taxis** Dunnaway ☎ (0243) 782403
**Car hire** Europcar at D Rowe Ltd ☎ (0243) 533537

*Further information* from Tourist Office, West Street, Chichester.

# Birdham Pool

**Harbourmaster** ☎ (0243) 512310          **Daily charge £££**

Birdham Pool, in its beautiful surroundings at the north-eastern end of Chichester Harbour, was one of the first marinas in the country. It is operated by a local family in conjunction with Birdham Shipyard. It is well run and anything but a high-powered leisure complex.

Visitors' berths are limited in number, but for those who appreciate an intimate marina with a management that understands boats, this is just the spot. Boats can safely be left in the care of Birdham Shipyard.

See Chichester Yacht Basin for *Shore Leave.*

### STEP ASHORE

**Nearest payphone** In road at head of Pool
**Toilets, showers** In Birdham Shipyard – almost always open
**Launderette** Chichester Yacht Basin, across the canal
**Clubhouse** Birdham Yacht Club welcomes visitors
**Shopping** Birdham Stores in Birdham
Village, one mile from the yacht harbour, open 0700–2100 Mondays to Fridays and 0830–2030 Sundays. Birdham Village has a good post office and general stores, but for banks and building societies it is necessary to go to Chichester four miles away

### SHIPS' SERVICES

*Water* On berths
*Electricity* On some berths
*Fuel* (diesel and petrol) From pumps on lock
*Gas* (Camping and Calor), *chandler, boatyard, engineer* From Birdham Shipyard adjoining Birdham Pool
*Sailmaker* Seahorse Sails on-site

# Littlehampton

Littlehampton does not rank among the great names of the Sussex coast, but its livelihood has always been gained from the sea and its harbour, so it has an independence and self-sufficiency that comes from having a real natural resource. It is a pleasant town to stroll around, but time should also be found to visit Arundel for its many interesting houses, its castle and, at the end of August, the Arundel Festival.

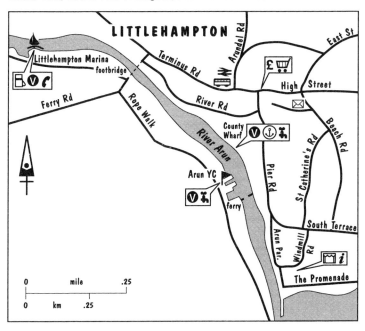

## SHORE LEAVE

### Food and drink
The marina café, open in the daytime, is suitable for filling a hungry crew. The Seahorse Restaurant is in a floating vessel where you can have drinks on the upper deck – better on a rising tide. Wimpy in Surrey Street is open till midnight.

### Entertainment
The **Windmill Theatre Complex** includes cinemas and theatres and a fun-fair with dodgems and water chutes.

### What to see
**Littlehampton Museum** in River Road houses a collection of paintings and other exhibits relating to the maritime interests of the town. The building itself incorporates a number of ships' timbers and dates from the late nineteenth century. The Littlehampton Civic Society publishes a leaflet called A *Littlehampton History Trail* which describes listed buildings and other places of interest; it is available from the tourist office.

*Excursions*

It is easy to get to **Arundel**, four miles north of Littlehampton, by bus, train or ferry. A day can easily be filled seeing **Arundel Castle**, home of the Duke of Norfolk, and enjoying the ancient town, its museum and antique shops. The castle at **Amberley** is now a hotel with fourteenth-century remains. Close to the railway station is the **Industrial Chalkpits Museum.** A ferry from near the Littlehampton Harbour Authority Office goes up river to Arundel or Amberley and gives you over an hour ashore.

*Exercise*

You can walk up the river bank, along the footpath on the west side, to Arundel and beyond or down Rope Walk and along the footpath to **Climping**, or stroll along the greensward between South Terrace and East Beach.

Littlehampton's beaches are the sandiest in Sussex: West Beach has the only sand dunes in West Sussex and is a site of special scientific interest; ferries cross to the east bank of the Arun for more beaches. Arun Windsurfing School is at 31 Beach Road, but if you do not fancy the sea, try the swimming pool in Sea Road.

## TRANSPORT AND TRAVEL

**Buses** From the Market Lanes bus stop in East Street to Arundel and to other parts of Sussex

**Trains** To Worthing, Portsmouth, Brighton, Gatwick and London. Littlehampton railway station is within a quarter of a mile of the marina via the footbridge, but the footbridge may be open for river traffic, so allow plenty of time

**Planes** From Gatwick airport

**Ferries** From Newhaven and Portsmouth. A local ferry crosses the Arun river at Littlehampton

**Taxis** Arun Taxis, 1 Bayford Road ☎ (0903) 717200. It is best to meet taxis on the east side of the footbridge, as otherwise it is a two-mile drive to the marina

**Car hire** Mida Vehicle Rentals, 4B Terminus Road

*Further information* from Tourist Office in the Windmill Complex in Coastguard Road. To get there, walk down Rope Walk, which is opposite the marina entrance, and take the ferry across to the east bank.

# Littlehampton Marina

| Harbourmaster ☎ (0903) 713553 | VHF Channels 80, M |
|---|---|
| Callsign Littlehampton Marina | Daily charge £££ |

Littlehampton Marina, on the west bank of the River Arun above the swing footbridge, is one of the few where you sail into the countryside and can see the masts of yachts across green fields. It has a marvellous view northwards to the hills of the South Downs where Arundel Castle guards the Arun Valley. The marina is clean and well maintained but the footpath along the river bank means that anyone can walk through the marina, so security cannot be relied upon. If you use a dinghy for transport, remember that the Arun is the second fastest river in the country.

## STEP ASHORE

**Nearest payphone** Opposite marina exit
**Toilets, showers** By marina office
**Shopping** About half a mile away; walk over the footbridge and turn right – all the usual high-street shops are there, including banks with outside cash dispensers, building societies, a post office, and bureaux de change in the Midland and NatWest banks. No early closing day. Gateway and Safeway supermarkets stay open till 2000 and are open on Sundays 0900–1500. Market on Fridays and Saturdays

### SHIPS' SERVICES

**Water and electricity** On pontoons
**Fuel** (diesel and petrol, including unleaded) From fuelling berth in marina
**Gas** (Camping and Calor) From Ockenden
Garden Centre, St Martins Lane, off shopping precinct
**Chandler, boatyard, engineer, sailmaker** In marina

---

*Alternative moorings*
**County Wharf** on the east side of the river has two alongside berths. There are also berths at **Hillyards** and **Arun Yacht Club Ltd** on the west bank below the footbridge.

# Shoreham

Shoreham Harbour is a small but busy commercial harbour where you can watch at close quarters comparatively big ships going through the locks. The town, at the western arm of the harbour, has many old Sussex flint houses and fine views up the River Adur of Lancing College. Shoreham is a useful place to come to for restocking supplies, but not really somewhere to visit in its own right.

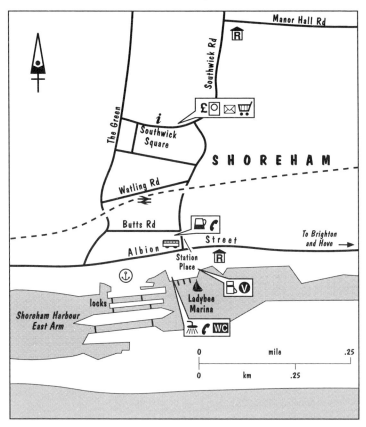

### SHORE LEAVE

**Food and drink**

Waves pub/restaurant in the marina also serves food outside on a patio, or try The South Coast Tavern, immediately across the road in Southwick Street. For a more upmarket meal, the Schooner Inn in Albion Street, with a dining-room overlooking the marina, is worth the price. The Cricketers on The Green, which serves good, quite reasonably priced food, overlooks both The Green and the attractive houses of what is left of the old village of Southwick. There is a fish and chip shop in Manor Hall Road. The Crown and Anchor in Shoreham High Street is recommended. La Gondola, 90 High Street, is an Italian restaurant featured in *The Good Food Guide 1992*.

### Entertainment

The Southwick Community Centre, Southwick Street is lively and includes the **Barn Theatre**. The nearest cinemas are in Worthing and Brighton.

### What to see

The **Marlipins Museum** in Shoreham High Street is an archaeological museum run by the Sussex Archaeology Society; it is an attractive Norman building and contains relics from bygone days when Shoreham was a large trading port. Admission is free.

### Excursions

Buses run from outside the marina to **Hove** and **Brighton** and it is as easy to see the sights of Brighton from here, only six miles away, as from Brighton Marina. Buses also run to **Worthing**. There is about one bus a day to the inland villages of **Steyning** and **Bramber**; worth seeing, but check the time of the return trip before setting out.

### Exercise

To reach the footpaths on the **South Downs** it is necessary to walk for about a mile through residential streets. You can walk across the locks, on the south side of which is a café, and down the east breakwater. Swim from the beaches at Shoreham or use the sports centre at Old Barn Way, off Manor Hall Road, Southwick. The King Alfred Leisure Centre, Kingsway, Hove, has three swimming pools, water slides, a ten-pin bowling alley and two sports halls.

### TRANSPORT AND TRAVEL

**Buses** Frequently from near the marina entrance to Hove, Brighton and Worthing
**Trains** Good train service to Brighton, Gatwick and London and to Portsmouth; Southwick railway station is 100 yards from the marina
**Planes** From Gatwick airport
**Ferries** From Newhaven and Portsmouth
**Taxis** Flaxley Cabs, 178 Old Shoreham Road, Southwick ☎ (0273) 591834

*Further information* from the public library at the back of Southwick Square.

# Ladybee Marina

Harbourmaster ☎ (0273) 593801          **Daily charge £££**

Ladybee Marina, owned by Shoreham Port Authority, is through the lock-gates on the north side of the canal. In spite of the commercial feel – the marina offices are in a small industrial estate – the welcome is warm and every effort will be made to accommodate yachts. The marina is very close to Southwick railway station and so is ideal for crew changes.

## STEP ASHORE

**Nearest payphones** At Waves pub and 50 yards east of entrance to marina
**Toilets, showers** In marina; berthholders MUST obtain key from marina office
**Launderette** In Southwick Square

**Shopping** Circle K in Southwick Square is open until 2000 (2100 on Fridays). Southwick Square, about 300 yards north of the marina, has a good selection of high-street shops, a bank with outside cash dispenser and a sub-post office

### SHIPS' SERVICES

*Water and electricity* On pontoons
*Fuel* (diesel) Available in marina; (petrol) 400 yards to the west
*Gas* (Camping and Calor) From chandler

*Chandler* G P Barnes in marina
A O Muggeridge, half a mile to the east
*Boatyard, engineer* in marina
*Sailmaker* Through G P Barnes

---

*Alternative moorings*

As well as Ladybee there are private moorings called **Riverside**, which will fit visitors in if there is room. Between Ladybee and Riverside in the canal are **Sussex Yacht Club** moorings with some visitors' berths. The main part of Sussex Yacht Club in Shoreham, one-and-a-half miles from the harbour, welcomes members of other clubs and provides a very good meal on a Saturday night. 1992 marks its centenary.

# Brighton

Once the marina is finally completed it will be unnecessary to go outside it during a visit, but it would be sad not to do so. To paraphrase Doctor Johnson, if you can't find something to interest you in Brighton, you must be very hard to please. This eighteenth-century watering place adopted by the Prince Regent has never looked back. From the Royal Pavilion and the elegant Regency crescents to the seedy backstreets, from the antique shops of the Lanes to the fair on the pier, it has something for everyone.

## SHORE LEAVE

### Food and drink
There are two pub-cum-steakhouse eating establishments and one restaurant in the marina village, all of a similar run-of-the-mill standard. Go into Brighton for a real meal in one of many top-quality restaurants: plenty are recommended in *The Good Food Guide 1992* and *Out to Eat*.

### Entertainment
The largest of several cinemas in Brighton are the Cannon Film Centre in East Street and the Odeon Film Centre in West Street. The **Theatre Royal** in New Road often presents pre-West End productions.

### What to see
Visiting Brighton's sights could fill a whole holiday; start with this selection. The **Royal Pavilion** was built by George IV in the style of the Moghul palaces of India; it remains furnished to his original taste and contains many items on loan from Buckingham Palace. The **Palace Pier** has traditional diversions and entertainments, ranging from clairvoyants to dodgems to refreshments. Off Nevill Road in Hove the **British Engineerium** is a beautifully restored nineteenth-century water-pumping station which houses full-sized and model engines, as well as a huge 1876 Beam Engine put under steam on Sundays. The **aquarium and dolphinarium**, near the Palace Pier, is one of the largest in Britain.

### Excursions
Brighton is within easy reach of many interesting diversions. The **Bluebell Railway**, eight miles away near Uckfield, is fun for a scenic five-mile ride pulled by steam locomotives. **Parham House**, near Pulborough – a little further afield – is an Elizabethan house with gardens set in a deer park; it houses collections of portraits, furniture, china tapestries and rare needlework. **Glyndebourne**, the internationally renowned opera house in the grounds of a beautiful Tudor house, is about 10 miles from the marina.

### Exercise
You can walk along the cliffs towards **Rottingdean** and **Beacon Hill windmill**, swim from the main beaches or from the small beach just outside the marina by the west pedestrian gate. The Prince Regent Swimming Pool is in Church Street just up from the Old Steine. At the King Alfred Leisure Centre Kingsway, Hove, there are three swimming pools, giant water slides, a ten-pin bowling alley and two sports halls.

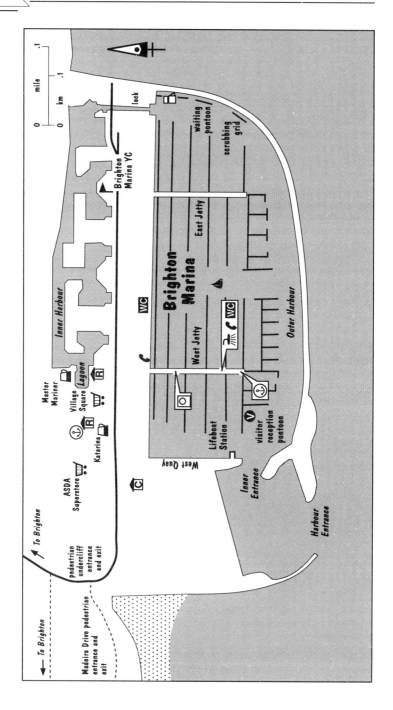

## TRANSPORT AND TRAVEL

**Buses** Frequent buses run into Brighton from the marina entrance
**Trains** To London frequently, taking just under an hour; 40 minutes to Gatwick. Also a coastal service. Volk's electric railway runs behind the beach from just outside the marina pedestrian gate to the Palace Pier
**Planes** From Gatwick airport
**Ferries** From Newhaven to Dieppe
**Taxis** Freefone by west jetty ramp
**Car hire** Europcar; freefone as above

*Further information* from Tourist Office, Old Steine.

# Brighton Marina

| | |
|---|---|
| Harbourmaster ☎ (0273) 693636 | **VHF Channels** 80, M, 16 |
| **Callsign** Brighton Control | **Daily charge** ££££ |

One of the first large modern marinas to be built in England, Brighton Marina is now coming to completion after many years of financial problems. The Marina Village has a variety of shops including a full-sized supermarket and three pub/restaurants varying in price more than in quality. An eight-screen cinema opened in 1991. The marina staff are most welcoming to visitors and the facilities are adequate and well kept. The high sea wall and the cliffs at the back of the marina give a rather claustrophobic feeling of detachment from the world outside.

## STEP ASHORE

**Nearest payphone** On the 'root' pontoon
**Toilets, showers, launderette** On the 'root' pontoon
**Clubhouse** Brighton Marina Yacht Club at the eastern end of the marina

**Shopping** Food and small necessities can be obtained in the marina shopping area – a convenience store is open 0700–2300 every day

## SHIPS' SERVICES

*Water and electricity* On pontoons; you need your own hose for water; cable for electricity is supplied on deposit
*Fuel* (diesel and petrol) From fuelling pontoon at east end of harbour
*Gas* (Camping and Calor) From fuelling pontoon
*Chandler, boatyard, engineer* All available in marina
*Sailmaker* Mrs Wilkinson, c/o Day Dawn in the marina

# Newhaven

The first steamer to cross the Channel left Newhaven for Le Havre in 1816, but Newhaven only became a port of substance when docks and shipyards were built just over a hundred years ago. For yachts it is the last port before the long haul eastward to Rye or Dover and for this reason it is a tempting stopping place. Basic facilities and supplies are available in or near the marina, but the main town is nearly a mile away down an unattractive road, and unexciting when you reach it.

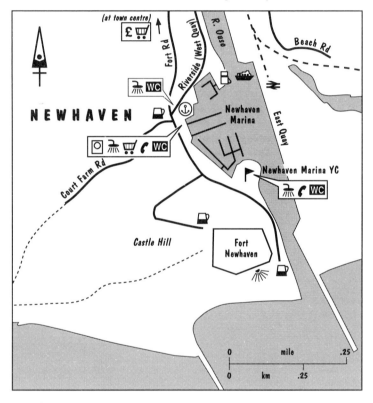

SHORE LEAVE

Restaurant meals can be had in the clubhouse, and pub food from several pubs nearby. There are more pubs and restaurants in the town.

The Victorian fortifications to the south of the marina house a museum, the largest in Sussex. In the town, the twelfth-century **Church of St Michael**, and the **Bridge Hotel**, where King Louis Philippe took refuge after fleeing France in 1848, are of interest.

Visit **Piddinghoe**, a pretty flint-walled village about a mile north-west of Newhaven. A bus runs there, or you could row a dinghy up the Ouse on the flood tide. Walk towards **Peacehaven** along the cliffs.

## TRANSPORT AND TRAVEL

**Buses** From South Way in the town centre to Brighton, Lewes and Eastbourne

**Trains** Good train service to London

**Ferries** To Dieppe

**Taxis, car hire** Ask in club or office

*Further information* from Tourist Office in ferry terminal car-park across the river.

# Newhaven Marina

| | |
|---|---|
| **Harbourmaster ☎** (0273) 513881 | **VHF Channels** 80, M |
| **Callsign** Newhaven Marina | **Daily charge** ££££ |

Although the welcome is warm enough, Newhaven is not a comfortable place to visit and if possible you should try to use Brighton. The visitors' berths are on the edge of the main channel used by the cross-Channel ferries and nights are disturbed by the noise and bad wash caused by their manoeuvres.

### STEP ASHORE

**Nearest payphones** Near marina shop and in clubhouse

**Toilets, showers, launderette** To north of marina entrance near boat-park

**Clubhouse** Newhaven Marina Yacht Club, on hill to south of pontoons

**Shopping** Small shop with very basic supplies by the marina entrance. Banks, bureau de change, post office, supermarket and a range of high-street shops in town centre, nearly one mile away

### SHIPS' SERVICES

*Water and electricity* On pontoons

*Fuel* (diesel and petrol) From fuelling berth

*Gas* (Camping and Calor), *chandler, boatyard, engineer* All near marina entrance

# Rye

In Saxon times Rye was an island; today it is almost two miles from the coast and surrounded by marshland. Much of the iron produced in the Weald of Kent during the Middle Ages was shipped from the port which later became one of the Cinque Ports, granted certain privileges in return for providing protection against French invasion. Much of Rye's charm lies in its narrow cobbled streets and timbered and Georgian houses. There is plenty to see of historical interest in and around the town and hiring a car gives access to places like Hastings and Eastbourne.

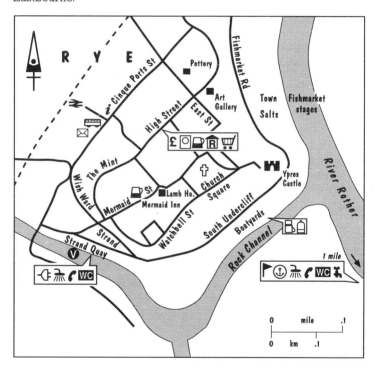

SHORE LEAVE

### Food and drink
The town is full of good pubs and restaurants, all within five to ten minutes' walk of the Strand. Landgate Bistro, 5–6 Landgate, is a busy restaurant, which welcomes children, recommended in *The Good Food Guide 1992*. Also featured is Flushing Inn, 4 Market Street, with good seafood and friendly service.

### Entertainment
Hastings, 12 miles away, is the nearest town for cinemas and theatres.

*What to see*

The **Rye Museum**, 4 Church Square, contains archives of Rye's long history. Mermaid Street is the home of the 700-year-old **Mermaid Inn**, and in a house at the bottom of the street there is a scale model of Rye, with light and sound effects. **Lamb House**, in West Street, is where Henry James wrote some of his best novels; part of the house, with some of his personal possessions on view, and the walled garden are open to the public. **Ypres Castle** built about 1250 and once a prison, houses the town museum. Rye is well known for its pottery, and numerous potteries sell traditional items.

*Excursions*

The wildlife park at **Hythe** and another near **Canterbury** are both easy to reach by bus, train or car. **Bodiam Castle**, 14 miles from Rye, is well worth a visit. Built in 1385 against a French invasion which never came, it remains remarkably intact and is the best example of its type in the country. Based at Tenterden, the **Kent and East Sussex Railway** has steam trains running through the Kent countryside to Northiam; the **Romney, Hythe and Dymchurch Railway**'s narrow gauge system crosses **Romney Marsh** to **Dungeness** lighthouse.

*Exercise*

The nature reserve and bird sanctuary on the riverside makes a good walk. Swimming and windsurfing are popular from Camber Beach, three miles down river on the coast. A holiday camp there has facilities which can be used by non-resident children.

### TRANSPORT AND TRAVEL

**Buses** From Rye town centre to Folkestone, Hastings, Tenterden and Ashford

**Trains** From Rye to Folkestone and Hastings

**Ferries** From Folkestone to Boulogne

**Taxis, car hire** From Rye Motors, 57 Winchelsea Road ☎ (0797) 223176

*Further information* from Tourist Office in Cinque Ports Street.

# Rye Harbour

| | |
|---|---|
| **Harbourmaster** ☎ (0797) 225225 | **VHF Channels** 16, 14 (0900–1700) |
| **Callsign** Rye Harbour Radio | **Daily charge** ££ |

Rye is a must on the list of any yachtsman passing up or down the Channel; it really is a delightful place. Some nautical almanacs give a false picture, making it seem less accessible than it really is, but navigation into the river is fairly easy provided that the rules are obeyed. As there is no marina at Rye, visitors are berthed at a stone jetty at Strand Quay, almost in the centre of the town. Fin-keeled boats must be secured to take account of the large tidal difference and should be supervised until settled in the mud. Visitors are made most welcome and security on the whole is fairly good.

## STEP ASHORE

**Nearest payphone** At Strand Quay and at harbourmaster's office

**Toilets, showers** At Strand Quay, harbourmaster's office and Rye Harbour Sailing Club

**Clubhouse** Rye Harbour Sailing Club is across the river from the harbourmaster's office, about one-and-a-quarter miles from Strand Quay; there are visitors' moorings on trots

**Shopping** The town centre is five minutes' walk from Strand Quay, and has the usual range of banks and building societies, a post office, bureau de change facilities and high-street shops. Budgen supermarket is opposite the railway station. Early closing Tuesdays

### SHIPS' SERVICES

*Water* Available from harbourmaster's office and Strand Quay

*Fuel* (diesel and petrol) Available from Sandrock Marine on the river between the harbourmaster's office and the Strand

*Gas* (Camping and Calor) From Sandrock Marine or Sea Cruisers ☎ (0797) 222070

*Chandler* Sea Cruisers

*Boatyard, engineer* Phillips Boat Yard Services ☎ (0797) 223234

# Dover

Dover is the nearest port to mainland Europe and a staging post for yachts as well as a vast amount of cross-Channel traffic. The town is some way from the harbour – a good 15-minute walk down rather tatty streets with a general impression of neglect. The centre of the town has a despondent air, though an attempt has been made to create the feel of a seaside resort on the seafront, to the disgust of the local fishermen who have been edged away to the east. However, if you find yourself weatherbound here or have the time to spare, take a look round and you will find there is enough of interest to make you feel the stay was worthwhile.

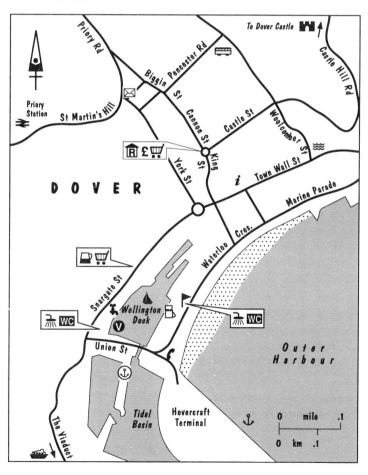

# SHORE LEAVE

## Food and drink

Snargate Street, which runs along the west side of Wellington Dock, is the first stop for pubs and take-aways, and there are plenty more pubs and restaurants in town.

## Entertainment

There is a cinema in the town.

## What to see

**Dover Castle** and the **Roman Pharos** on the hill are the main attractions – the Norman castle houses a museum with sound and smell effects of the Queen's Regiment in battle. The Pharos, built in the second century AD as one of two lighthouses on the cliffs, is the tallest Roman structure surviving in Britain. In New Street, in the centre of the town, there is an exceptionally well-preserved **Roman town house** with unique wall-paintings and elaborate under-floor heating system. The **Town Hall**, founded in 1203, has interesting stained glass windows, and armour and weapons on display; beneath the building is a fully restored Victorian gaol. **St Edmund's Chapel**, near the Town Hall, was consecrated in 1253 and is the smallest church in use in England.

## Excursions

The **Pines Garden**, with a lake and waterfall, is an attractive modern garden at Beach Road, St Margaret at Cliffe — you could walk or bus the four miles there. If you don't have time to sail across the Channel, you could take a day trip to Calais.

## Exercise

Swimming off the beach is safe, or use the swimming pool at the sports centre, along Town Wall Street to the east. Walk on the 'white cliffs of Dover'; it is easy to return by bus from St Margaret at Cliffe, Kingsdown or Deal. See the *Holiday Which? Good Walks Guide* walk 43.

## TRANSPORT AND TRAVEL

**Buses** Along the coast to Folkestone and to Deal
**Trains** From Priory station, half a mile from the docks, to Canterbury, London and along the coast to Folkestone and to Deal
**Ferries** To Oostende, Zeebrugge, Calais and Boulogne
**Taxis** Rank near Wellington Dock at the Hoverport. Crown Taxis, Castle Street ☎ (0304) 204420
**Car hire** Budget Rent-a-car ☎ (0304) 211200

**Further information** from Tourist Office in Townwall Street.

# Dover Harbour

| | |
|---|---|
| **Harbourmaster** ☎ (0304) 240400 | **VHF Channels** 74, 12 |
| **Callsign** Port Control | **Daily charge** £££; anchorage in outer harbour is free |

Yachts are usually berthed on the south and west side of Wellington Dock – contact harbour control for instructions. Arrangements are pleasant but business-like. The dock itself looks rather abandoned but is quite safe, although beware of grit from the aggregate works in the adjoining basin when the wind is in the west.

If you are only staying for a very short time it is possible to anchor in the outer harbour to the east of the Hoverport, but it is restless, exposed to winds from the north-east through south to south-west; in gales a heavy sea and swell can build up. You can land on the beach near the Royal Cinque Ports Yacht Club but the boat should not be left for long.

## STEP ASHORE

**Nearest payphone** 100 yards to the left outside dock gate

**Toilets, showers** In building on north side of dock, by gate

**Clubhouse** Royal Cinque Ports Yacht Club in Waterloo Crescent provides **showers**, a bar and hot and cold meals

**Shopping** Half a mile to the north-east; a wide range of high-street shops as well as the usual banks, building societies and bureau de change facilities. Early closing Wednesdays

**Food and drink** Pubs and take-aways in Snargate Street along west side of Wellington Dock

## SHIPS' SERVICES

*Water* On quay

*Fuel* (diesel and petrol) Dover Yacht Co to the left over the road bridge, on the east side of the dock (Cruising Association Boatman)

*Gas* (Camping and Calor) From chandler opposite Commercial Quay

*Chandler* Dover Marine Supplies, 158 Snargate Street

*Boatyard, engineer* Dover Yacht Co

# Ramsgate

Ramsgate is a pleasant and fairly unspoilt Victorian resort. The building of Ramsgate harbour was begun in 1748 and took nearly 40 years to complete, but proved its worth because it was there, in June 1815, that Wellington embarked with his army for Europe and his victory over Napoleon at Waterloo. Later, George IV used the port when travelling to Hanover and bestowed the right to call the harbour 'Royal'.

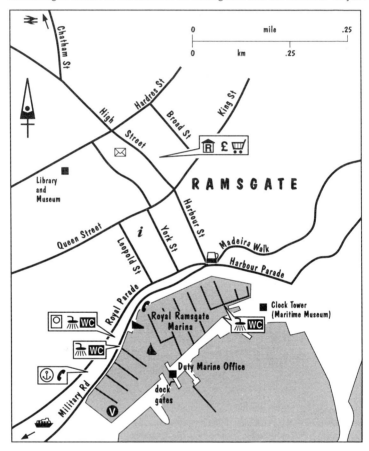

SHORE LEAVE

### Food and drink
Harvey's Oyster House is a pub/restaurant with a good atmosphere and cheerful service; it is personally recommended. There is a fairly wide choice of places to eat, and plenty of take-aways including a whelk stall.

### Entertainment
Ramsgate has both a cinema and a theatre.

*What to see*
The **Maritime Museum**, by the harbour, is housed in an early nineteenth-century Clock House and has four galleries: one includes the original clock mechanism, another has a photographic display of the development of the harbour. *Sundowner*, a Dunkirk little ship, has been restored by the East Kent Maritime Trust and is on display in the harbour; the steam tug *Cervia* is being restored and so is the fishing smack *Vanessa*. The intention is to exhibit both these vessels in the eighteenth-century dry dock, itself undergoing restoration.

*Excursions*
**Broadstairs** is a short bus ride away. Above Broadstairs Harbour, on the cliff top, you can visit **Bleak House** where Charles Dickens once lived. It includes a maritime exhibition of the Goodwin Sands and the cellars contain a display of smuggling.

*Exercise*
Swimming and windsurfing from the beach are popular.

### TRANSPORT AND TRAVEL

**Buses** To Broadstairs and Margate
**Trains** To Canterbury, London, Sandwich and Dover
**Ferries** To Dunkerque

**Taxis** Arrow Taxis, Station Approach ☎ (0843) 226688. Also a rank at the railway station
**Car hire** Enquire at marina office

*Further information* from Tourist Office, Argyle Centre, Queen Street.

# Royal Ramsgate Marina

| | |
|---|---|
| **Harbourmaster** ☎ (0843) 592277 | **VHF Channel** 14 |
| **Callsign** Ramsgate Harbour Port Control | **Daily charge** £££ |

In the mid-1970s the marina was built in the inner basin of the Royal Harbour. It is reached through a lock and is well organised and secure. Visitors' berths are on the port hand as you enter. Ask for a berth in the outer harbour if you are not staying long.

### STEP ASHORE

**Nearest payphone** By the harbour office
**Toilets** on floating pontoons (these leave room for improvement) and ashore, with **showers** and **launderette**, near the harbour office

**Clubhouse** Royal Temple Yacht Club
**Shopping** By the marina and to the north; all the usual shops to be expected in a medium-sized town
**Food and drink** Plenty of take-aways

### SHIPS' SERVICES

*Water and electricity* On pontoons
*Fuel* (diesel and petrol) From fuel pontoon in outer harbour
*Gas* (Camping and Calor) From chandler
*Chandler* Bosun's Locker & Seagear,

Military Road
*Boatyard, engineer* Marine Centre, Military Road
*Sailmaker* Straits Marine Association ☎ (0843) 592944

# Faversham

Faversham stands at the end of a long, narrow but navigable creek which wends its way through a marshland nature reserve noted for its birdlife; the surrounding fertile ground supports many orchards. To the south, beyond the A2 and the M2 motorway, the land rises through farmland and open countryside to the North Downs. Of all towns on navigable water Faversham is closest to the real Garden of England.

The town is an architectural gem: it is well preserved and has many ancient and interesting buildings – over 400 are listed. Abbey Street, which leads from the harbour to the town centre, and Court Street, with its Guildhall, are the oldest parts of Faversham and particularly attractive. Much of the centre of the town is pedestrianised. Faversham is well worth a visit if you like historic buildings, gentle countryside and bird life.

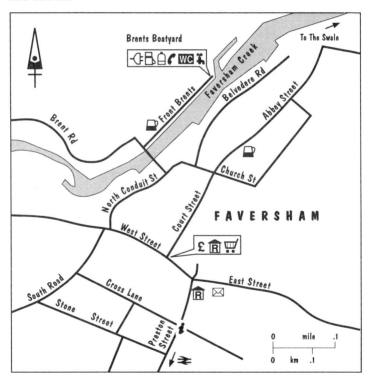

SHORE LEAVE

*Food and drink*
There are many cafés and restaurants of all varieties. Recommended are the Phoenix in Abbey Street both for pub food and for the restaurant, and the Shipwrights' Arms at Hollowshore for pub food.

*Entertainment*

Faversham has the **Arden Theatre**. Canterbury, 15 minutes away by train, offers a wider choice, including cinemas and the **Marlowe Theatre**.

*What to see*

The **Fleur de Lis Heritage Centre** is a fifteenth-century inn with displays of the history of the town. The **Guildhall** retains its original Elizabethan arcade. **Arden's House**, 80 Abbey Street – a restored sixteenth-century street – is a picturesque house which includes the remains of an ancient abbey gatehouse, scene of Mayor Thomas Arden's murder in 1551.

*Excursions*

Go to **Canterbury** to see the cathedral and much else, including several museums. At **Sittingbourne**, six miles away, you can see the **Dolphin Yard Sailing Barge**, a working museum with sail loft, shipwright's tools and forge, and two barges in the course of restoration. **Belmont**, an eighteenth-century mansion four miles south-west of Faversham, is in its original state, with family mementoes of Indian connections, and fine gardens. **Maison Dieu**, at Ospringe, three miles away, houses displays of Norman and Saxon pottery, glass and jewellery.

*Exercise*

Walk inland over the Downs. To seaward are the **South Swale Nature Reserve** to the east and the **Saxon Shore Way** to the west; both are reached over marshlands with plenty of wildlife. There is an open-air swimming pool in the town centre.

### TRANSPORT AND TRAVEL

**Buses** From town centre to Oare
**Trains** From the station at the top of Preston Street, a 10-minute walk, to Sittingbourne, Sheerness, Rochester, London, Margate, Ramsgate, Canterbury and Dover

**Ferries** From Sheerness to Vlissingen and Dover to Oostende, Zeebrugge, Calais and Boulogne; both are less than an hour away by train
**Taxis** A1 Taxis ☎ (0795) 533869
**Car hire** Invicta Motors, West Street

*Further information* from Tourist Office, Fleur de Lis Heritage Centre, 13 Preston Street.

# Faversham

| **Harbourmaster** ☎ (0795) 663025 | **VHF Channel** 74 |
|---|---|
| **Callsign** Medway Radio | **Daily charge** ££ |

The harbour is industrial rather than smart. There are drying moorings in soft mud at Brents Boatyard up river from Faversham but their facilities are limited.

## STEP ASHORE

**Nearest payphone** At taxi office by gate to Brents Boatyard
**Toilets** At yard and in central car-park
**Clubhouse** Hollowshore Cruising Club, Hollowshore
**Shopping** It is only 500 yards into town, where there is a full selection of shops, banks, building societies and a post office. Early closing Thursdays. Markets are held in Market Place on Tuesdays, Fridays and Saturdays

### SHIPS' SERVICES

**Water** Brents Boatyard
**Fuel** Diesel from boatyard; petrol from garage
**Gas** (Camping and Calor) At boatyard

**Chandler** At Oare (weekends only)
**Boatyard, engineer** Brents Boatyard
**Sailmaker** The nearest is at Conyer or Whitstable

---

*Alternative moorings*

For those wishing to remain afloat, there are a few visitors' moorings at **Harty Ferry** with shore access at all times except low water springs. From the landing it is a 20-minute walk to the village of Oare, with a village shop (in Russell Place), chandlery (weekends only), boatyard (with crane and diesel) and an old attractive pub, the Three Mariners, which serves food. There is an hourly bus service to Faversham.

Down river at **Hollowshore**, at the confluence of Faversham and Oare Creeks, there is limited space to anchor and a yard with most facilities. The pub, the Shipwright's Arms, is popular with yachtsmen and provides good pub food, including breakfasts.

---

# Gillingham

Gillingham is an excellent base from which to visit the surrounding area, which must be of interest to all those who know something of Britain's maritime history and tradition. Gillingham itself does not have a great deal to offer.

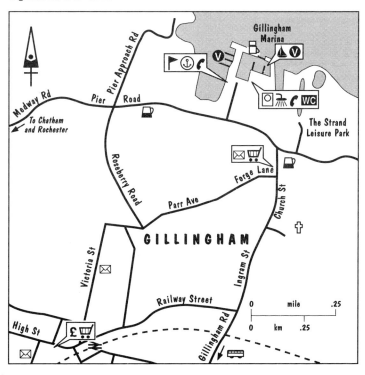

SHORE LEAVE

*Food and drink*
The marina office recommends The Ship pub, but there are various other pubs nearby, too. You will find a Chinese take-away at the end of Church Street.

*Entertainment*
Gillingham has a cinema.

*What to see*
Gillingham Strand, half a mile to the east of the marina, offers excellent views. The **Royal Engineers Museum** at **Brompton Barracks** traces the history of military engineering since 1066 and has a large gallery showing the life and work of the Royal Engineers during the Second World War. The ancient **parish church** on Gillingham Green is mentioned in the Domesday Book and is worth a visit to see how it has been changed over the centuries.

At **Chatham** you can visit the **Historic Dockyard** which takes you back to the days of English seapower and shows you the crafts and skills by which a ship of the line was built. **Fort Amherst**, also open to the public, was built in the late eighteenth century to defend the Dockyard.

*Excursions*

**Rochester**, only a short distance away, has a magnificent **Norman castle** with a great view from the top of the keep over the rivers and countryside of Kent, so that one understands its strategic position. Not to be missed in Rochester is the impressive **cathedral**. Rochester is also the scene of many Dickens novels and his admirers will enjoy the **Dickens Centre**. The town still has many shops dating from his time.

*Exercise*

All kinds of water sports are enjoyed on the river, including waterskiing, windsurfing and canoeing; there are sandy beaches, too. The Strand Leisure Park is almost immediately to the east of the marina, with a large open-air swimming pool among its numerous attractions. Many other sports, such as ice-skating and indoor bowls, are catered for in Gillingham. The shore path makes an interesting walk.

## TRANSPORT AND TRAVEL

**Buses** From Beresford Road in the town centre, half a mile to the south-west, to Chatham and Rochester

**Trains** To London, Dover and Ramsgate
**Taxis, car and bicycle hire** Ask in marina office

*Further information* from Tourist Office, Eastgate Cottage, High Street, Rochester ☎ (0634) 43666.

# Gillingham Marina

| | |
|---|---|
| **Harbourmaster** ☎ (0634) 280022 | **VHF Channel** 80 |
| **Callsign** Gillingham Marina | **Daily charge** £££ in locked basin; ££ in tidal basin |

The marina is very modern and clean with purpose-built facilities and security is very good. The outlook from the marina to seaward is pleasant and open, but the power-station is an eyesore; inland the view is somewhat dreary.

## STEP ASHORE

**Nearest payphone** In the car-park or opposite the entrance gate to marina
**Toilets, showers, launderette** In marina
**Clubhouse** Available for berth holders, with a bar and a restaurant
**Shopping** The marina shop has food and an off-licence; the late-night shop is a

15-minute uphill walk away in the main shopping area, where you will find most major chain-stores, banks and a post office in the pedestrianised High Street. Hempstead Valley Shopping Centre has a full range of shops under cover

## SHIPS' SERVICES

*Water and electricity* On pontoons
*Fuel* Diesel at fuelling point; petrol from garage at entrance to marina
*Gas* Camping from chandler, Calor

from berthing staff
*Chandler, boatyard* On-site
*Sailmaker* Elliots at Chatham Historic Dockyard

# London –
# St Katharine Yacht Haven

St Katharine Yacht Haven is in the old dock built by Telford. The Ivory House, headquarters of the Cruising Association, and the Dickens Inn stand between the basins which are surrounded on their other sides by less inspiring examples of modern architecture.

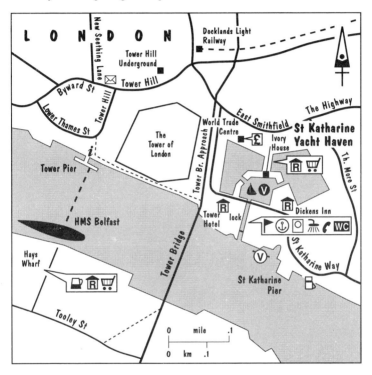

## SHORE LEAVE

### Food and drink
In St Katharine Dock the Dickens Inn offers a Victorian atmosphere and ale brewed on the premises; the building is an old, but rebuilt, timber warehouse. The Tower Hotel Carvery serves a standard hotel meal. In Ivory House the Riverside Café serves food (as well as being a mini-supermarket) and the Patisserie serves snacks to eat on the premises. The Mala Indian Restaurant is near the Dickens Inn. They are all good, but expensive. If you want a cheaper Indian meal go to Brick Lane. *Out to Eat* and *The Good Food Guide 1992* both recommend a large number of restaurants in London.

### Entertainment
The whole of London is before you. The *Evening Standard* entertainments

page is a daily guide to what's on and various listing magazines give weekly coverage.

### What to see

The **Tower of London**, where the crown jewels are kept, and Tower Bridge, with its own museum, are a few minutes' walk from St Katharine Dock. **HMS** *Belfast*, reached from Tooley Street across Tower Bridge, is a floating museum. In Tooley Street itself is the **London Dungeon**, a medieval horror museum. Guides to what to see further afield in London can be obtained from the information desk in the Tower Hotel foyer.

### Excursions

Take the Docklands Light Railway to Island Gardens and walk through the tunnel under the Thames to **Greenwich** to visit the **National Maritime Museum**, Elizabeth I's **Queen's House** and the **Royal Observatory**. You can visit the **Thames Barrier** by boat and see its history illustrated at the Visitor Centre — telephone for details ☎ 081-854 5555. **Wapping Market** and **Brick Lane** in Shoreditch are large general markets; **Petticoat Lane** in Spitalfields, which is nearer, sells mainly clothes and has a craft market on Sundays.

### Exercise

There is a swimming pool, Wapping Baths, at The Highway in Wapping, 10 minutes' walk to the north-east.

### TRANSPORT AND TRAVEL

**Buses** To the West End from Tower Hill
**Trains** The nearest underground station is Tower Hill on the District and Circle Lines. It is two stops on the Circle Line to Liverpool Street Station and a 10-minute walk to London Bridge station. Docklands Light Railway leaves from Tower Gateway

**Planes** The Piccadilly Line from King's Cross runs to Heathrow Airport; Gatwick is serviced by trains from Victoria
**Taxis** From outside Tower Hotel
**Car hire** Europcar-Docklands, 249–251 East India Dock Road ☎ 071-538 2066

**Further information** from Tourist Office by West Gate of Tower of London. Some information is available in the Tower Hotel foyer.

## St Katharine Yacht Haven

| Harbourmaster ☎ (071) 488 2400 | VHF Channels 80, M |
|---|---|
| Callsign St Katharines | Daily charge £££ |

Bringing your boat up the Thames to St Katharine for a few days is ideal as a cheap and central base from which to explore London.

## STEP ASHORE

**Nearest payphone** In the Tower Hotel foyer
**Toilets, showers, launderette** In Marine Centre on side of lock
**Clubhouse** The Cruising Association welcomes visitors and there is also a proprietary club
**Shopping** Late-night shop on the north side of the basin in Ivory House. The nearest bank and bureau de change is in the World Trade Centre in East Smithfield; the nearest post office is near Tower Hill underground station. There is a post box in the Tower Hotel. For more comprehensive shopping, take the Docklands Light Railway from Tower Gateway near Tower Hill underground station to Shadwell for Sainsbury supermarket and Wapping market

### SHIPS' SERVICES

*Water and electricity* On pontoons
*Fuel* (diesel and petrol) From fuel barge in the river
*Gas* From Pumpkin Marine in The Highway

*Chandler* Pumpkin Marine and Kelvin Hughes (in The Minories)
*Boatyard, engineer* Ask in Yacht Haven Office

# EAST ANGLIA

# Burnham-on-Crouch

The town of Burnham began to develop in 1253 when a market charter was granted to the Fitzwalter family. By the nineteenth century there was a flourishing oyster fishing industry and when the railway reached the town, yachting became very popular. Burnham is now a busy yachting centre and a reasonable-sized town. It has often been described as the Cowes of the east coast and a lot of racing goes on, especially at weekends and on Wednesday evenings. Many residents of the town commute to London and there is a more cosmopolitan atmosphere than in any other east coast sailing centre; this is a lively place with a wide variety of places at which to eat and drink.

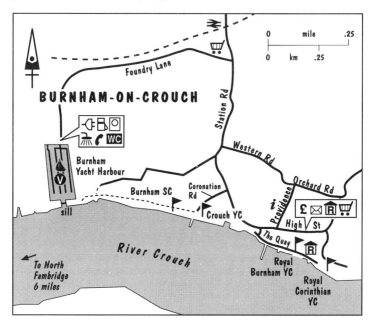

## SHORE LEAVE

*Food and drink*
The best and most expensive restaurant is the Contented Sole. Chinese, Italian and Indian restaurants vie for business in the High Street, although you could opt for fish and chips. The best pub is probably the White Harte on the quayside – it has a wide range of bar food and a restaurant and children are allowed in the eating areas – but there are at least half a dozen others. Polash, 169 Station Road, is a popular tandoori restaurant featured in both *Out to Eat* and *The Good Food Guide 1992*.

*Entertainment*
There is a cinema in the High Street.

### What to see

**Burnham Week** is the last week of August or the first week in September, when there are events for a wide range of sailing craft. **Burnham Carnival** is in September. The **Clock Tower** in the High Street was built in 1877; access to it can be arranged by appointment with the Information Officer, Maldon District Council ☎ (0621) 854477. **Burnham Museum**, Providence, contains exhibits of local interest, with maritime and agricultural connections.

### Excursions

**Mangapps Farm Railway Museum** on the Southminster Road has a large display of railway relics, including one of the largest collections of signalling equipment in Britain, with a demonstration line.

### Exercise

No visit to Burnham would be complete without a walk along the sea wall, at least as far as the Royal Corinthian Yacht Club. You could walk 15 miles along the sea wall to Bradwell Nuclear Power Station. There is a sport and leisure centre five minutes' walk from the marina and a squash court at the Royal Corinthian Yacht Club. On the bank of the river, to the west of Burnham, there is a large country park which is pleasant to walk in.

## TRANSPORT AND TRAVEL

| | |
|---|---|
| **Buses** To Woodham Ferrers and Maldon | **Taxis** B & H Taxis ☎ (0621) 784878 |
| **Trains** To London, taking one-and-a-quarter hours | **Car hire** Two local firms |

*Further information* from Tourist Office in Providence off the High Street.

# Burnham Yacht Harbour

| | |
|---|---|
| **Harbourmaster** ☎ (0621) 782150 | **VHF Channels** 80, M |
| **Callsign** Burnham Yacht Harbour | **Daily charge** ££ |

Burnham Yacht Harbour is a small, go-ahead marina with all facilities. It is a pleasant and safe place to stop, just outside the town, which can be reached by an enjoyable riverside walk. Some of the yards along the river have swinging moorings for visitors. If you use them, beware of the strong current in the river if you want to get ashore by dinghy.

## STEP ASHORE

**Nearest payphones** In amenities block, or up to main road and turn left over railway bridge

**Toilets, showers, launderette** In amenities block; there is a security code lock on the doors

**Clubhouses** None in the marina, but to the east along the sea wall are several: Crouch Yacht Club, Royal Burnham Yacht Club and Royal Corinthian Yacht Club. It is half a mile to Crouch Yacht Club, which is very friendly and serves food at weekends in the season; Royal Burnham Yacht Club is slightly further east and has a bar overlooking the river; Royal Corinthian Yacht Club is an unusual building, recently extensively refurbished

**Shopping** The Co-op supermarket (open until 2100 on Fridays and 1900 on Saturdays) is one mile away at the end of Foundry Lane, the road into the marina. Several other shops are in this area, as well as along both sides of the High Street into the town. If you like wine, Davisons in the High Street opens late and has a particularly wide selection. All the usual banks and building societies are represented in Burnham and there is a post office. Early closing Wednesdays. Local herring and fresh oysters can be bought at a stall near the war memorial, along with other fresh fish

### SHIPS' SERVICES

**Water and electricity** On pontoons
**Fuel** Diesel only in the marina
**Gas** (Camping and Calor) From the chandler

**Chandler, boatyard, engineer** All in the marina
**Sailmaker** Cranfield Sails, The Sail Loft, Burnham Business Park
☎ (0621) 782108

---

*Alternative moorings*
On the other side of the river is **Essex Marina** which has good facilities but is on the wrong side for the town and station.

# North Fambridge

This reach of the River Crouch, well up river from Burnham, is a great place to commune with nature and really get away from the world, yet the railway line to Liverpool Street is less than a mile away. The people in the yard and at the club are very hospitable and willing to help out with any problem. Security is excellent. The only sign of civilisation is the very old Ferry Boat Inn with its wholesome food and village atmosphere. Don't be surprised if you find yourself taking part in an organised quiz.

Apart from a few modern houses which have grown up round the railway station, the area is mainly farmland on low rolling hills. Mike Peyton, the celebrated nautical cartoon artist, is a local resident, so be careful or you may find your antics on the water appearing in a yachting magazine.

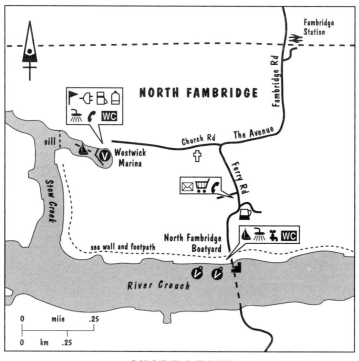

SHORE LEAVE

Fambridge is a very tranquil backwater. Peace, quiet and wildlife are the principal attractions. The Ferry Boat Inn, just outside the boatyard gate, is the only pub. It is a very old building with a good atmosphere and quite famous locally, serving food at lunchtimes and in the evenings. For exercise, walk three miles along the sea wall to Althorne and return by train – or vice versa, depending on the wind direction.

## TRANSPORT AND TRAVEL

**Trains** From Fambridge station, three-quarters-of-a-mile from the boatyard, to London, take one-and-a-quarter hours

**Taxis** Elite Taxis ☎ (0621) 741487

*Further information* from Tourist Office in Providence, off the High Street in Burnham-on-Crouch ☎ (0621) 856503.

# Westwick Marina

| | |
|---|---|
| **Harbourmaster** ☎ (0621) 740370 | **VHF Channels** 80, M |
| **Callsign** Westwick Marina | **Daily charge** in marina ££; on swinging moorings £ |

The swinging moorings at North Fambridge are controlled by North Fambridge Boatyard. There is a substantial floating pier (with water) where boats can tie up temporarily to make enquiries. The entrance to Westwick Marina, also run by North Fambridge Boatyard, is another three-quarters of a mile up river. It must be one of the quietest marinas in the country.

Entry to the marina is possible at all times except for an hour either side of low water. In summer a launch service runs from the swinging moorings to the landing stage on Saturdays, Sundays and Bank Holidays, 0830–1800. Several clubs make a group visit to Westwick during the year and enjoy the hospitality. It is the apparent isolation of the place which makes it an interesting marina to visit.

## STEP ASHORE

**Nearest payphones** On the wall of the clubhouse of Westwick Marina or outside Fambridge Stores, less than 200 yards from North Fambridge Boatyard
**Toilets, showers** In boatyard and in marina
**Clubhouse** Westwick Yacht Club is open at weekends; barbecues are held on alternate Saturday evenings in the summer
**Shopping** North Fambridge Stores and post office – early closing Thursdays. Otherwise shop at Burnham

### SHIPS' SERVICES

*Water* From the end of the floating pier at the boatyard and on pontoons in the marina
*Electricity* On pontoons in marina
*Fuel* Diesel only, at marina
*Gas* (Camping and Calor) At both yard and marina

*Chandler, boatyard, engineer* All available from North Fambridge Boatyard
*Sailmaker* Cranfield Sails, The Sail Loft, Burnham Business Park
☎ (0621) 782108

# Bradwell-on-Sea

In fine weather this marina and the surrounding area have much to offer, although its main appeal is to walkers and those who are interested in history and pleasant pubs; it might not suit families. On the other hand, in really bad weather it is an excellent place to leave a boat, along with Tollesbury Marina or Burnham Yacht Harbour, which offer similar security. If you like the countryside, wildlife, pleasant walks along the sea wall and unspoilt villages, you might want to spend two days here.

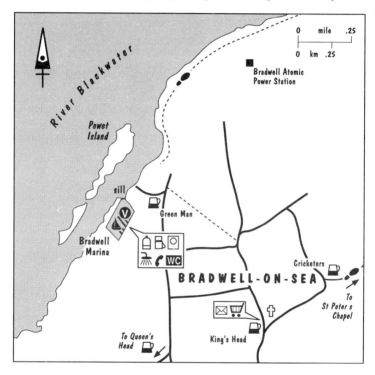

SHORE LEAVE

### Food and drink
The Green Man, the pub at Bradwell Waterside, has better food and beer than the marina clubhouse. The King's Head in Bradwell Village has excellent food and beer, and the landlord keeps a llama in the field at the back.

### Entertainment
The nearest cinema is at Burnham-on-Crouch.

### What to see
**St Peter's Chapel**, a short walk from Bradwell Village, is a Saxon chapel built in AD 654 which has had many uses through the ages, from barn to lighthouse. It was re-consecrated in 1920. Close by is **Linnett's Cottage**, once a coastguard

station and subsequently home of a renowned wildfowler; it is now derelict. There is a **nature reserve** and **bird observatory** nearby. **Bradwell Village Church** is an interesting medieval building added to and restored over the years; a lock-up, not used since their abolition in the 1850s, still remains in the churchyard. Guided tours of **Bradwell Nuclear Power Station** take place from time to time.

*Exercise*
The Wymarks beach, along the sea wall towards the power station, is the best beach. Windsurfing is a possibility there if you have your own board. Try one of the walks suggested in the leaflet available from the Tourist Office in Maldon.

## TRANSPORT AND TRAVEL

Ask for detailed information about transport at Tower office in the marina.

**Buses** Nearest at Maldon
**Trains** Nearest station is Southminster
**Taxis** Banyard's Taxis, Maldon
☎ (0621) 853569

**Car hire** Tavern Hire, Maldon
☎ (0621) 858773
**Bicycle hire** High Street Cycles, Maldon
☎ (0621) 853188

*Further information* from Tourist Office in the Maritime Museum, Hythe Quay, Maldon.

# Bradwell Marina

| | |
|---|---|
| **Harbourmaster** ☎ (0621) 76235 | **VHF Channels** 80, M |
| **Callsign** Bradwell Marina | **Daily charge** ££ |

Bradwell Marina, on the south shore of the Blackwater River, is a very friendly marina, well-run and with helpful staff. It is a safe place to leave a boat but not particularly easy to get to by land, especially by public transport.

## STEP ASHORE

**Nearest payphone** At the side of the clubhouse
**Toilets, showers, launderette** New showers, toilets and a washing machine have recently been installed in clubhouse. There are public toilets below the Tower office

**Clubhouse** Bradwell Cruising Club is open for drinks and meals every day during the season
**Shopping** Bradwell Village is just over one mile from the marina — it has a post office/general store

## SHIPS' SERVICES

*Water and electricity* On pontoons
*Fuel* (diesel and petrol) From fuelling jetty
*Gas* From chandler (closed Mondays and Tuesdays) or from garage on main road about one mile away
*Chandler* At Bradwell Waterside 200 yards from marina, open 0900–1700

*Wednesday to Sunday*
*Boatyard, engineer* Normally available Monday to Friday; ask at the Tower Office in an emergency
*Sailmaker* Cranfield Sails, The Sail Loft, Burnham-on-Crouch ☎ (0621) 782108

# Maldon

Maldon's history extends beyond the Roman invasion, and commerce and shipbuilding on the River Blackwater go back hundreds of years. The town is one of the most attractive in East Anglia with its focus on Hythe Quay, its weatherboarded pubs and the fleet of Thames barges – in beautiful condition – to delight the eye when they are not away racing.

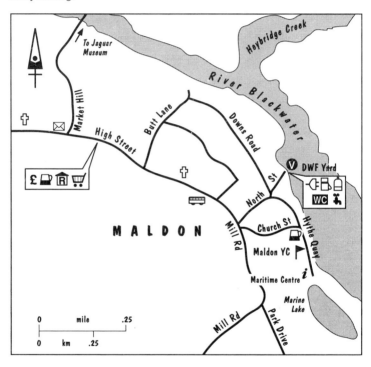

## SHORE LEAVE

### Food and drink
The pubs on the riverside serve good beer and excellent seafood. The town has many other eating and drinking places to suit all tastes. Wheelers fish and chip shop, 13 High Street, is recommended in both *Out to Eat* and *The Good Food Guide 1992*.

### Entertainment
There are two cinemas and a theatre in the town.

### What to see
Visit the **Plume Library,** St Peter's Tower, Market Hill. The tower is all that remains of thirteenth-century St Peter's Church after its collapse in 1665. The nave was rebuilt by Dr Thomas Plume, presented to the town in 1704 and contains his sixteenth and seventeenth-century library. A Medieval Garden has

recently been opened alongside the Tower. The **Maritime Museum** on Hythe Quay contains exhibits connected with barge building. **Moot Hall** in the High Street is worth seeing for its original fifteenth-century spiral brick staircase and eighteenth-century court-room. The **Jaguar Museum** in Mill Lane has a collection of Jaguar cars dating back to the very first to be built.

*Excursions*
**St Peter's Chapel** at Bradwell-on-Sea, is one of the earliest surviving churches in England. Worth a visit to appreciate the isolated setting and perhaps do some bird spotting is the nearby **nature reserve. Chelmsford** is within easy reach. See the cathedral, once a medieval church; the interior has been restored to enhance the old structures. If you would enjoy a view of rural Essex, try a boat trip along the **Chelmer and Blackwater Navigation Canal.** Northey Island, now a nature reserve owned by the National Trust, is believed to have been the base camp for the Viking army defeated by the Saxon Earl of Essex at the Battle of Maldon in AD991 – it is occasionally open to the public or can be visited by appointment ☎ (0621) 853142. (24 hours' notice is required.)

*Exercise*
There is a leisure centre and swimming pool in Promenade Park. Walk downstream along the river to the site of the Battle of Maldon. Walk upstream through lush meadows to **Beeleigh Falls**, passing swans-in-residence, and on to the lock where the Blackwater and the Chelmer join. You will find many public footpaths from which to enjoy the countryside. A long distance path, **St Peter's Way**, runs for 45 miles between Chipping Ongar and St Peter's on the Wall at Bradwell-on-Sea. Other routes include the **North Blackwater Trail** which follows the sea wall along the banks of the river.

### TRANSPORT AND TRAVEL

**Buses** From the bus station in High Street to Chelmsford, Hatfield Peverel and Witham
**Trains** From Hatfield Peverel to London

**Taxis** Banyards Taxis ☎ (0621) 853569
**Car hire** Tavern Hire ☎ (0621) 858773
**Bicycle hire** High Street Cycles in High Street

*Further information* from Tourist Office in the Maritime Museum, Hythe Quay.

# Maldon Moorings

| | |
|---|---|
| **Harbourmaster** ☎ (0621) 740264 | **VHF Channel** M |
| **Callsign** Danwebb | **Daily charge** £ |

There is limited accommodation for visiting yachts to dry out in soft mud at the jetties in Dan Webb and Feesey's yard.

### STEP ASHORE

**Nearest payphone** In the boatyard
**Toilets** In the boatyard
**Clubhouse** Maldon Little Ship Club on Hythe Quay
**Shopping** Just up the hill via North Street

to the High Street where there is a very good range of facilities: all you would expect in a country town. Early closing Wednesdays

## SHIPS' SERVICES

**Water** Quayside and boatyard
**Fuel, gas, chandler, boatyard, engineer**
All at Dan Webb and Feesey

**Sailmaker** Taylors, next door to Dan Webb
and Feesey, make and repair sails for
barges and cruising yachts

---

### Alternative moorings

For those who want a really Dickensian experience, **Downs Road Boatyard**, a little further up stream, is full of character and would repay a visit. ☎ (0621) 853330 first to make sure there is room.

# Heybridge

Heybridge Basin is at the seaward end of the Chelmer and Blackwater Navigation Canal, which was built in 1797 to take boats to and from Chelmsford. The canal itself has a long history, as do the warehouses at Heybridge and the older houses. The largest warehouse was built in 1863 by Edward Bentall, a Victorian ironfounder and agricultural engineer who also built some of the earliest cars.

No other place in the area is quite like Heybridge: it is somewhere time has forgotten. Nostalgic excitement takes charge as you lock through into the old canal and find yourself surrounded by mainly wooden boats of all shapes and sizes. If you like peace and quiet and are a lover of traditional boats, it's a must.

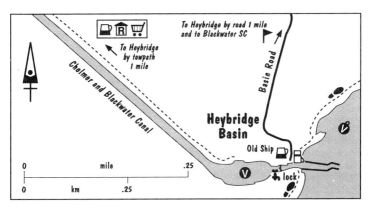

SHORE LEAVE

### Food and drink
Two pubs are within three minutes' walk of the basin: the Jolly Sailor and the Old Ship. The Old Ship is particularly recommended for its good food at lunch and in the evening. Oriental Glory in Bentall's Centre in Heybridge serves excellent Indian food. The alternatives are the Bembridge Hotel, The Anchor and The Half Moon pubs, Pizza Time, and Trevor's Fish and Chips (take-away).

### Entertainment
A folk club enlivens the Old Ship on Thursday evenings.

### What to see
The area is rich with bird life, especially in winter. The **Heybridge Basin Regatta** is held in July.

*Excursions*
Visit **Maldon** to see the old town wharf and sailing barges; it is within easy reach.
**Colchester** is also very accessible – it is a most interesting old town dating from
before Roman times.

*Exercise*
Walk along the canal towpath, which eventually brings you to Chelmsford after
15 miles. It is possible to walk along the sea wall towards and past the
Blackwater Sailing Club and find the ancient causeway to Osea Island.
Alternatively, go waterskiing at Mill Beach.

## TRANSPORT AND TRAVEL

**Buses, trains** From Maldon ☎ (0621) 859822

**Taxis** Alouetta Taxis, Maldon ☎ (0621) 852212

**Bicycle hire** High St Cycles, Maldon ☎ (0621) 853569

**Car hire** Triangle Garage, Heybridge

*Further information* from Tourist Office in the Maritime Centre at Hythe Quay,
Maldon ☎ (0621) 782237.

# Heybridge Basin

**Harbourmaster** ☎ (0621) 853506

**Daily charge** first night (includes locking in and out) £££; extra nights £

If you have time, two nights are better value than one because of the
lock fees. The facilities are basic, but the two pubs within a three-
minute walk are friendly. It would be worth strolling into Heybridge one
evening; don't go bare-legged in summer because of the stinging
nettles on the towpath.

## STEP ASHORE

**Nearest payphones** In the pubs or at the entrance to the car-park

**Toilets** At the entrance to the car-park

**Clubhouse** Blackwater Sailing Club is a quarter of a mile away

**Shopping** The nearest shops are at Heybridge; allow 30 minutes to walk there along the canal towpath. There is a supermarket, baker, chemist, greengrocer, Chinese take-away and post office, but no bank. Early closing Wednesdays

## SHIPS' SERVICES

*Water* From standpipe near inner lock gates

*Fuel, chandler, boatyard* From Holt & James Ltd on the sea wall

*Engineer* The lock-keeper is a competent engineer who will help out if necessary

*Sailmaker* Taylors at Maldon ☎ (0621) 853456

# Tollesbury

This is a pleasant haven for those who seek peace and quiet in unsophisticated surroundings and will appeal to lovers of nature and village life. It is a good base for exploring the ancient towns of Maldon and Colchester, both of which have excellent shopping facilities and amenities.

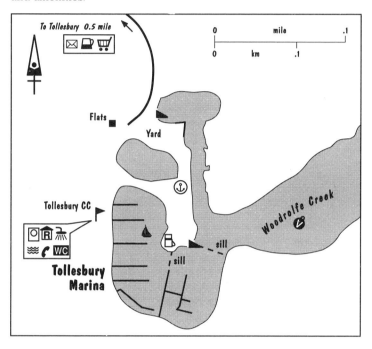

SHORE LEAVE

*Food and drink*
The club restaurant in the marina is recommended. There are also pubs in the village.

*What to see*
The **Old Hall Bird Sanctuary** on the north side of the harbour can be visited by road, or sea if you have shallow draught.

*Excursions*
Five miles away, at Layer de la Haye, you will find **Layer Marney Manor** and church. The Hall was started in the early fifteenth century but only the west wing and the gate-house were built – the latter is one of the great buildings of its time. There is a large **bird sanctuary** at Layer and nearby is **Abberton reservoir** and **nature reserve.**

*Exercise*
Walk from the marina to the south side of the creek, along the sea wall and

riverside. You can windsurf in 'The Leavings', down the creek, but there are no facilities. There is a leisure centre at Witham, five miles away.

### TRANSPORT AND TRAVEL

**Buses** Good bus services from Tollesbury Village to Maldon, Colchester, Witham and Hatfield Peverel

**Trains** The nearest station is Hatfield Peverel, with a regular service to London
**Taxis** Enquire at marina office

*Further information* from Tourist Office in the Maritime Centre at Hythe Quay, Maldon ☎ (0621) 782237.

# Tollesbury Marina

| | |
|---|---|
| **Harbourmaster** ☎ (0621) 869202 | **VHF Channel** M |
| **Callsign** Tollesbury Marina | **Daily charge** ££ |

Tollesbury Marina is at the head of the three-quarter-mile Woodrolfe Creek. There are five marina buoys where you can await high water. The marina is constantly being improved: it is newly rewired, the pontoons have been refurbished and a substantial new hauling-out area has been added. If you are not going into the marina there are deep-water moorings in the south channel near the entrance to Woodrolfe Creek and a rough hard where you can land your dinghy.

### STEP ASHORE

**Nearest payphone, toilets, showers, launderette** In the clubhouse (open 0700–2300)
**Clubhouse** Tollesbury Cruising Club, in the marina, welcomes visitors. It is a very well equipped and friendly club with a restaurant, a covered swimming pool and tennis courts
**Shopping** Tollesbury Village, one mile up the road, has village shops and a post office/general store open 0800–2100. There are banks and more shops at Tiptree, five miles away

#### SHIPS' SERVICES

*Water, electricity* On marina berths
*Fuel* (diesel and petrol) From fuelling wharf
*Gas* (Camping and Calor) From chandlery

*Chandler, boatyard, engineer, sailmaker* From the well-equipped Woodrolfe Boatyard in marina

# Brightlingsea

Brightlingsea has the distinction of being the only Cinque Port outside Kent and Sussex, and its ships and sailors have gone to sea from time immemorial. The Town Hard is where you can see all the waterfront comings and goings, including the activities of the Colne Smack Preservation Society which maintains a sea-going link with the past.

Perhaps it is because it is on the way to nowhere that Brightlingsea is so full of character – and so are the local inhabitants.

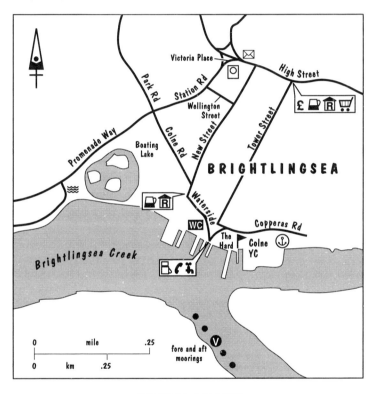

## SHORE LEAVE

### Food and drink
There is a restaurant in the Colne Yacht Club. The Anchor Hotel nearby and The Yachtsman's Arms in Waterside are personally recommended, as is Brightling Chinese Restaurant, 56 High Street, a 10-minute walk away.

### Entertainment
The nearest cinemas are in Clacton, Harwich and Colchester.

### What to see
Thirteenth-century **Jacobes Hall**, an old, timbered house in the High Street and now a restaurant, is one of the oldest occupied buildings in Essex, and well

worth a visit. The parish church, which is on the highest point around the town, contains ceramic tiles commemorating local people whose lives were lost at sea. There is an **Aviation Museum** in the Martello tower at Point Clear, across the harbour, with wartime memorabilia of the RAF and USAF.

*Excursions*

**St Osyth's Priory**, two miles from Brightlingsea, is in private hands but open to the public. The eleventh-century buildings are in parkland where deer roam – the lake, water-gardens and art collection are further attractions. The **East Anglian Railway Museum** at Chappel and Wakes Colne Station is 10 miles away, near Colchester. It is a collection of old railway buildings, steam trains, coaches, signal boxes and small exhibits in a very picturesque setting. **Colchester** is the oldest recorded town in Britain and there is plenty to see there. The main item of historical interest is the Castle Keep: it is the largest in Europe and is now a museum with a fine collection of Roman and other antiquities.

*Exercise*

Exploring is rewarding in Brightlingsea; try walking along the promenade and Ropewalk. Swimming and windsurfing from beaches at Point Clear or St Osyth are popular. There is a leisure centre in Clacton.

## TRANSPORT AND TRAVEL

**Buses** To Clacton and Colchester
**Ferries** From Harwich or Felixstowe
**Taxis** A1 Taxi ☎ (0206) 303998
**Car hire** Budget Rent-a-Car, Clacton

☎ (0255) 222444
**Bicycle hire** East Essex Cycles, 84 Pier Avenue, Clacton ☎ (0255) 434490

*Further information* from Tourist Office, 23 Pier Avenue, Clacton ☎ (0255) 423400.

# Brightlingsea Moorings

| Harbourmaster ☎ (0206) 302200 | VHF Channel 68 |
|---|---|
| Callsign Brightlingsea | Daily charge £ |

The harbour is clean and pleasant and security reasonably good. Mooring is on piles some way from the Colne Yacht Club and it can be a hard row ashore, so an outboard motor is an advantage. The waterside area is well supplied for nautical needs, but the high-street shops are a good 10-minute walk away.

## STEP ASHORE

**Nearest payphone** Near top of hard alongside wooden shelter with clock
**Toilets, showers** In Colne Yacht Club
**Clubhouse** Colne Yacht Club is on the waterfront near The Hard and welcomes visiting yachtsmen – a sign outside the door says so
**Shopping** The main shopping area is about half a mile to the north, with the usual high-street shops, banks, building societies and a post office. Early closing Thursdays

## SHIPS' SERVICES

**Water** Hose available from Colne Yacht Club pontoon, ask club steward for key
**Fuel** (diesel and petrol) From French Marine in Waterside
**Gas** Camping from French Marine; Calor from Morgan Marine in Waterside

**Chandler, engineer** French Marine and Morgan Marine
**Sailmaker** J Lawrence, 22–28 Tower Street and Malcolm Goodwin at Wivenhoe ☎ (0206) 826171

# Walton Backwaters

At the heart of the east coast rivers, deep in Arthur Ransome country, Titchmarsh Marina is in the area covered by *Secret Waters*; a study of the book on the spot will make fascinating reading, and the charts are as relevant today as in 1939. The Backwaters are designated a special landscape area and coastal protection zone. The undeveloped coastline and thousands of acres of saltmarsh, islands, creeks, intertidal mudflats and beaches make it a superb sailing area.

The seaside towns of Walton-on-the-Naze and Frinton-on-Sea are equidistant from Titchmarsh Marina. Walton is a family resort; the narrow and charming streets lead to an outstanding sandy beach and one of the longest piers in the country. Frinton is much grander, with tree-lined avenues and an extensive cliff-top greensward.

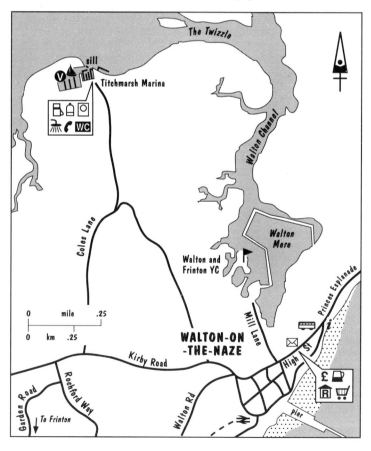

## SHORE LEAVE

*Food and drink*
Walton and Frinton both have a variety of eating places, but there are no pubs in Frinton.

*Entertainment*
There is a repertory theatre in Frinton and cinemas and theatres in Clacton-on-Sea and Colchester.

*What to see*
The pier at Walton has its own fun-fair, so there is no need to go to Clacton. **Walton Maritime Museum** in the old Lifeboat House, East Terrace, has a permanent collection illustrating the maritime history of the Tendring Peninsula.

*Excursions*
The many very charming inland towns and villages on the Tendring peninsula invite exploration. **Thorpe-le-Soken** is a village accessible by train from Frinton and Walton and worth a visit for its shopping attractions, particularly antique shops, good pubs and restaurants. The ancient town of **Colchester** is also within easy reach by train.

*Exercise*
Follow the nature trail in the **Naze Nature Reserve**, with over 100 acres of parkland and woodland on the edge of the cliffs and views across the Naze and Hamford Water. The eight miles of sandy beaches are good for walking, swimming and windsurfing. There is a leisure centre and swimming pool at Clacton.

### TRANSPORT AND TRAVEL

**Buses** Minibus service from Walton along the coast to Frinton and Clacton
**Trains** From Walton and Frinton to Colchester; change for London
**Planes** Ipswich airport is the nearest
**Ferries** From Harwich

**Taxis** Dancabs ☎ (0255) 675910
**Car hire** Budget Rent-a-Car, Clacton ☎ (0255) 222444
**Bicycle hire** East Essex Cycles, 84 Pier Avenue, Clacton ☎ (0255) 434490

*Further information* from Tourist Office, Princes Esplanade, Walton-on-the-Naze.

# Titchmarsh Marina

| Harbourmaster ☎ (0225) 672185 | VHF Channel M |
|---|---|
| Callsign Titchmarsh Marina | Daily charge ££ |

The marina lies in an area of flat, open landcape, adjacent to the wide expanse of the Backwaters and by their agricultural hinterland. It is sheltered from the sea by the Naze peninsula and is an excellent spot from which to explore the east coast or to set off for the Dutch coast.

## STEP ASHORE

**Nearest payphone** Beside marina office
**Toilets, showers** In marina car-park
**Launderette** Beside marina main office
0800–2000
**Clubhouse** Walton and Frinton Yacht Club
**Shopping** It is one-and-a-half miles to the
shops: half a mile down the road turn left
for Walton-on-the-Naze, turn right for
Frinton-on-Sea. Both have the usual
range of high-street shops, banks,
building societies and a post office.
No late-night shopping; early closing
Wednesdays

### SHIPS' SERVICES

*Water and electricity* On pontoons
*Fuel* Diesel only from marina fuel berth
*Gas* (Camping and Calor) from **chandler**,
Marine Traders, in marina

*Boatyard, engineer* Hall & Son, Mill Lane,
close to marina car-park
*Sailmaker* East Coast Sails, Hall Lane,
Walton

# River Orwell

As you enter through the dock area with Felixstowe to starboard and Harwich to port, the Orwell is ahead, the Stour to the west. The Orwell leads north to Ipswich, and, in spite of heavy commercial traffic, manages to present a serene and rural aspect; it is one of the most beautiful of the east coast rivers. The village of Pin Mill, half-way between the sea and Ipswich, is attractive in a somewhat faded way.

The lower reaches of the Stour are rather uninteresting although the upper reaches, painted by both Constable and Gainsborough, offer some of the most lovely landscapes in the country. Above the Parkeston Quay ferry terminals there is a bird sanctuary with, surprisingly, a waterskiing area alongside.

The ports of Harwich and Felixstowe are more oriented to commerce than to leisure, and though both are accessible by harbour ferry from Shotley Point, you will probably find little compulsion to visit them. Ipswich is a busy commercial port and town, and on the face of it not attractive. However, on a rainy day or after days spent among the Essex marshes, it can provide a very welcome change.

## SHORE LEAVE

*Food and drink*
There are plenty of places to eat in a relaxed way in Ipswich.

*Shopping*
Ipswich is a large town with all the usual facilities and has two modern shopping precincts.

*Entertainment*
The Odeon Theatre, St Helens Street, has live entertainment and two cinema screens. The Film Theatre, King Street, also has two screens. The Wolsey Theatre, Civic Drive, has monthly repertory shows. There are three nightclubs.

*What to see*
Ipswich is an ancient town with fine buildings from many periods, including twelve medieval churches. **Christchurch Mansion**, Christchurch Park, is a fully furnished Tudor house belonging to the town. **Wolsey Art Gallery**, Christchurch Park, has the most important collection of Gainsboroughs and Constables outside London. **Ipswich Museum**, High Street, has galleries devoted to natural history, geology, ethnography and archaeology.

*Excursions*
Visit Constable country: **East Bergholt**, **Flatford Mill** and **Dedham** where Constable went to school and **Sir Alfred Munnings' house**, which is open to the public. **Gainsborough's house** at Sudbury is beautifully furnished and has a museum and exhibition gallery.

*Exercise*
Crown Pools, Crown Street, has three swimming pools. Windsurf in the Stour and Orwell Rivers or walk along the riverbanks.

## TRANSPORT AND TRAVEL

**Buses** Services from all the marinas to Ipswich
**Trains** From Ipswich, Harwich and Felixstowe to London
**Planes** Ipswich
**Ferries** From Harwich to The Hook of Holland and from Felixstowe to Zeebrugge
**Taxis** Ipswich Cab Co ☎ (0473) 255555
**Car hire** Budget Rent-a-Car, 151 St Helen's Street, Ipswich ☎ (0473) 216149
**Bicycle hire** The Bicycle Doctor, 18 Bartholomew Street, Ipswich ☎ (0473) 259833

*Further information* from Tourist Office, Town Hall, Princes Street, Ipswich.

# Harwich — Shotley Point Marina

| | |
|---|---|
| **Harbourmaster** ☎ (0473) 788982 | **VHF Channels** 80, M |
| **Callsign** Shotley Point Marina | **Daily charge** £££ |

Shotley Point is the first marina you come to on entering the Orwell and is the most suitable if you are arriving late or wish to depart early. It is self-contained with all facilities on-site and the small village of Shotley Street just down the road. Ipswich is only nine miles away and Harwich and Felixstowe (for the continental ferries) can be reached by river ferry from the marina. The Shotley Peninsula is renowned for its natural beauty.

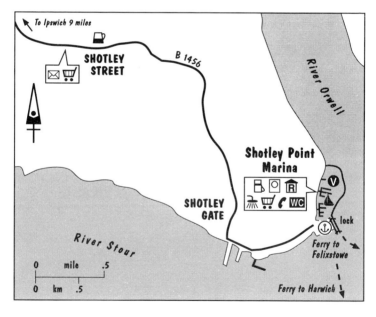

## STEP ASHORE

**Nearest payphone** Beside the marina control tower
**Toilets, showers, baths** In marina; always open
**Launderette** In the marina, open 0600–2200
**Clubhouse** Shotley Point Marina Yacht Club

**Shopping** The Admiral's Larder in the marina sells food and is also an off-licence; in Shotley, a quarter of a mile away, there are village shops and a post office
**Food and drink** The Flagship bar and restaurant in the Yacht Club

### SHIPS' SERVICES

*Water and electricity* At all berths
*Fuel* (diesel only), *gas* (Camping and Calor) Available 24 hours a day in marina

*Chandler, boatyard, engineer* Available 0900–1700 in marina
*Sailmaker* In marina 0800–1800

### TRANSPORT AND TRAVEL

**Buses** From Shotley to Ipswich

**River ferry** To Harwich and Felixstowe

# Woolverstone Marina

| **Harbourmaster** ☎ (0473) 780354 | **VHF Channels** 80, M |
|---|---|
| **Callsign** Woolverstone Marina | **Daily charge** £££ |

Woolverstone is a well-run marina with friendly and helpful staff who keep it tidy and clean; the security is good and surroundings very pleasant. For a short visit, most essentials are near at hand, but for a longer visit it would be a good idea to get to grips with the local bus service or a taxi firm. The Cat House, an old house by the entrance to the marina, is the subject of a legend that a china cat used to be put in the window to warn smugglers that the 'preventive men' were about.

## STEP ASHORE

**Nearest payphone** In the blue box opposite the pier
**Toilets, showers, launderette** In main block under flag, open 24 hours a day
**Clubhouse** Royal Harwich Yacht Club by the marina gate welcomes visitors
**Shopping** The Pantry in the marina is a store and off-licence; there are village shops at Chelmondiston, two miles from the marina

### SHIPS' SERVICES

*Water* On pontoons
*Electricity* By arrangement
*Fuel* (diesel and petrol) From the barge at the end of the pier

*Gas* (Camping and Calor) *chandler, boatyard, engineer, sailmaker* Hipperson Marine Services, on-site: very well stocked chandlery; boat and rigging repairs to a high standard

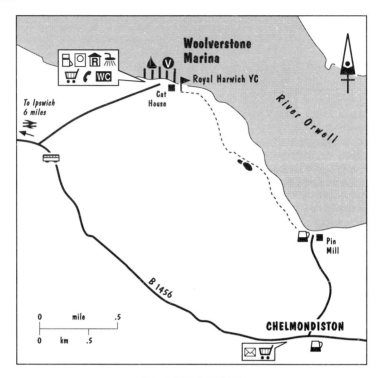

## SHORE LEAVE

### Food and drink

The Schooner in the marina has a bar and serves reasonably priced snacks and meals. The Butt and Oyster pub at Pin Mill, a mile to the south-east by water, a mile-and-a-half by pleasant riverside walk, or three-and-a-half miles by road, serves food and is deservedly famous. The Boot pub is about a mile to the west.

### What to see

The Orwell is a pretty river and the surroundings are very pleasant. The best walk is the one-and-a-half miles to **Pin Mill** under old oaks and past sandy arable fields. But often there are muddy patches, so wellies are advisable. The path is well looked after but poorly signposted.

### TRANSPORT AND TRAVEL

**Buses** From Shotley to Ipswich
**Taxis** ☎ (0473) 252222

**Car hire** Willhire ☎ (0473) 213344

# Fox's Marina

| | |
|---|---|
| **Harbourmaster** ☎ (0473) 689111 | **VHF Channels** 80, M |
| **Callsign** Fox's Marina | **Daily charge** ££ |

The marina is well run and the staff are friendly and very helpful. Security is low key and apparently not a problem. The site is sheltered and, although close to the commercial port, reasonably quiet. The main drawback is that the marina is not within easy walking distance of Ipswich town centre.

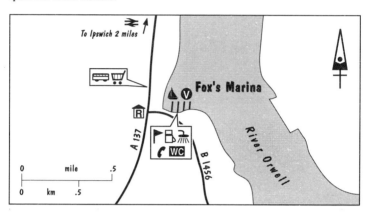

## STEP ASHORE

**Nearest payphone** Near marina office
**Toilets and showers** At marina; always open
**Launderette** One mile away, towards Ipswich
**Clubhouse** Fox's Marina Yacht Club welcomes visitors

**Shopping** Doubles' General Store on the main road outside the marina is the nearest shop; Ipswich is two miles away
**Food and drink** The Ostrich Inn and restaurant is opposite the marina gate

## SHIPS' SERVICES

*Water and electricity* On pontoons
*Fuel* (diesel only), *gas* (Camping and Calor) On-site

*Chandler, boatyard, engineer, sailmaker* All these on-site or ask at office

## TRANSPORT AND TRAVEL

**Buses** To Ipswich from outside the marina

**Taxis** Ipswich Cab Co ☎ (0473) 255555

# River Deben – Woodbridge

The River Deben is beautiful but slightly marred by the profusion of moorings. Woodbridge, nine miles from the mouth of the Deben, is a very pleasant, compact town with comprehensive shopping facilities. It has many ancient buildings, some half-timbered and some in the distinctive East Anglian style borrowed from the Netherlands just across the North Sea. Woodbridge has been a centre for building sea-going vessels since early in the seventeenth century.

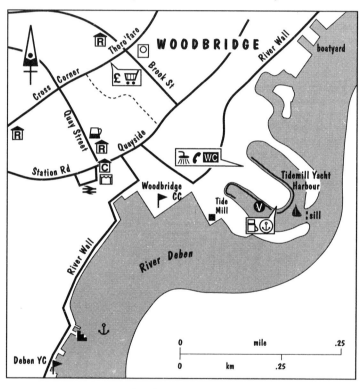

SHORE LEAVE

### Food and drink

Starting with The Anchor, there are pubs galore. Very good meals can be had from The Captain's Table, Quay Street, the Georgian House Restaurant, Thoro'fare, the Golden Panda, Cumberland Street, The Bull Hotel, The Square and most of the pubs, including The Horse and Groom at Melton. Seckford Hall, just outside Woodbridge, is very good but expensive. All are recommended. Royal Bengal is a good-quality 'curry house' Indian restaurant at 4–6 Quay Street; the Wine Bar, 17 Thoro'fare, is atmospheric and serves imaginative meals offering exceptional value for money. Both are featured in *Out to Eat* and *The Good Food Guide 1992*.

*Entertainment*
The Riverside Theatre, by the railway station, has a cinema and theatre.

*What to see*
**Woodbridge Tide Mill** overlooking the yacht harbour is the outstanding feature of the town. Built in 1790, it is the only surviving tide mill in the country and has been superbly restored. Across the river is the **Sutton Hoo** ship burial site. It is well worth a visit, though the original treasures are now in the British Museum; replicas are in Ipswich Museum.

*Excursions*
**Framlingham Castle** is 12 miles to the north. Built in the twelfth century, it is one of the finest examples of a curtain-walled castle. The ornate Tudor chimney pots on each tower are a whimsical addition, the more so because many of them are dummies. Inside is a pleasing range of buildings of all periods, including an eighteenth-century poorhouse, and a museum of local bygones. There are excellent views from the walls over Framlingham Mere and the town. There is also a vineyard at Framlingham which can be visited. **Saxtead Green Post Mill**, which is not far away, is in perfect working order and also worth a visit.

*Exercise*
Very pleasant walks on the river banks run both up and down river. There is a swimming pool near the railway station.

## TRANSPORT AND TRAVEL

**Buses** From town car-park, two minutes' walk from the yacht harbour, to Ipswich
**Trains** From station beside Yacht Harbour – railcar to Ipswich for main lines

**Taxis** M & R Taxis ☎ (03943) 6661/6191
**Car hire** Smithfields, Melton Road ☎ (0394) 380398

# Tidemill Yacht Harbour

| | |
|---|---|
| **Harbourmaster** ☎ (0394) 385745 | **VHF Channel** 80 |
| **Callsign** Tidemill Yacht Harbour | **Daily charge** £££ |

The yacht harbour is clean and well-maintained, secure and close to the shops, and is under constant improvement. There are holding moorings to use while waiting to go over the sill.

## STEP ASHORE

**Nearest payphone** In Yacht Harbour office and at the railway station
**Toilets, showers** In Yacht Harbour
**Clubhouses** Deben Yacht Club and Woodbridge Cruising Club

**Shopping** The main shops are five minutes' walk from the Yacht Harbour and are excellent; there is the usual selection of banks, building societies and a post office. Early closing Wednesdays

## SHIPS' SERVICES

**Water and electricity** On pontoons
**Fuel** (diesel and petrol), **gas** (Camping
and Calor) In Yacht Harbour
**Chandler** At boatyard

**Boatyard, engineer** In Yacht Harbour
**Sailmakers** M & B Covers, for dodgers
and so on, in Yacht Harbour; Suffolk Sails
in Quayside Buildings, just outside
Yacht Harbour

---

**Alternative moorings**

The Deben has several anchorages in the lower reaches, where you can lie afloat. They are far from the few quays and the shoreline is only accessible at high water. You should be warned that the dinghies which race in these waters positively refuse to give way and can be a serious hazard to larger yachts, which are forced to take all way off in the narrow fairways and strong tides.

The harbourmaster at **Ramsholt** is an old river-hand and is most helpful. He is there at weekends and most weekdays. There is only the quay and hard, and the Ramsholt Arms, a first-class pub with really excellent local beer and very good meals. There is no public transport.

**Brown's Boatyard** at **Waldringfield** is good and helpful and can usually find you a mooring. Otherwise, anchor at the end of the moorings, clear of the fairway. Brown's Boatyard can provide diesel, petrol, Camping and Calor gas and chandlery. The well-stocked village store opens long hours and on Sundays; there is also a post office, a public phone and a bus service to Woodbridge. The Maybush Inn at the water's edge does good food.

# Aldeburgh

Aldeburgh is a quiet, unspoilt resort with a long, steeply shelving beach. Many years ago it was a thriving port centred around the fine Tudor Moot Hall — the hall still stands as a museum and council offices, but because of coastal erosion it is now nearly on the beach, along with the old cottages and houses which line the High Street. Fishermen still ply the waters along the Aldeburgh shoreline and sell their daily catches direct to the public from their huts on the beach.

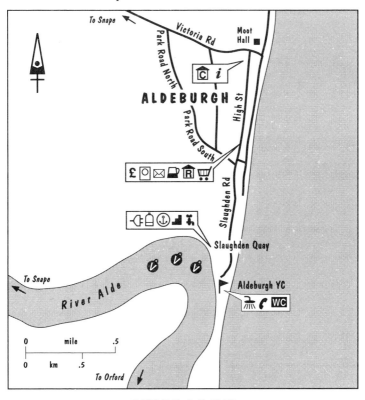

SHORE LEAVE

### Food and drink

There are several pubs: the Cross Keys is recommended for its food. Fish and chips in Aldeburgh are exceptionally good. The Aldeburgh Fish and Chip Shop, 226 High Street, is in both *Out to Eat* and *The Good Food Guide 1992*. Both books also feature Regatta, 171–3 High Street, a bustling wine bar. *The Good Food Guide 1992* adds Austins, 243 High Street, a hotel with restaurant.

### Entertainment

The cinema is excellent. **Snape Maltings Concert Hall** is nearby and well worth a visit.

*What to see*

The museum in **Moot Hall**, Sea Front, gives a history of the town and its maritime affairs through prints, paintings, photographs, and relics from Anglo-Saxon ship burials. The sixteenth-century timbered hall is interesting in its own right. The Aldeburgh Music Festival is held at nearby Snape every June, but cultural offerings aren't confined to music — the town is a great draw for art enthusiasts who visit the galleries and shops in the High Street. There is wonderful estuary birdlife to enjoy and not far away is **Minsmore Bird Sanctuary**. Seals are often to be seen at the mouth of the Alde.

*Excursions*

Aldeburgh is an excellent base for exploring east Suffolk, with Constable country to the south and beautiful coast to the north up to Dunwich. **Dunwich** was once a Saxon cathedral city and the capital of East Anglia, but the city disappeared into the North Sea because of erosion of the cliffs on which it stood. The story of its disappearance is vividly displayed in Dunwich museum with pictures and maps showing the ever-decreasing size of the town.

*Exercise*

A good sea walk takes you south towards **Orford Ness**. You can also walk along the riverbank to **Snape**. The numerous opportunities for walking include the **Suffolk Coast Path**, which runs for 50 miles from Lowestoft to Felixstowe. The *Holiday Which? Good Walks Guide* walk 120 describes a route north to Thorpeness. Aldeburgh has a good, uncrowded, shingle beach. There is a leisure centre at **Leiston**, and a swimming pool at **Thorpeness**. Both towns are three miles from Aldeburgh and interesting places to visit.

### TRANSPORT AND TRAVEL

**Buses** To Thorpeness, Leiston and Saxmundham

**Trains** Nearest railway station is at Saxmundham, six miles away

**Planes** From Norwich airport, 35 miles away

**Ferries** From Felixstowe, 15 miles away

**Taxis** Crisp Taxis ☎ (0728) 830509

**Car and bicycle hire** Ask at the Tourist Office

*Further information* from Tourist Office in the cinema, High Street.

# Slaughden Quay

**Harbourmaster** ☎ (0728) 453047                    **Daily charge** £

Aldeburgh is a famous and popular sailing centre and the river up to Snape from here is excellent for sailing on the tide and for windsurfing. Yachts must approach it along a 10-mile reach of the Rivers Ore and Alde; the entrance into the Ore from the sea is not easy, except at high water, because of shifting bars. Pick up a swinging mooring in the river and contact the harbourmaster.

## STEP ASHORE

**Nearest payphone** At Aldeburgh Yacht Club
**Toilets, showers** Aldeburgh Yacht Club; public WC on Slaughden Quay
**Clubhouses** Aldeburgh Yacht Club and Slaughden Sailing Club are open at weekends

**Shopping** The nearest shops are in Aldeburgh, half a mile from the moorings. Aldeburgh is a tourist centre and has a comprehensive shopping area with the usual banks, building societies and a post office. Early closing is on Wednesdays

### SHIPS' SERVICES

*Water* At Aldeburgh Yacht Club, Slaughden Sailing Club and Slaughden Quay
*Fuel* (diesel and petrol), *gas* (Camping and Calor) from **chandler** Aldeburgh Chandlers (Peter Wilson) at Slaughden Quay
**Boatyard, engineer** Russell Upson on quay
**Sailmaker** See chandler

# Orford Quay

Orford is four miles downstream from Slaughden Quay. Three hundred years ago large ships were built here, but it is now a sleepy anchorage. Facilities ashore are virtually non-existent, but stop for a peaceful night tucked in behind the long sandspit and protected from the sea.

## STEP ASHORE

**Nearest payphone** In the car-park behind the quay
**Toilets** In the car-park behind the quay

**Shopping** Village shops and a post office at Orford, half a mile up the lane from the quay

## SHORE LEAVE

Visit **Orford Castle**, built by Henry II in the twelfth century for coastal defence. There are lovely views across the River Alde to Orford Ness from its fine, 90-foot-high Norman keep. Inside there is an exhibition describing the ever-changing Suffolk coastline, which will interest navigators of these treacherous shores.

The Old Warehouse restaurant and the Jolly Sailor pub are just behind the quay. In Orford itself is the Butley Oysterage famous for seafood either in the restaurant or to take away. It is recommended in both *The Good Food Guide 1992* and *Out to Eat*, which also include the King's Head for its fish and its puddings.

# Southwold

Southwold itself is nearly a mile from the moorings, across the marshy flats. It is an attractive East Anglian town with an ancient history and many old houses showing the Dutch and Flemish influence on the region. The Elizabethan house in the High Street, where the Duke of York had his headquarters during the battle of Sole Bay in 1672, can still be seen, with its Jacobean plaster ceilings intact. Southwold is also a popular seaside resort, complete with pier and entertainments.

On the other side of the harbour, reached by ferry or the old railway bridge, is Walberswick – a charming small town popular with artists.

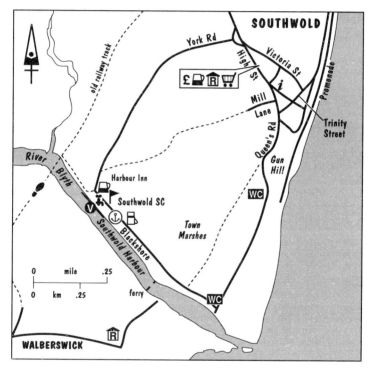

## SHORE LEAVE

***Food and drink***

There is a pub on the quayside, the Harbour Inn, and many pubs and restaurants in town; the Dutch Barn Restaurant in Ferry Road is recommended. The Crown, 90 High Street, is recommended for serving excellent food in the bar as well as the restaurant in both *Out to Eat* and *The Good Food Guide 1992*. *Out to Eat* also includes Squiers, 71 High Street, as a good place for breakfasts, light lunches and cream teas, while *The Good Food Guide 1992* adds the Swan, Market Place, which is a sister establishment to the Crown.

### What to see
The sixteenth-century painted screen in St Edmund's church (1460) is one of the finest in England. **Southwold Museum** has reminders of the old Southwold Railway and there is an **RNLI museum**.

### Exercise
Southwold is surrounded by a designated area of Great Natural Beauty, with sand and salt marshes backed by large ares of woodland – a paradise for the walker and birdwatcher. Take the ferry to Walberswick and walk back through the marshes and over the old railway bridge. The *Holiday Which? Town and Country Walks Guide* walk 104 describes this area in detail.

## TRANSPORT AND TRAVEL

**Buses** To Halesworth and Lowestoft
**Trains** From Halesworth
**Planes** From Norwich
**Ferries** From Felixstowe
**Taxis** ☎ (0502)724104

**Car hire** Bettahire Ltd, 18 Victoria Street ☎ (0502) 723331
**Bicycle hire** 2 Blyth Road, at Southwold end of the old railway track

**Further information** from Tourist Office, Town Hall, Market Place.

# Southwold Harbour

| | |
|---|---|
| **Harbourmaster** ☎ (0502) 724712 | **VHF Channels** 16, 12 |
| **Callsign** Southwold Harbour Radio | **Daily charge** £££ |

If you are intrepid enough to put into the Blyth you will find a narrow river lined with small craft of all kinds on a variety of pontoons and stagings. The visitors' moorings are about half a mile inland at the far end of the harbour near the lifeboat house.

## STEP ASHORE

**Nearest payphone** At chandlery on quay
**Toilets** In car-park at river mouth
**Clubhouse** Southwold Sailing Club, near the moorings welcomes visitors
**Shopping** The nearest shops are one mile away in Southwold: usual range of high-street shops, a bank and a post office. Early closing Wednesdays, though some shops stay open. Markets are held on Mondays and Thursdays

### SHIPS' SERVICES

**Water** On quay
**Fuel** (diesel and petrol) From chandler on quay

**Gas** Camping Gaz from Mumford, 66 High Street
**Chandler** On quay

# Lowestoft

Lowestoft is a typical British seaside resort, but not over-commercialised. It is nothing to get excited about, but is well situated for exploring Suffolk villages and countryside and it has very good beaches. It is an entry point to the Norfolk Broads, though the formalities and cost imposed by the Port Authority will deter all but the most determined skipper. It is far better to go via Great Yarmouth if you want to sail on the Broads.

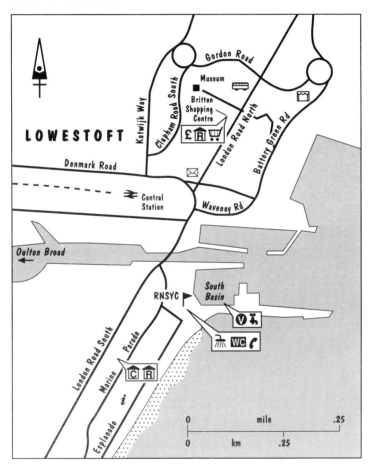

SHORE LEAVE

### Food and drink

There are pubs and restaurants of all sorts. Mr Leung's Chinese Restaurant is recommended.

*Entertainment*
The Hollywood Cinema is in London Road, a theatre in Battery Green Road.

*What to see*
The **Maritime Museum** is in a converted fisherman's cottage in Sparrows Nest Gardens below the lighthouse – it tells the story of the Lowestoft fishing fleet. **Lowestoft Museum**, Broad House, Oulton Broad, has collections of porcelain, archaeology, costume and local history.

*Excursions*
**Somerleyton Hall**, five miles away, is a stately home with state rooms, gardens, maze, miniature railway and deer park – great for a day out with children.

*Exercise*
Many walks lead through lovely Suffolk villages and along the coast; get details from the tourist office. Swim or windsurf from the excellent beach, or swim indoors at the Waveney Leisure Centre.

### TRANSPORT AND TRAVEL

**Buses** From High Street to Beccles
**Trains** The station is four minutes' walk from the harbour; trains to Norwich and Ipswich
**Planes** From Norwich

**Ferries** From Great Yarmouth
**Taxis** Lowestoft Cab Co ☎ (0502) 572690
**Car hire** John Grose (Ford Rent-a-Car) ☎ (0502) 565659

*Further information* from Tourist Office, The Esplanade, South Beach.

# Lowestoft Harbour

| | |
|---|---|
| **Harbourmaster** ☎ (0502) 572286 | **VHF Channel** 14 (no VHF to Club) |
| **Yacht Club** ☎ (0502) 566264 | |
| **Callsign** Lowestoft Harbour Radio | **Daily charge** ££ |

Visitors are accommodated on moorings in the South Basin. Contact the bosun of the Royal Norfolk and Suffolk Yacht Club for a berth. The South Basin is very convenient for the town, the clubhouse is at the landward end.

### STEP ASHORE

**Nearest payphone, toilets, showers** In the clubhouse
**Clubhouse** Royal Norfolk and Suffolk Yacht Club

**Shopping** Over the bridge from the yacht club is a full selection of shops, banks, building societies and a post office

### SHIPS' SERVICES

*Water* On quayside
*Fuel* Ask at Yacht Club
*Gas* (Camping and Calor) From Combined Gas Services, Norwich Road ☎ (0502) 513052
*Chandler* At Oulton Broad

*Boatyard* At Oulton Broad
*Engineer* M J Slack Yachts, Commercial Road ☎ (0502) 569332
*Sailmaker* Jeckells & Son Ltd, Battery Green Road

# Great Yarmouth

Having made your way up the two-mile-long channel among the commercial dock and shipping serving the fishing and North Sea gas industries, and past all the 'no mooring' signs, you may wonder why Great Yarmouth is included in this guide. The reason is that it is far easier to enter the Broads from here than from Lowestoft because the bridges open more frequently and the charges levied are much lower. Unless you have a good reason for stopping, it would be better to go on into the Broads where there are proper facilities for yachts. In spite of all this, quite a number of foreign yachts visit Great Yarmouth, and most are satisfied with what they find.

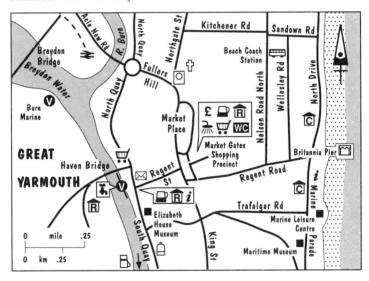

## SHORE LEAVE

### Food and drink

The Star Hotel, Regent Road, Mr T's Restaurant, Southtown Road (over Haven Bridge) – reasonable prices and bar – Allen's Bar and the Ship pub in Hall Plain are all recommended. Mastersons, a fish and chip shop attached to a wet fish shop at 113 Regent Road, is recommended in *Out to Eat*. *The Good Food Guide 1992* features an upmarket fish restaurant, the Seafood Restaurant at 85 North Quay.

### Entertainment

There are three cinemas and a theatre in Marine Parade, and other theatres on Brittania and Wellington Piers.

### What to see

Apart from being an industrial town and a brash seaside resort, Yarmouth has a history stretching back 900 years, with much to interest the visitor. Nelson was a Norfolk man and his monument on South Denes was built many years before that in Trafalgar Square. Anna Sewell, the author of *Black Beauty*, was born in Great Yarmouth. There are eight museums, including the **Maritime Musuem**, the **Tollhouse** and the **Elizabethan House**. Visit the town walls, built in the thirteenth and fourteenth centuries to protect what was one of the wealthiest towns in Britain – they are among the best-preserved in the country. Children will enjoy the **Sealife Centre** and **Marina Pleasure Centre**, both on Marine Parade.

*Excursions*
All of Norfolk and the **Broads** are accessible from here but since it is not a place to leave your boat for long, you would do better to go on into the Broads before setting off ashore.

*Exercise*
Swim from the three miles of golden sand or at the leisure centre on Marine Parade.

### TRANSPORT AND TRAVEL

**Buses** From Wellington Road; comprehensive local service
**Trains** From North Quay to Norwich
**Planes** From Norwich

**Taxis** Star Taxis, 12b Bridge Road (over Haven Bridge) ☎ (0493) 603071
**Car hire** Gapton Car Hire, Morton Peto Road ☎ (0493) 650373

*Further information* from Tourist Office, Marine Parade.

## Great Yarmouth Harbour

| | |
|---|---|
| **Harbourmaster** ☎ (0493) 855151 | **VHF Channels** 12, 16 |
| **Callsign** Port Control | **Daily charge** ££ |

Once the premier herring fishing port in the world, Great Yarmouth is now mainly used by oil-rig supply vessels servicing the rigs in the southern North Sea. The entrance is very busy. Yachts moor to Town Hall Quay just below the Haven Bridge. There are no facilities and the wall can be uncomfortable due to the tidal range and the shortage of ladders. Beware of vandals.

### STEP ASHORE

**Nearest payphone** Across the road from the quay outside the post office
**Toilets, showers** In Market Gates Precinct (go up Regent Street) – close at 2100
**Shopping** Nichols Stores on North Quay is the nearest shop and is open until 2100.

Go up Regent Street to the Market Gates shopping precinct where you will find all shops, banks, building societies and post office. No early closing. Late-night shopping Wednesdays, Thursdays and Fridays

### SHIPS' SERVICES

*Water* On quay
*Fuel* (diesel and petrol) From P Williment, downstream on west bank at Gorleston
*Gas* (Camping and Calor) From J Carter, Long Lane, Bradwell

*Chandler* Yarmouth Stores, Friars Lane, off South Quay
*Boatyard, engineer* Bure Marine, on west bank, through Haven Bridge
*Sailmaker* Kirklands, 16 Southgates Road ☎ (0493) 843060

# SOUTHERN HOLLAND
## and
# BELGIUM

# Veere

Veere is a small but colourful town in the Veerse Meer, on the north-east coast of the former Island of Walcheren. Veere was a fishing village when the estuary was open to the sea; it was also a flourishing port in the sixteenth and seventeenth centuries, enjoying considerable trade links with Scotland, until the outlet to the sea silted up and put an end to the entry of deep-draught, sea-going craft. When the dam was built in 1961 the fishing fleet sailed away with sad ceremony – bands played, flags were at half mast, and there were lumps in every throat. 'The heart left the town,' said one old lady. Now Veere is a tourist trap, and a delightful little one. Coachloads of visitors come for a few hours.

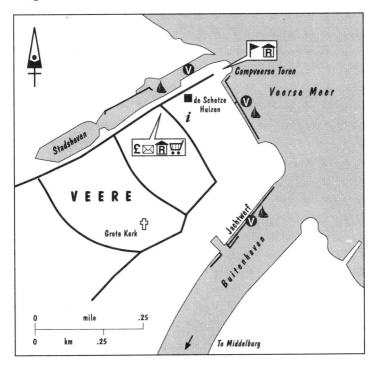

SHORE LEAVE

### Food and drink
On the quay there are two restaurants, a hotel and a van selling food, including the special Dutch herrings called *hollandse nieuwe haring*. The Campveerse Toren, the imposing former look-out tower on the waterfront, has a restaurant which is recommended, as is Waepen van Veere, Markt 23.

## What to see

By modern standards Veere is little more than a big village and any energetic person can see the whole place in an hour. Two magnificent waterfront houses, both built in 1561, are still called **de Schotse Huizen** (the Scotch Houses) from the days of Veere's trading connections with Scotland. They now contain attractive folklore and fishing museums. Another fine building is the fifteenth-century **Stadhuis** (Town Hall) where statues adorn the façade – it has a famous carillon of bells. The **Grote Kerk**, a vast, domed church, where Napoleon once stabled his horses, is now a museum where concerts, lectures and exhibitions are held regularly. The view from the church tower is excellent. Veere is very popular with artists – their work can be seen in the many galleries around the town.

## Excursions

A large excursion ship, the *Madeleine*, offers day trips round the **Veerse Meer**.

## Exercise

Every sort of water sport is catered for nearby, including windsurfing – sailboards can be hired. There is a leisure centre at Kamperland, a mile away. Swimming in the Veerse Meer is enjoyable, with several good beaches and warm water. Gliding and flying are on offer at Arnemuiden airport.

### TRANSPORT AND TRAVEL

**Trains** From Middelburg (which has a good train service), a four-mile taxi ride away

**Planes** From Arnemuiden, near Middelburg, to Amsterdam-Schipol

**Ferries** From Vlissingen to Sheerness

**Taxis** Telephone numbers are posted in telephone kiosks

**Car and bicycle hire** Enquire at tourist office

*Further information* from tourist office, VVV-Veere, Oudestraat 28.

# Veere Harbour

| Harbourmaster ☎ 01181-246 | VHF Channel 10 (same for whole of Veerse Meer) |
|---|---|
| Callsign Veere | Daily charge £ |

Veere's old harbour, Stadshaven, is very small and gets very full in the high season – you should not leave a yacht unattended for more than a few hours. The marina in the Walcheren canal, at the back of the town, caters only for small craft.

Just outside the harbour you can tie up to the quay, or anchor off if the quay is crowded, for an hour or two without charge while you do any necessary shopping.

### STEP ASHORE

**Nearest payphone** On the quayside in Stadshaven (the old harbour)
**Toilets, showers** In the club on the quay
**Clubhouse** W V De Arne Yachtclub, on quay

**Shopping** Shops near the quay as well as a selection of high-street shops in the town; these include antique and gift shops and a good small supermarket. Banks, a bureau de change and a post office are on the quay

## SHIPS' SERVICES

**Water** On quay
**Fuel, gas** Not available on the quay but can be obtained from other marinas on the Veerse Meer
**Chandler** On quay

**Boatyard, engineer** Jachtwerf Oostwatering, Polredijk 138, 4351 RT Veere, a marina one-and-a-half miles to the west
**Sailmaker** Scaldis Sails ☎ 01181-1775

# Veerse Meer

This 5,000 acre lake was created by two dams – the Veersegatdam in the west and the Zandkreekdam in the east – as part of the Delta plan to close off estuaries that had been the cause of disastrous flooding.

The Veerse Meer is over seven miles long and has several excellent marinas on both the north and the south shores. It winds round a series of natural and man-made islands, some with mooring facilities, some restricted to wildlife. There are pontoons and recommended anchoring places on the edges of the islands but many shallow to three feet or less. At various islands staging has been placed with barbecue sites and dustbins. It is possible to tie up securely for the night at these, with perhaps only another yacht or two for company, and it costs nothing.

This is a wonderful sailing area and offers unrivalled facilities for every water sport. Barges and deep-draught craft use the buoyed channel but there are acres of tideless shallow water for others, sympathetically administered so that sailors, waterskiers, fishermen, sailboarders and birdwatchers can co-exist. Good walking is to be had around the Veerse Meer, too.

# Middelburg

Half-way down the Veere–Vlissingen Canal, Middelburg is in the middle of Walcheren, which was once an island in the North Sea, but is now joined to the other five islands of the province of Zeeland by roads, bridges and reclaimed land. Middelburg is the capital of Zeeland and an important market town for the surrounding rural area. The narrow streets and old houses lie in an unusual pattern of roughly concentric circles inside a star-shaped moat called the Vest.

The town is full of character, with such a wealth of wonderful buildings that it is a feast for the eye of a photographer or artist. In former times the sea came to its doors, so old quaysides and grand merchants' houses now sit in the middle of an inland city. There is much, both ancient and modern, to explore. It is an excellent place for a crew change, because transport is so good, and also for exploring further afield, as yachts may be left safely in the basin inside the bridge, under the harbourmaster's care.

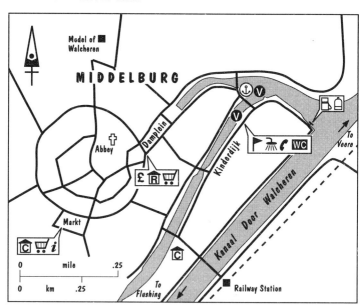

SHORE LEAVE

### Food and drink

There are plenty of places of every sort to eat and drink. De Ploeg in the Markt is recommended for good, inexpensive food.

### Entertainment

Middelburg has cinemas and theatres. The Lang Jan, the high tower dominating the town, is part of the **Nieuwkerk**, the church in the Groenmarkt where organ recitals and concerts are held.

## What to see

The **abbey** is adjacent to the Nieuwkerk, with the **Zeeland Museum** in its north-west wing. As well as displays of both natural and local history, there is a video film of the history of Walcheren, including the Second World War and the 1953 floods. The fifteenth-century **Stadhuis** (Town Hall), overlooking the Markt Square, was razed during the war but has been rebuilt as it was originally. As with many old buildings, the stones were preserved and used in rebuilding, and in this case the 25 original statues on the façade were, too. **Miniature Walcheren** is a scale model of the island, with 200 buildings, covering half an acre; having seen this you will be enticed to explore further afield.

## Excursions

A bus-ride away there are Roman remains at **Domburg**. Moored in the main canal is the iron-clad ship, the Ramschip *Scorpion* built in about 1875. **Arnemuiden**, four miles to the east, has preserved something of its ancient costume. The particular feature of the Zeeland women's costumes is the *beuk* (square chest-covering) and the different forms of cap – every village has its own.

## Exercise

Cycling is one of the best ways of both getting around and enjoying some exercise. A walk round the moat is pleasant, with gardens, some old walls and interesting gates to look at.

### TRANSPORT AND TRAVEL

**Buses** To Vlissingen frequently
**Trains** From the railway station on the east side of the Walcheren canal, one-and-a-half miles from the yacht harbour, go to Vlissingen – it is a 20-minute train ride to the ferry terminal – and to Amsterdam

**Planes** From Arnemuiden to Amsterdam-Schipol
**Taxis** ☎ 01189-1995
**Car and bicycle hire** From the chandler, Nautic Ring, by the yacht club

**Further information** from tourist office, VVV, Markt 65a, on the west corner of the square.

# Middelburg Harbour

**Harbourmaster** ☎ 01180-27180               **Daily charge** £

Middelburg is easily reached from Veere: the canal has only one lock between the two towns. There is a marina in the inner harbour and moorings in the canal and in the arm leading to the harbourmaster's office. Anyone arriving should find a berth easily; otherwise the harbourmaster will arrange for you to go on into the marina or small basin, where yachts may be left safely, when the bridges are opened.

## STEP ASHORE

**Nearest payphone** In the yacht club
**Toilets, showers, launderette** All at the yacht club
**Clubhouse** Yacht Club W V De Arne on the Kinderdijk, open 1000–1200, 1500–1800 and 2000–2359
**Shopping** The yacht harbour is close to the centre of Middelburg and every facility is within a five or ten-minute walk, including a full selection of high-street shops, banks with outside cash dispensers, a post office and a bureau de change. Some food shops stay open late. Market every Thursday, where many of the stallholders wear traditional local costume

### SHIPS' SERVICES

*Water and electricity* On pontoons
*Fuel* (diesel and petrol), *gas* (Camping and Calor) Available at the fuel barge/chandler Winkelship Helena Maria Jos Boone
*Chandler* The Winkelship is excellent; also Nautic Ring, Kinderdijk, by the yacht club
*Boatyard, engineer, diver, sailmaker* Available via the harbourmaster

# Vlissingen

Vlissingen is a small town but an important commercial port on the north side of the entrance to the Westerschelde. Although often bypassed by yachtsmen on their way to more historic places, it is well worth taking a little time to get to know: perhaps spend a day in the town and a day exploring the wild dune and forest areas by bicycle.

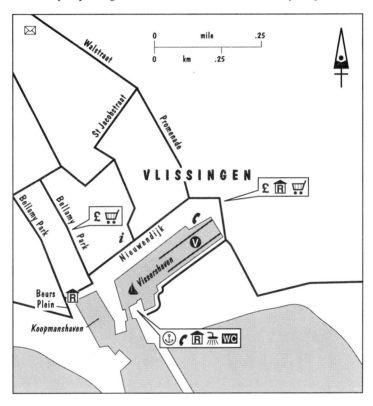

SHORE LEAVE

### Food and drink
There are many good pubs and restaurants in the nearby town centre, ranging from Italian to Indonesian food and including some theme bars. The harbourmaster will advise, after first trying to persuade you to eat in his own café-bar.

### Entertainment
There is a cinema, the Alhambra, on the corner of Spuistraat and Coosje Buskenstraat. The Nestzak theatre is at 5 Bellamy Park.

### What to see
Vlissingen is not a typical old Dutch town, as it was rebuilt following war-time destruction. There are, however, a few old buildings, many statues and enough

atmosphere to give some flavour of Holland to those unable to travel further. The **Stedelijk Museum** in Bellamy Park is the municipal museum; it highlights Vlissingen's maritime past with paintings, model ships and archaeological finds, and contains memorabilia of the famous naval hero Admiral de Ruyter. The **Zeeuws Planetarium**, at Boulevard Evertsen 4, runs five performances each day.

The **Westerschelde** is probably the third busiest waterway in Europe and contains every conceivable form of shipping – it is fun to watch the big ships come and go and to speculate on their cargoes and destinations.

*Excursions*

Unless you are going on to **Middelburg** or **Veere** by boat (check that your insurance is valid for Dutch inland waters) it is well worth visiting these delightful old towns by bicycle or by bus (Line 57 or 58).

*Exercise*

There is an exercise track (free of charge) in the Westduin area, by Van Wolderenlaan. The beaches are also free. During the summer swimming is superintended – watch for safety flags. The town bathing beach is safe for swimming. At Nollebeach, closer to the dunes, the swimming is safe but without the refinements of changing rooms. The views from the dunes over the sea and over the countryside of Walcheren are typical of so much of Holland: a low-lying coastline broken only by the occasional lighthouse and equally flat hinterland with church spires showing where the towns are. Windsurfing is possible, and permitted, in limited areas, but justifiably forbidden in many places due to strong streams and heavy shipping. The Boulevard de Ruyter and the Boulevard Bankert lead north-west to a beautiful beach. The swimming pool at Baskenburgplein has modern indoor and outdoor baths with every facility. There are several cycling routes from Vlissingen – ask at the tourist information office for advice.

## TRANSPORT AND TRAVEL

**Buses** Three bus lines run from the town centre, all go to Middelburg; buses run every 30 minutes from the yacht harbour to the railway station and to Middelburg

**Trains** The station is one mile north-east of the yacht harbour – Bus 56 to Roosendaal takes you there. Trains run to Middelburg and to Amsterdam

**Planes** From Arnemuiden, near Middelburg, to Amsterdam-Schipol

**Ferries** From the Buitenhaven near the railway station, one-and-a-half miles from the town centre, to Sheerness

**Taxis** Several firms: telephone numbers are posted in phone boxes

**Car hire** Enquire at the tourist office (VVV), 15 Nieuwendijk

**Bicycle hire** Available from harbourmaster, also from most cycle dealers and the cycle-shed at the railway station

*Further information* from tourist office, VVV, 15 Nieuwendijk, by yacht harbour.

# Vlissingen Marina

**Harbourmaster ☎ 01184-14498**          **Daily charge ££**

The new marina, in the old Visserhaven, is a cheerful, friendly place, much more convenient than the old marina through the locks. It is accessible direct from the sea, through a lifting bridge, and at any state of the tide. The harbourmaster runs the local café-bar and is quite likely to welcome you whilst wearing a chef's hat and apron. It is claimed that every yachting problem can be solved here – you only have to ask. Security is good, but if you are leaving a yacht for any length of time, Middelburg, three miles up the canal, is preferable since it is half the price.

The old yacht marina, through the locks and by the first bridge in the canal, is still in full operation and cheaper, but it is far less convenient for shopping and services although it is better placed for customs and the internal waterways system.

## STEP ASHORE

**Nearest payphone** Downstairs in harbour toilet block (open 24 hours a day)

**Toilets, showers, launderette** Harbour building contains excellent toilets, showers and washing facilities (open 24 hours a day), plus a first-class café-bar and staff who speak good English

**Clubhouse** None as such but the café-bar fulfils this function

**Shopping** No late-night shop but the small family grocery in Nieuwstraat will be helpful in an emergency – the owner lives over the shop. The main shops are 100 yards from the yacht harbour entrance.

Many shops are closed on Monday mornings and most close by 1800 every day, except some larger shops which stay open until 2100 on Fridays. There are banks with cash dispensers, some of which accept international cards, bureaux de change (the one open the longest hours and with the best rates is at the bank in the railway station) and a post office. Market on Fridays in Lange Zelke and on Spuistraat; market for fruit, fish and other local produce on Spuistraat on Saturdays

### SHIPS' SERVICES

*Water and electricity* On yacht harbour pontoons

*Fuel* Diesel only, available in the yacht harbour

*Gas, chandler, boatyard, engineer, diver, sailmaker* Available from 'big ship' firms

*in the dockyard area or from private individuals working from home. In all cases it is advisable to approach the harbourmaster and ask him to arrange whatever it is you need*

# Breskens

If the tide is wrong for getting into Vlissingen or you need a good start for going westwards, Breskens is very useful for an overnight stay, particularly as you don't have to lock in. The town is not much of a place for its own sake: there is not a lot to do or see. If you are caught here by weather or other circumstances, a visit to ancient Brugge makes an interesting excursion.

## TRANSPORT AND TRAVEL

**Trains** To Brugge
**Ferries** To Vlissingen
**Taxis** Telephone numbers are posted in
phone box
**Car and bicycle hire** Enquire at marina office

## Breskens Marina

**Harbourmaster** ☎ 01172-1902          **Daily charge** ££

Opposite Vlissingen, on the south side of the Westerschelde, Breskens is a port and fishing harbour. The harbour is well sheltered from all winds, although a swell develops if strong north-westerlies combine with high-water spring tides. Yachts are not allowed in the ferry port but there is plenty of room for them in the yacht harbour. It is an old-fashioned harbour, where you tie up fore and aft, but highly organised.

### STEP ASHORE

**Nearest payphone, toilets, showers** In toilet block
**Clubhouse** Modern clubhouse in the south-east corner of the marina with a bar and a restaurant

**Shopping, food and drink** It is a bit of a walk into the town, but it has a selection of high-street shops, banks, a post office and several good restaurants

### SHIPS' SERVICES

*Water and electricity* On pontoons
*Fuel, gas, chandler, boatyard, engineer*
*In marina; visitors report that the best boatbuilder in Holland is here, the*
*sailmaker is very good and the chandler has an exceptionally wide-ranging stock including Dutch charts at low prices; the chandler is a Volvo agent*

# Zeebrugge

The Belgian coast is an all-but-unbroken belt of sand stretching for 40 miles from the Netherlands to the French border. The country behind is mostly polder country – it lies below sea level – to a large extent relying for its protection on the line of reeded sand-dunes between the coast road and the sea and on the large dike which adds to the protection of the main built-up areas.

Zeebrugge is an important commercial port with heavy ferry traffic at the terminals. You will also see the occasional North Sea oil-rig undergoing a refit and several of the oddly-shaped ultra-modern oil-rig support vessels – a source of endless fascination.

The town is of little interest to the tourist, but a small resort area, Zeebrugge Bad, lies beyond the foot of the mole. There would not be much to say in favour of a prolonged stay in Zeebrugge were it not for the proximity of Brugge, only a 15-minute journey by train. It would be a pity not to visit this medieval city while in Zeebrugge.

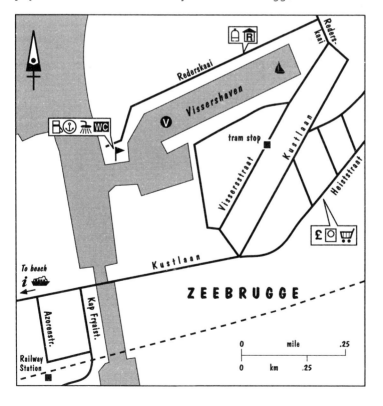

## SHORE LEAVE

*Food and drink*
There are several restaurants near the harbour, about seven of them on the Rederskaai which is only a five-minute walk from the pontoons.

*What to see*
**Zeebrugge Bad** is a small seaside resort and has few attractions apart from good sandy beaches. However, the water is shallow and there can be strong currents, so watch out for the warning flags if you intend to swim. There is windsurfing at Heist and Duinbergen and a swimming pool at Brusselstraat 13 in Zeebrugge Bad.

*Excursions*
Visit **Brugge** by railway or travel to **Oostende** by tram.

### TRANSPORT AND TRAVEL

**Trams** The tram stop is a 15-minute walk from the yacht harbour towards Zeebrugge Bad
**Trains** The railway station is a 30-minute walk towards Zeebrugge Bad
**Ferries** Just beside Zeebrugge Bad, about

45 minutes on foot from the yacht harbour, to Dover, Felixstowe and Hull
**Taxis** Richard ☎ 050/54.42.59
**Car hire** Inseco Rent-a-Car ☎ 050/54.64.59
**Bicycle hire** At the railway station

*Further information* from tourist office, Dienst voor Toerisme, Zeedijk, Zeebrugge Bad, open only during summer.

# Zeebrugge Yacht Harbour

| | |
|---|---|
| **Harbourmaster** ☎ 050/54.32.11 | **VHF Channel** 71 (lock to inner harbour: 13) |
| **Callsign** Zeebrugge Port Control | **Daily charge** ££ |

The yacht harbour is contained within the fishing harbour; it provides excellent shelter and although often crowded, the harbourmaster always finds room for one more. The Royal Belgian Sailing Club, which has authority over the pontoons, welcomes visitors and keeps everything as ship-shape as possible (including security). It is a good harbour to leave your boat if necessary: it is secure, prices are reasonable and travel to England is easy by ferry.

## STEP ASHORE

**Nearest payphone** In the Alberta Clubhouse, open until midnight
**Toilets, showers** Beside clubhouse – they remain open all night during summer
**Launderette** In the main street in the village

**Clubhouse** Alberta Clubhouse, just above the pontoons
**Shopping** At Zeebrugge Village, about 20 minutes' walk away. Shops are open until 1830, 2000 on Fridays; no early closing day

### SHIPS' SERVICES

*Water and electricity* On the pontoons
*Fuel* Diesel is available at the club shed; the nearest petrol station is about 20 minutes' walk

*Gas* Camping Gaz at chandler
*Chandler, boatyard, engineer* Neels Jean Pierre (Marine Technics), Rederskaai 17 ☎ 050/54.60.31

# Blankenberge

Blankenberge is one vast holiday resort, all tower-block apartments, hotels, eating-houses, beefburgers, fizzy drinks and sweaty bodies. It is an experience, but not a beauty spot. The countryside is flat and uninteresting, but there are good beaches. It is thanks to these that Blankenberge has been a seaside resort since 1860 and still rates among the best in Belgium.

Because of tidal characteristics the harbour has changed over the last 20 years from being mainly a fishing port to including an attractive yachting harbour. The entrance to the harbour is protected against silting by a vast breakwater. It is here that the mile-long dike promenade, lined with hotels and villas, begins.

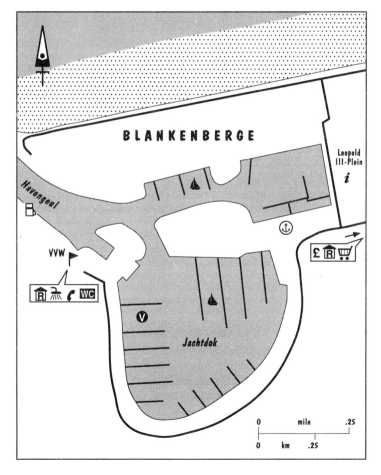

## SHORE LEAVE

### Food and drink

Of the several places to eat nearby, you will do best if you wander two to three hundred yards on from the south-east corner of the fishing harbour. Blankenberge is one mass of eating houses, bars and cake shops!

### Entertainment

There are cinemas, amusement arcades and a casino in the middle of the dike promenade.

### What to see

A large, elegant, wrought-iron windbreak – the **Paravang** – overlooking the harbour offers a sheltered view of the activities. There is a mile-and-a-half, pedestrians-only promenade with many cafés, a British-style pier, a modern aquarium complete with model ships, plus camping sites and full provision for all the usual seaside sports. Steps up to the dike are at the north end of Kerkstraat, the main street. Opposite the station in Kerkstraat is the **Gothic church** of St Antonius, consecrated in 1358.

### Excursions

**Brugge** and **Ghent** are easily accessible by coastal tram to Zeebrugge and then by train. Both are ancient cities with recorded histories going back to the seventh century.

### Exercise

The beaches are crowded, but less so to the west of town; small buoys denote the limit of safe bathing. Windsurfing is popular. The small indoor swimming pool at the sports stadium has a sauna.

## TRANSPORT AND TRAVEL

**Trams** To Zeebrugge or Oostende
**Trains** From Zeebrugge to Oostende
**Planes** From Oostende to Heathrow
**Ferries** From Oostende to Dover, or

Zeebrugge to Dover, Felixstowe and Hull
**Taxis, car and bicycle hire** Enquire at marina office

**Further information** from tourist office at Leopold III-plein.

# Blankenberge Marina

| Harbourmaster ☎ 050/47.75.36 | VHF Channel 8 |
|---|---|
| Callsign Blankenberge | Daily charge ££ |

The old yacht harbour, used by local people, lies at the end of the port arm, but the marina is reached through a narrow passage to starboard after passing the quays of chandlers and engineers. The marina is large and very adequate and the harbourmaster cheerful and helpful. The main advantage of Blankenberge is that berthing is quieter than at Zeebrugge.

## STEP ASHORE

**Nearest payphone** Beside the fishing harbour
**Toilets, showers** Behind the clubhouse
**Clubhouse** VVW (Vlaamse Vereniging voor Watersport) has a bar and restaurant

**Shopping** Lots of late-night shops, and the main shopping centre is close by, with a full selection of shops including banks with outside cash dispensers, a post office and bureaux de change

### SHIPS' SERVICES

**Water and electricity** _On pontoons_
**Fuel** _(diesel and petrol) Available from fuelling pontoon_

**Gas** _(Camping and Calor) Obtainable from_ **chandler** _in marina_
**Boatyard, engineer** _See chandler_

# Oostende

Oostende is the oldest settlement on the Belgian coast; its history goes back to the tenth century. It was from here that the Crusaders sailed to the Holy Land. Originally a village at the east end of the coast stretch called Ter Streep, today it is the most important seaport in Belgium. Oostende acquired the title 'Queen of the Seaside Resorts' because of substantial Royal patronage in the nineteenth century. It has also been a favourite haunt of many artists and writers, including Victor Hugo, Lord Byron and Georges Simenon.

The harbour contains several docks, large and small, and extends about a mile inland, as far as the opening of the Oostende-Brugge Canal.

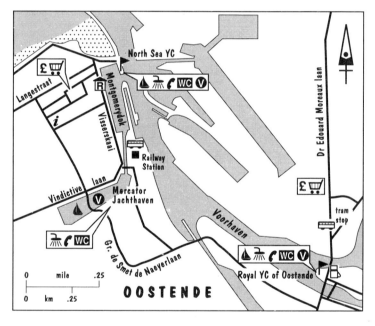

SHORE LEAVE

### Food and drink

Belgium is well known for its good food. In Oostende there are more than 200 restaurants, 50 of which are on Visserskaai; they offer a wide variety of fish and seafood, all bought in the auction held every morning at the fish market. Oostende specialises in gastronomic marathons.

### Entertainment

Oostende offers a great variety of entertainment throughout the year – ask at the tourist office to find out what is going on when you visit. There are lectures, film and slide shows, concerts, theatrical and other performances in the **Kursaal** on the dike.

*What to see*

The twin spires of the **Church of St Peter and Paul** are the first things a yacht's crew sees on the approach to Oostende. A brick tower next to the church is all that remains of its fourteenth-century origins. The **festival hall** in Wapenplein has a belfry over 200 feet high with a 49-bell carillon; it is open to the public in July and August. Inside the festival hall is a **library** and a **museum of fine arts** which includes paintings by English-born James Ensor.

A high and wide sea-dike lines the shore for nine miles as far as Westende. Above the main bridge in the bend of the dike stands the **Kursaal** with a large concert hall, exhibition rooms, a casino and a restaurant. Further west on the dike is the restored **Chalet Royal** built by Leopold II in the early nineteenth century. Two piers, built to protect the entrance to the harbour, extend from the dike – the western pier is a popular promenade with a café.

The three-masted *Mercator*, a former Belgian training ship lying in the Mercator Yacht Harbour, is open to the public. Further east, beyond the Naval docks and Tijdok is the fishing harbour with the fish market on the west side; the morning fish auction is an entertainment in itself.

*Excursions*

Ask at the tourist office about guided visits by coach to **Brugge, Ghent, Brussels** and **Antwerp**, among other places. Regular tram services along the coast stop at all the seaside resorts, north to the Dutch border and south to the French border.

*Exercise*

There is a municipal swimming pool and solarium at Koninginnelaan 1. Swimming and windsurfing are popular from the beaches which border the coast to the east.

### TRANSPORT AND TRAVEL

**Trams** From the railway station to Brugge and Nieuwpoort
**Trains** The railway station, with boat connections to Dover, is on the outer harbour, east of the old commercial port and south of the old town
**Planes** From Oostende airport to Southend and Heathrow
**Ferries** To Dover
**Taxis** Taxi rank at the railway station ☎ 059/70.28.88
**Car Hire** Budget Rent-a-Car, Groentemarkt 22 ☎ 059/50.35.08

*Further information* from tourist office, Wapenplein 3 (in the south-east corner of Wapenplein).

# Royal Yacht Club of Oostende

**Harbourmaster** ☎ 059/70.36.07          **Daily charge** ££

The Royal Yacht Club of Oostende has pontoon moorings at the south-east end of the Voorhaven with good facilities. Finger pontoons make berthing easy. One advantage of the Royal Yacht Club of Oostende marina is the friendly, helpful, English-speaking harbourmaster. More peaceful nights can be guaranteed in this marina than in other Oostende marinas. For those who like to be a little out of town, this is the place.

## STEP ASHORE

**Nearest payphone** Upstairs near the bar in the clubhouse
**Toilets, showers** In the clubhouse
**Clubhouse** Royal Yacht Club of Oostende – an impressive modern building
**Shopping** 10 minutes' walk north-east from the marina is a bank, baker, grocer and a tram stop: five minutes on the tram takes you into the centre of the town to the main shopping area. Most of the shopping streets in the centre of Oostende are pedestrian precincts. Most shops stay open till 1800, 2100 on Fridays. On Thursday mornings markets are held in three squares: Wapenplein, Groentemarkt and Mijnplein. On summer evenings markets selling handicrafts can be found all over Oostende
**Food and drink** The food in the clubhouse is good but there is a better choice in Oostende

### SHIPS' SERVICES

**Water and electricity** On the pontoons
**Fuel** (diesel and petrol), **gas** (Camping and Calor) From the garage in front of the clubhouse
**Chandler** Three minutes' walk over bridge
**Boatyard** There is a boat lift at the club
**Engineer** Ask harbourmaster

# North Sea Yacht Club – Montgomery Dock

| Harbourmaster ☎ 059/70.27.54 | Daily charge £££ |
| --- | --- |

There are tidal berths at the North Sea Yacht Club at the seaward end of the Montgomery Dock but they are liable to disturbance from scend from the harbour channel and the entry and departure of fishing vessels.

# Mercator Yacht Harbour

| Harbourmaster ☎ 059/70.57.62 | VHF Channel 14 |
| --- | --- |
| **Callsign** Mercator Yacht Harbour | Daily charge ££ |

The Mercator Yacht Harbour, in the centre of the town by the central station, is reached through a lock. It has limited facilities but is cheaper and quieter than the Montgomery Dock, so is worth considering if you are staying for more than one night.

# Nieuwpoort

Three miles south of Oostende and two miles from the mouth of Yser River, Nieuwpoort was founded in the twelfth century as a fortified new port for Ypres after the Yser had changed its course. In the First World War it held a key position because of its six locks by which the entire area could be flooded: the sluice-gates were opened, the polder country made impassable and a decisive role played in the defence of Ypres and the Channel ports – a bust in the town commemorates the water-control expert, Geeraert, who directed the flooding.

It is now an important fishing port and a centre for fish-processing, metal and chemical industries as well as tourism. Tourism is concentrated at Nieuwpoort-Bad, which is two miles north of Nieuwpoort-Stad, the town. The attraction of Nieuwpoort-Bad is largely its nearness to the estuary, which makes it a good yachting centre.

Of the two marinas, Vlotkom on the western bank is the smaller; Novus Portus is further up on the eastern bank. Yachts may not tie up in the channel.

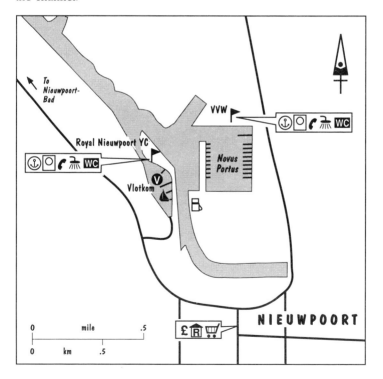

SHORE LEAVE

*Food and drink*
There are six or seven hotels and three restaurants in Nieuwpoort-Bad, but only two restaurants of any note in Nieuwpoort-Stad.

*Entertainment*
Carillon concerts are held on Wednesday and Saturday evenings from July to September; a programme of entertainments is available from the tourist office.

*What to see*
**The Cloth Hall** in Grote Markt, partly preserved from the original built in 1280 and partly rebuilt, is interesting in itself as well as for what is inside. In the lower hall the **ornithological museum** has a collection of sea birds and crustaceans. In the upper hall there is a First World War museum and the **Pieter-Braecke Museum** of sculptures. Behind the Town Hall is the **Church of Our Lady**, destroyed in both wars but each time rebuilt in the original Gothic style. In a separate tower is a carillon of 67 bells. To the north-west of the Grote Markt at 18 Kokstraat is the **municipal museum of ethnography**. There are frequent art exhibitions in the fish market and permanent exhibitions at a number of galleries.

*Exercise*
Walks along the sea wall, good beaches and windsurfing provide plenty of opportunity for exercise. A variety of organised sports is also available.

**TRANSPORT AND TRAVEL**

**Trams** To Oostende, also stop near Oostende airport, and to Zeebrugge
**Trains, planes, ferries** From Oostende

**Taxis** Phone numbers are posted in phone boxes
**Car hire** Ask at tourist office, Marktplein 7

*Further information* from tourist office, Marktplein 7.


# Vlotkom Yacht Harbour

| | |
|---|---|
| **Harbourmaster** ☎ 058/23.33.53 | **VHF Channels** 9, 16 |
| **Callsign** Nieuwpoort | **Daily charge** ££ |

The facilities in this small yacht harbour on the west side of river are excellent and the berthing quiet.

STEP ASHORE

**Nearest payphone** By the inner corner of the yacht basin, or at the club bar
**Toilets, showers** In toilet block, open 0800–2100
**Launderette** In toilet block, open 0900–1600
**Clubhouse** Royal Yacht Club (Koninklijke Yacht Club de Nieuwpoort) is very comfortable and welcoming; it offers

good meals and the steward is helpful and informative. Bonded stores can be ordered from the club bar
**Shopping** Quite a good supermarket 300 yards from the south-west corner of the yacht basin; it is a 15-minute walk to the shops in Nieuwpoort-Stad
**Bicycle hire** From yacht club

### SHIPS' SERVICES

**Water and electricity** On all pontoons
**Fuel** (diesel and petrol) From fuel jetty
up river
**Gas** (Camping and Calor) Obtainable from

**chandler** near yacht harbour
**Boatyard** Two near yacht harbour
**Engineer** Near yacht harbour (Volvo
agent)

# Novus Portus Yacht Harbour

| | |
|---|---|
| **Harbourmaster** ☎ 058/23.52.32 | **VHF Channels** 77 |
| **Callsign** Argus | **Daily charge** ££ |

This marina is one of the largest on the North Sea coast, occupying the outer harbour and Novus Portus yacht harbour itself; it provides quiet berthing and has excellent facilities. Visiting yachts moor in front of the white building in the outer harbour.

### STEP ASHORE

**Nearest payphone** In clubhouse
**Toilets, showers, launderette** In white
pyramid building

**Clubhouse** VVW (Vlaamse Vereniging voor
Watersport) has bars and restaurants

### SHIPS' SERVICES

**Water and electricity** On pontoons
**Fuel** (diesel and petrol) Available in
marina

**Chandler, boatyard, engineer, sailmaker**
All in marina
**Bicycle hire** Free for a shopping trip or
hire for longer; ask harbourmaster

# NORTH-EAST FRANCE

# Dunkerque

From its origins as a small village, Dunkerque grew into a small port in about the tenth century, and was fortified at around the same time. It has been successively Flemish, Burgundian, Spanish and English. It was bought by Louis XIV from Charles II to become definitively French in 1662.

Dunkerque is now a commercial port, the third largest in France. Situated on the North Sea, it is 12 miles from the Belgian border and 25 miles from Calais. The western outer harbour is very busy with ferries, container ships and tankers on their way to and from the oil refinery. The town is substantial, with some interesting buildings, especially the St Eloi church, the war damage to which has finally been repaired in the last year or two. You will find plenty of shops and some good fish stalls.

There are two yacht harbours – one in the Port d'Echouage, the other in the Bassin du Commerce. Both offer good shelter and have a wide range of facilities. Dunkerque is a port of entry to the canal system through the Canal de Bergues.

## SHORE LEAVE

### Food and drink
The choice of restaurants in Dunkerque ranges from the sophisticated to the bourgeois, with the selection of specialist restaurants and fast-food outlets usual in a large town. Aux Ducs de Bourgogne, 29 Rue de Bourgogne, is a French family restaurant where food is more important than flashy décor.

### Entertainment
Dunkerque is a popular conference centre and as such offers a wide range of entertainments, many of which are held in the Palais des Congrès on the seafront. There are several cinemas and a municipal theatre.

### What to see
The **Belfry**, once the bell-tower of St Eloi Church, dates from the fifteenth century. It is 200 feet high, has a 48-bell carillon and is open to the public; a War Memorial is set in the west wall; the tourist information office is on the ground floor, its entrance also on the west side. The **Leughenaer Tower**, for centuries a landmark for sailors, is the oldest building in Dunkerque and the last of the 28 towers built during the Burgundian fortifications in 1405.

The **Museum of Contemporary Art** is set in gardens appropriately land-scaped with modern sculptures. The **Fine Arts Museum** in Place du Général de Gaulle contains several hundred paintings from the sixteenth to the twentieth centuries — part of the museum is dedicated to local and naval history. There is an **aquarium** in Malo Park. The tourist office has a booklet describing guided visits of Dunkerque, including tours of the harbour by boat.

### Excursions
Because of its excellent communications, Dunkerque is a good base for visiting places inland. **Lille**, with its citadel – one of Vauban's finest and best preserved – and a fine arts museum generally acknowledged to be one of the best in provincial France, would be a good choice.

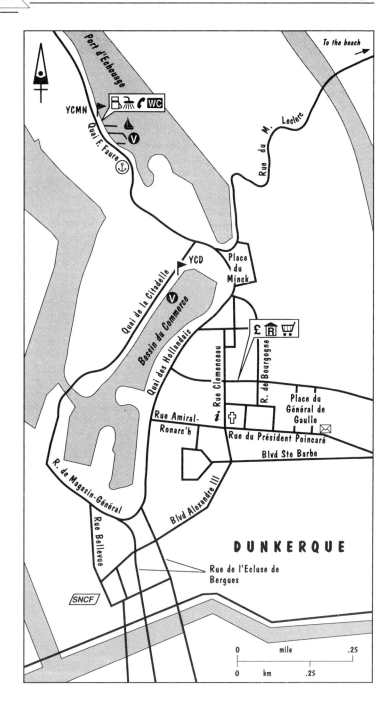

*Exercise*
Dunkerque's four miles of fine sandy and safe beaches are popular with holiday-makers. The promenade has restaurants and shops and at the western end a memorial dedicated to those who fell during May and June 1940. There are several swimming pools, indoor and out, and many tennis courts.

## TRANSPORT AND TRAVEL

**Buses** To Lille, Gravelines and Calais
**Trains** To Arras (change there for Paris), to Lille, to Calais and along the coast to Boulogne
**Ferries** To Ramsgate. The ferry terminal is seven miles to the west (yachts are forbidden to enter except in an emergency). The Cross-Channel Tourist Office is in Rue des Fusiliers-Marins ☎ 28.66.28.84
**Taxis** From the railway station taxi rank ☎ 28.66.73.00
**Car hire** Europcar, 1–3 Rue du Chemin de Fer ☎ 28.66.45.61

*Further information* from tourist office on the west side of the Belfry in Rue Clemenceau.

# Yacht Club de la Mer du Nord

| | |
|---|---|
| **Harbourmaster** ☎ 28.66.56.14 | **VHF Channels** 12, 73 |
| **Callsign** Yacht Club de la Mer du Nord | **Daily charge** ££ |

This is a tidal marina on Quai F. Faure, and very much in dockland.

## STEP ASHORE

**Nearest payphone, toilets, showers** In marina
**Clubhouse** Yacht Club de la Mer du Nord
**Shopping** No shops on the quay, but there are fish stalls at the end of the dock past the dock harbour. The main shopping area is 15 minutes' walk: turn left outside the yacht harbour

### SHIPS' SERVICES

*Water and electricity* On quay
*Fuel* (diesel and petrol) From Yacht Club
*Gas* (Camping and Calor) From chandler across the road
*Chandler* Opposite yacht harbour
*Boatyard, engineer* Opposite yacht harbour

# Yacht Club de Dunkerque

| | |
|---|---|
| **Harbourmaster** ☎ 28.66.11.06 | **Daily charge** ££ |

This is the municipal marina in the Bassin du Commerce, accessible through the Trystram Lock. It is advisable to book if you want to come here during the first week in June because there are racing meets. The harbour office is in the *bateau feu* (fireship) *Le Dyck*.

## STEP ASHORE

**Nearest payphone** On Quai du Risban
**Toilets, showers** On quay
**Clubhouse** Yacht Club de Dunkerque, Quai du Risban

**Shopping** The main shopping area for the town comes down to this quay

### SHIPS' SERVICES

*Water and electricity* On quay

*Fuel, gas, chandler, boatyard, engineer* See Yacht Club de la Mer du Nord

# Calais

The name Calais appears for the first time in a charter drawn up in 1181. The nearest port to England, it became the port most frequently used by the English and French from the end of the twelfth century. In 1347 Edward III captured Calais for England, in whose possession it stayed for over 200 years, but few relics of the English occupation now remain.

Calais' growth and prosperity have been linked to its British connections – the lace industry introduced from Nottingham in the nineteenth century took over from fishing as the main occupation of Calais. In this century Calais has become the largest passenger port on the European mainland, with the majority of people travelling to and from Britain.

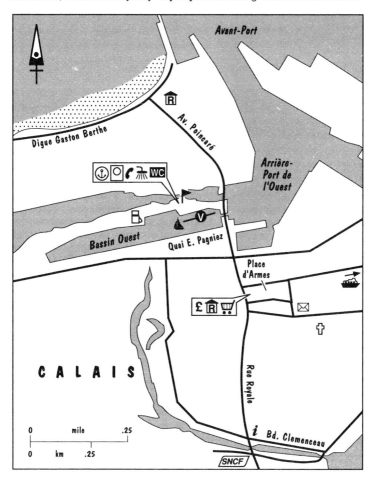

# SHORE LEAVE

*Food and drink*

Many of the restaurants in Calais are specifically geared to British visitors and, like the similarly minded shops, these display a 'Calais Shopping Circle' label. British foods and beverages are often in evidence in Calais, but they tend to be expensive compared with French equivalents. The honorary local representative of the Cruising Association is French and recommends, among others, the following restaurants: Au Côte d'Argent, 1 Digue Gaston Berthe, La Sole Meunière, 1 Boulevard de la Résistance and A l'Assiette, 2 Place de Suède.

*Entertainment*

The nearest cinema to the yacht harbour is the Alhambra, 122 Boulevard Jacquard. There is a municipal theatre in Boulevard Léon Gambetta.

*What to see*

Most places of interest can be reached comfortably on foot in about 15 minutes.

The **Town Museum (Art and Lace)**, 25 Rue Richelieu, is well worth visiting to see Flemish paintings, Rodin sculptures, samples of Calais lace and other relics of the town's history. Outside the **Town Hall** (built in Flemish Renaissance style) in Boulevard Jacquard, is **Rodin's** largest and most famous statue, cast in bronze, marking the attempt by six Calais citizens in 1347 to prevent a massacre by Edward III – their lives were spared as a result of the Queen's intervention. The **War Museum**, in Parc St Pierre, was formerly the German navy's main telephone exchange in northern France.

The **Watch Tower** in the Place d'Armes is the oldest building in Calais; it was built in the thirteenth century to observe shipping movements in the Channel. The **church of Notre Dame** is believed to be the only example of the English Perpendicular style of architecture on the continent – its oldest parts dates from the thirteenth century. The **Citadel** is a tranquil place with attractive gardens beside all that remains of Calais' ancient fortifications.

*Excursions*

Buses run along the coast to fishing villages such as **Audresselles** and **Ambleteuse** and to **Wissant**, once a port with the same status as Calais – it has a large beach ideal for water sports. Nearer Calais is **Sangatte**, the site of the Channel tunnel works, where there is an exhibition. Also to the west are the high chalk cliffs of **Cap Blanc Nez**, the closest point to England, once part of the southern fringe of the North Downs of Kent.

*Exercise*

The beach is a short walk from the yacht harbour; the sand is fine and the bathing safe. A good view of shipping in the port and across the Channel can be had from the beach and on a clear day you can see Dover.

## TRANSPORT AND TRAVEL

**Buses** To Dunkerque and Boulogne

**Trains** To Paris and Basel

**Planes** From Calais International Airport at Marck, four miles east of Calais, to Gatwick

**Ferries** Frequent service to Dover; ferry takes 75 minutes, hovercraft 30 minutes.

Hovercrafts also go to Ramsgate

**Taxis** Radio Calais ☎ 21.97.13.14; Union Calais ☎ 21.96.29.29

**Car hire** Hertz and Avis, Place d'Armes

**Bicycle hire** Ebaïme, Boulevard de la Résistance

*Further information* from tourist office at 12 Boulevard Clemenceau.

# Port de Calais

| | |
|---|---|
| **Harbourmaster** ☎ 21.34.55.23 | **VHF Channel** 12 |
| **Callsign** Calais Port | **Daily charge** on pontoon ££; on quay £ |

Despite the fact that Calais is an extremely busy port, with its cross-Channel ferries and hovercraft traffic, yachts are made very welcome. There are mooring buoys in the Arrière-Port for vessels waiting to enter Bassin de l'Ouest; yachts may remain there for up to 24 hours. Bassin de l'Ouest, through the sea lock, has good facilities and good all-round shelter, although strong north-west and north-east winds create quite a surge when the lock gates open. It is usual for yachts to be given a berth beside the Yacht Club – when it is busy the yachts may be three or more deep. Larger yachts may be directed to the quay opposite the yacht club. This is cheaper and closer to town but further from the yacht club facilities and less secure; moreover, the quay is used by commercial traffic and you may be asked to move. Calais is a port of entry into the French canal system through the lock into Bassin Carnot.

## STEP ASHORE

**Nearest payphone** At yacht club
**Toilets, showers, laundry facilities** In yacht club
**Clubhouse** The clubhouse in the yacht harbour has a bar and takes orders for duty-free goods
**Shopping** The main shops are within 10 minutes' walk of the yacht harbour. A bus service runs from the central station to the two hypermarkets on the outskirts of the town. Under-cover market on Wednesdays in Place d'Armes and markets on Thursdays and Saturdays in Boulevard Lafayette. Shops which display a 'Calais Shopping Circle' label provide a special welcome to British visitors. Plenty of banks and bureaux de change, and two post offices

### SHIPS' SERVICES

**Water, fuel** From yacht club
**Gas** (Camping and Calor) From Deregnaucourt, 25 Place d'Armes
**Chandler** Ebaïme, Boulevard de la Résistance
**Boatyard** Enquire at yacht club
**Engineer** Rogliamo – contact through yacht club
**Sailmaker** Ebaïme

# Boulogne

Colourful, functional and efficient rather than attractive, Boulogne, as you would expect from a port of its size, can provide everything for the yachtsman. It's worth climbing up to the old town where there are some lovely old buildings, a museum, some unusual shops and bars and restaurants. You can walk round the ramparts, getting an excellent overall view of the town.

Boulogne is all right for a night, some shopping and a good dinner but not recommended if you are looking for a quiet night and a pretty backcloth. It is good for serious restocking of supplies: there are a couple of hypermarkets a short taxi-drive away.

## SHORE LEAVE

*Food and drink*
Boulogne is France's most important fishing port and has fish restaurants for all pockets. Very good seafood is to be had in L'Huîtrière, 11 Place Lorraine.

*Entertainment*
Cinéma Les Arcades is in Rue Nationale. Casino, Rue Félix Adam, has boules, roulette, baccarat and dancing.

*What to see*
The **ramparts** of the old town are impressive and enclose handsome eighteenth-century houses in the attractive streets. The **Château d'Aumont Museum** is in the old town and so is the cathedral with its Italianate dome that is such a landmark.

*Excursions*
There are two **hypermarkets** at La Capelle on the outskirts of Boulogne; an hourly bus service from the Commercial Centre, south of the pontoons and on the other side of the basin, goes to Auchan hypermarket on the road to St Omer. Leclerc hypermarket is on the N1 to Paris.

A less prosaic excursion is to the seventeenth-century walled city of **Montreuil-sur-Mer**, now nearly nine miles from the sea; you can explore the cobbled streets or walk round the ramparts of this hill town, or go further up the Canche valley to picturesque **Hesdin**, near the battlefield of Agincourt.

*Exercise*
There are beaches at Boulevard Ste Beuve for swimming and windsurfing.

## TRANSPORT AND TRAVEL

**Buses** The bus station is just across the bridge on Quai de la Poste; buses go along the coast road to Wimereux and inland to a number of villages
**Trains** From SNCF Gare Maritime nearby, or Boulogne-Ville, Boulevard Voltaire to Amiens and on to Paris, a fast and frequent train service

**Ferries** From behind the Gare Maritime, every two or three hours to Dover
**Taxis** Radio taxis ☎ 21.91.25.00; or from the rank at Gare Maritime
**Car hire** Hertz, Rue Victor Hugo
**Bicycle hire** At SNCF Gare Boulogne-Ville – in season

*Further information* from tourist office 50 yards from the berths, across the bridge on Quai de la Poste.

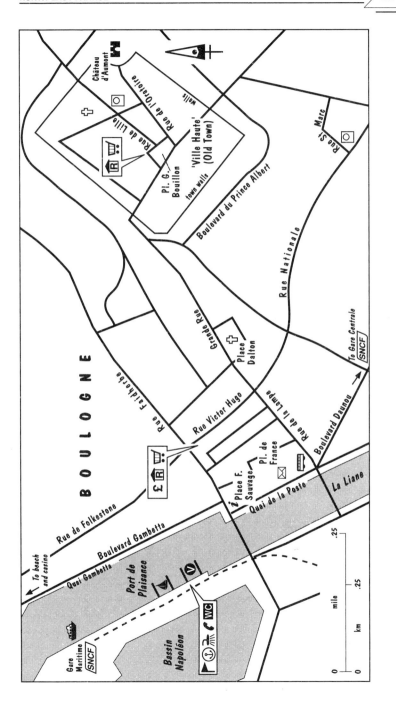

BOULOGNE

Château d'Aumont

Rue de l'Oratoire

Rue de Lille

'Ville Haute' (Old Town)

town walls

Pl. G. Bouillon

Boulevard du Prince Albert

Rue Nationale

Rue St-

Mare

Grande Rue

Place Dalton

To Gare Centrale
SNCF

Rue Faidherbe

Rue Victor Hugo

Rue de la Lampe

Boulevard Daunou

Place F. Sauvage

Pl. de France

Quai de la Poste

La Liane

Rue de Folkestone

Boulevard Gambetta

Quai Gambetta

To beach and casino

Port de Plaisance

Bassin Napoléon

Gare Maritime
SNCF

WC

km    mile    .25

0    0    .25

# Port de Boulogne

| | |
|---|---|
| **Harbourmaster** ☎ 21.31.70.01 | **VHF Channel** 9 |
| **Callsign** Port de plaisance | **Daily charge** ££ |

Boulogne is France's largest fishing port and one of the busiest cross-Channel ferry terminals, but the small boat fraternity is still appreciated. Once you're past the massive and protective harbour walls and have dodged P&O and Sealink ships, you will find the marina in a sheltered basin just past the ferry terminal.

The position is not idyllic – central to the town, the marina lies between the industrial centre, with its two miles of quays, warehousing and boat-train facilities, and the residential, shopping and tourist centre. You look across the fairly colourful fishing boats moored along the harbour wall to four grim blocks of flats sticking up above the quay. The motor boat marina is beyond the bridge and rather scruffy and dirty compared with the yacht marina. Visitors can use a small, though not very beautiful, clubhouse with bar, toilets and showers. The town is only a short walk away where bars, good restaurants and shops are plentiful.

## STEP ASHORE

**Nearest payphone** Behind the clubhouse (*carte* only)
**Toilets, showers** Unisex, beside the berths, open 0800–1800
**Clubhouse** Yacht Club Boulonnais, just by the pontoons
**Shopping** Late-night shop on corner of Rue de Brequerecque and Rue du Chanoine, open till 2100. The main shops are only about 100 yards from the berths; the main shopping streets are Victor Hugo, Thiers, Faidherbe and de la Lampe. Most shops shut on Sundays and Monday mornings. Plenty of banks and bureaux de change, and a post office. Nouvelles Galeries, 57 Rue Thiers and Prisunic, 39 Rue de la Lampe are department stores with food supermarkets; don't miss Philippe Olivier, 45 Rue Thiers where a wide range of excellent cheeses is available from the master *fromagier*. A good selection of dried fruit at Idriss, 24 Grande Rue; market in Place Dalton is on Wednesday and Saturday mornings. Fresh fish every day on Quai Gambetta

## SHIPS' SERVICES

*Water and electricity* On pontoons
*Fuel* (diesel and petrol) Available in cans from Mory SA, Place des Capucins; if you need more than 100 litres they will deliver
*Gas* (Camping and Calor) 200 yards from the berths, same side of bridge
*Chandler* Angelo, Rue du Pot-d'Etain is very good; others on Rue de Folkestone and Rue Coquelin
*Boatyard, engineer* Opale Marine, Place de Capécure
*Sailmaker* Benmangen opposite berth area

# St Valéry-sur-Somme

One of St Valéry's claims to fame is that it is the town from which William the Conqueror set sail for England. (Rather touchingly St Valéry's twin town is Battle in Sussex.) Joan of Arc was imprisoned here, too, and you can see the remains of the gate she was led through.

The town is built into the hillside with houses and streets ranged down towards the banks of the Somme. The promenade runs practically the whole length of the town, passing some unusual houses with the wide, wild, bleak but attractive area of low-lying salt marshes stretching out on the other side of the river. At low tide you can walk across the estuary as endless sandy expanses emerge, and with the incoming tide it is fun to watch boys in waders fishing.

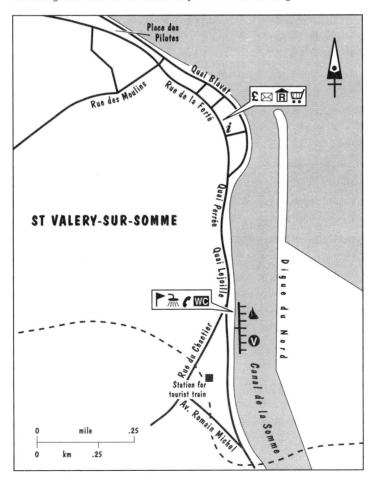

Most of the shops, restaurants and local activity centre around the main one-way street. High above stands the old town, well worth a visit, with its old abbey, private château, walls and gateways. There is a busy Sunday market in the main square and along the streets. St Valéry has great charm and is generally a delightful place to be.

## SHORE LEAVE

**Food and drink**
The restaurant in the clubhouse looks good, and there is a café just across the green. B. Martell, in Rue de la Ferté, is a coffee/tea-shop with delicious pâtisseries. Le Connoisseur restaurant in Hôtel Les Pilotes, Rue de la Ferté, looks promising, though some of the menus are quite expensive.

**Entertainment**
There is a disco and a cinema.

**What to see**
The **Musée Picarvie Rétro** has a reconstruction of village life. It is lovely to walk around the town, up to the old abbey and ancient gate through which Joan of Arc passed. From the **Calvaire des Marins** you will have a good view of the bay and the town.

**Excursions**
Take the little tourist steam train to **Le Crotoy** or **Cayeux-sur-Mer.**

**Exercise**
A leaflet describing walks is available from the tourist office. There are beaches all around which emerge at low tide. Windsurfing and swimming are probably better at Le Crotoy.

### TRANSPORT AND TRAVEL

| | |
|---|---|
| **Buses** To Le Crotoy and Abbeville | **Ferries** From Dieppe and Boulogne |
| **Trains** The small tourist railway with steam train goes to Le Crotoy and Cayeux-sur-Mer and links with SNCF | **Taxis** Ask at clubhouse |
| | **Car hire** Ask at tourist office |
| **Planes** From Le Touquet | **Bicycle hire** Ask at tourist office |

**Further information** from tourist office, 2 Place Guillaume le Conquérant.

# Port de St Valéry-sur-Somme

| | |
|---|---|
| Harbourmaster ☎ 22.26.91.64 | **VHF Channel** 9 |
| **Callsign** Directeur du port | **Daily charge** ££ |

The long entrance to the small fishing port through the dredged channel needs care and settled weather. Once inside the well-maintained marina, however, you can be sure of a totally secure, hospitable and enjoyable stay. The clubhouse was built in 1988 and is a smart, well-equipped brick and wood construction with a comfortable-looking bar and restaurant. The club members have invested heavily to make the facilities the best in the area. There is a large chandlery 100 yards away and the extremely attractive town is only five minutes' walk. It's a lovely place to spend a few days.

## STEP ASHORE

**Nearest payphone** Across the green opposite the club or in the clubhouse (*carte* only)
**Toilets, showers** In clubhouse, very high standard
**Clubhouse** Sport Nautique Valéricain on Quay, open 0700–1200 and 1300–2100; this is also the capitainerie. The clubhouse is new, well-kept and very clean
**Shopping** The main shops, banks and the post office are in the main street, Rue de la Ferté, five minutes' walk across the green; late-night shop open until 2000

### SHIPS' SERVICES

*Water and electricity* On pontoons
*Fuel* (diesel and petrol) Available in cans from the town half a mile away
*Gas* (Camping and Calor) In town
*Chandler* Latitude 50, 100 yards from the clubhouse
*Boatyard* On quay
*Engineer* Ask at club

# Le Crotoy

| | |
|---|---|
| **Harbourmaster** ☎ 22.27.82.24 | **VHF Channel** 9 |
| **Callsign** Le Crotoy | **Daily charge** £ |

Le Crotoy is smallish and an odd mixture of attractive old buildings and some very modern constructions. Its main industry is fishing and the majority of shops and restaurants offer daily-catch dishes. It isn't as sophisticated or as pretty as St Valéry-sur-Somme just across the bay, but it does have a certain charm. The two places make a pair: if you were staying in St Valéry it would be worth dropping into Le Crotoy for lunch and a walk around. The beach here is particularly good and windsurfing is popular. The marina is tucked in at the north end of the harbour behind groynes, but still exposed – flattish dunes provide little shelter and it is not suitable in strong winds. The pontoons are well kept and modern.

## STEP ASHORE

**Nearest payphone** A few hundred yards away in the town (*carte* only)
**Toilets, showers** In marina, open all the time
**Clubhouse** The small clubhouse has a bar and a couple of scruffy chairs and tables; it is only open at high tide
**Shopping** Only a five-minute walk from the marina, just round the edge of the harbour to Rue de la Porte du Pont: all necessary shops, banks and a post office. Early closing day varies from shop to shop

### SHIPS' SERVICES

*Water and electricity* On pontoons
*Fuel* (diesel and petrol) From town in cans
*Gas* (Camping and Calor) From town

### TRANSPORT AND TRAVEL

**Buses** Run to St Valéry-sur-Somme, Abbeville and Amiens
**Trains** Tourist train to St Valéry-sur-Somme
and Cayeux-sur-Mer connects with SNCF to Abbeville

# Dieppe

Dieppe is the oldest French seaside resort and the nearest to Paris. In the late nineteenth century it was taken up by the English and became very fashionable. Aubrey Beardsley holidayed here and Oscar Wilde is said to have written *The Ballad of Reading Gaol* in the café next to the ferry. The fine casino and gardens on the seafront are reminiscent of the Edwardian era.

A working port, Dieppe is blessedly free of seaside amusement arcades and tawdry knick-knacks. See the fish market by the yacht harbour and wander through the old back streets, or sit in a bar on the quayside. The north-east corner near the ferry terminals is run-down but picturesque – the inspiration of Georges, Simenon's Newhaven-Dieppe thrillers. Dieppe is a ferry terminal, so useful for leaving a yacht or for crew changeovers.

## SHORE LEAVE

### Food and drink

There are over 100 restaurants in Dieppe, ranging from haute cuisine to fast-food: a good selection can be found on the Quai Duquesne. You won't have to look far to find restaurants specialising in Norman dishes made with cider and cream or delicious fresh fish and shellfish. The crêperie in Rue de la Marinière is recommended for a light lunchtime snack.

### Entertainment

Dieppe has three cinemas, as well as a theatre and cinema in the **Jean Renoir Cultural Centre** (Le CAC). The new casino, modelled on the Crystal Palace, is lively.

### What to see

Visit the **Castle Museum** where sixteenth and seventeenth-century navigational instruments and maps are displayed. There is also a unique collection of fourteenth to seventeenth-century ivories and a permanent exhibition of paintings, including some by Pissarro, Renoir and Sickert. You can visit the sixteenth-century **Tourelles**, the last remaining part of the old ramparts, the fourteenth-century **St Jacques Church** and the **Canadian Monument.**

### Excursions

Just over a mile to the west, opposite Dieppe golf club, is a museum describing the devastating air-raid of 19 August 1942. **Varengeville**, six miles away, is worth visiting to see the **Manoir d'Ango**, a sixteenth-century manor house, the old church and also **Les Moutiers**, a house designed by Sir Edwin Lutyens with gardens by Gertrude Jekyll. **Rouen** is less than an hour away by train, and has a fine cathedral, old timbered houses and a whole panoply of other sights. A bus ride will take you to **Le Tréport**, a bustling port with seafood restaurants on the quay.

### Exercise

The best walks are around town and along the promenade and cliffs to the west. You can swim safely from the beaches; they are pebbly, but wet sand appears at low tide. The most sand is at the western end of the beach, where there is also a

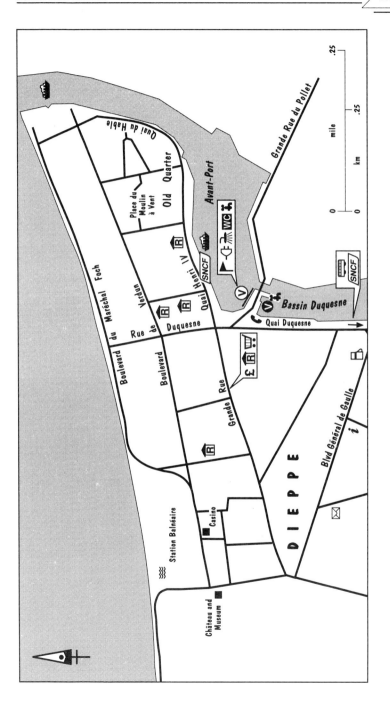

heated open-air swimming pool. There are several indoor swimming pools in the resort area. Windsurfing is popular off the beach.

## TRANSPORT AND TRAVEL

**Buses** To Le Havre, Rouen, St Valéry-en-Caux and Fécamp from the railway station
**Trains** To Rouen and Paris
**Ferries** To Newhaven, taking four hours, four times a day

**Taxis** ☎ 35.84.20.05
**Car hire** Europcar, Rue Thiers; Avis, Boulevard Général de Gaulle (nearest)
**Bicycle hire** From SNCF

*Further information* from tourist office in Boulevard Général de Gaulle.

# Port de Dieppe

| | |
|---|---|
| **Harbourmaster** ☎ 35.84.32.99 | **VHF Channel** 12 |
| **Callsign** Dieppe Port | **Daily charge** ££ |

The moorings in the Avant-Port and Port de Pêche (Bassin Duquesne) are not very attractive, being surrounded by busy and grubby streets, traffic, ferries and trains. There is a heavy swell in the Avant-Port in strong onshore winds. The yacht club is by the lock and has well-appointed showers and toilets; the bar and club room is welcoming but rather empty in the week.

## STEP ASHORE

**Nearest payphone** One outside the yacht club (by the lock) and another inside
**Toilets, showers** In the yacht club
**Clubhouse** Open 0800–1900 every day

except Wednesdays (0800–1200 and 1400–1900)
**Shopping** The main shopping streets are directly to the west of the yacht club

### SHIPS' SERVICES

*Water* Available on pontoons
*Electricity* On the quay in the outer basin north of the yacht club
*Fuel* (diesel and petrol) Available from the

garage in Boulevard Général de Gaulle, but has to be collected in cans
*Chandler* Co-op Maritime in Rue Pierre Pocholle

# St Valéry-en-Caux

St Valéry was destroyed in the desperate rearguard action of 1940, when the 51st Highland Division and the French 2nd Cavalry Division held out against the Nazi advance. Two monuments on the cliffs and a cemetery commemorate them.

Despite being rebuilt post-war, St Valéry is a very pleasant resort with particularly attractive floral displays everywhere, and an interesting modern church. Old buildings still stand in odd corners as a reminder of what the town was once like. The restored Maison Henri IV dates from the sixteenth century and makes an impressive setting to the harbour.

Among the attractions of St Valéry are cliff walks and bus or car trips to villages along the coast and inland. Dovecotes (*colombiers*) are a feature of the region and a tour of them is organised by the tourist office. Tours to see cheese and cider being produced are also recommended.

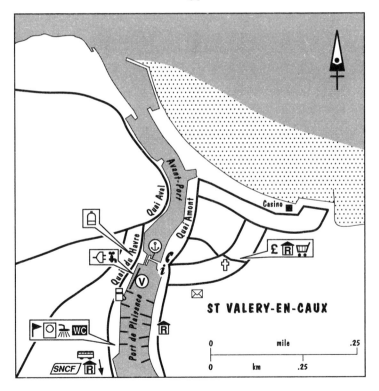

SHORE LEAVE

*Food and drink*
There are many restaurants, crêperies and pizzerias both on the quay and across the bridge. Recommended are the Hôtel des Bains, the Catamaran and Belle Epoque crêperie.

*Entertainment*
There is a cinema in the casino.

*What to see*
Visit the cloister of the **Hospice des Pénitents** (1640), **Maison Henri IV** (1540), the twelfth-century parish church and sixteenth-century chapel on the hill.

*Excursions*
Several châteaux, including **Château de Cany** and **Château de Valmont**, are easily reached by bus. The **Nuclear Power Station** at **Paluel** opens on Mondays, Tuesdays and Wednesdays from 1500, Saturdays from 0930. Visit the attractive seaside village of **Veules-les-Roses**, or travel the **Route des Colombiers** to see the dovecotes of the region.

*Exercise*
This is a good centre to set off on cliff walks. Swimming is safe; the beaches are good, but stony except at low tide. You can windsurf off the beaches, too. The leisure centre has a swimming pool and tennis courts.

## TRANSPORT AND TRAVEL

**Buses** To Dieppe, Fécamp and Rouen from the railway station
**Trains** To Paris (four a day)

**Taxis** Simper ☎ 35.97.19.87
**Bicycle hire** Vélocation is out of town but will deliver ☎ 35.97.05.28

*Further information* from tourist office on corner of bridge opposite Hôtel de Ville, open 1000–1230 and 1500–1900 every day.

# Port de St Valéry-en-Caux

| Harbourmaster ☎ 35.97.01.30 | VHF Channel 9 |
|---|---|
| Callsign St Valéry | Daily charge £££ (third night free) |

Waiting for the stream of boats coming out of the lock can be a little worrying as it looks as though the gates will shut before you can get in. However, once you're inside the basin is pleasant and comfortable, though surrounded by busy roads. The harbourmaster is friendly and co-operative over the choice of locking times to leave. If you stay two nights, the third is free.

## STEP ASHORE

**Nearest payphone** Outside Hôtel de Ville, east of lock

**Toilets, showers, launderette** At yacht club on the Quai du Havre, the west quay, open 24 hours a day; the harbourmaster gives you your own key when you arrive

**Clubhouse** On west quay, open at weekends only

**Shopping** Main shopping centre is over the bridge with a small selection of high-street shops with banks, a post office and bureaux de change; also a few shops on the west side. Fresh fish from stalls at the outer harbour

### SHIPS' SERVICES

**Water** Available on pontoons

**Electricity** Available on residents' berths; by arrangement with harbourmaster, it may be possible to move to a spare resident's berth

**Fuel** (diesel and petrol) In cans from garage on west quay

**Gas** (Camping and Calor) At top of steps

**Chandler, boatyard, engineer, sailmaker** All on west quay

# Fécamp

At first sight, especially on a hot and dusty summer day, Fécamp may not seem attractive, but persevere. There is the beach, with large pebbles – so you need to wear shoes – though a little sand shows at low water. To the north the high cliff is surmounted by the semaphore station and Notre Dame de Salut, dedicated to the safe return of fishermen. In town, a pleasant hour or so can be spent in the Benedictine Museum. La Trinité church on the other side of town is one of the greatest and most beautiful in France – don't be put off by the unfortunate eighteenth-century west front. The Municipal Museum in Rue Alexandre-Legros is a charming eighteenth-century building entered from a narrow street through an archway which opens into a pleasant garden. On the seafront there is also a modern museum of the Newfoundland fishing industry: Fécamp's fishing fleet sails regularly to the Newfoundland Banks.

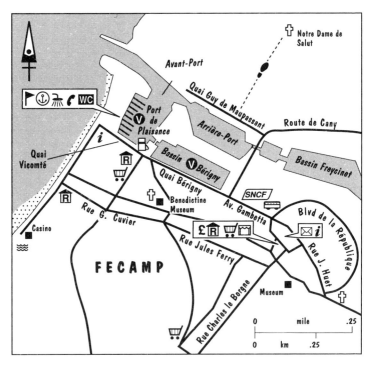

# SHORE LEAVE

*Food and drink*

Various take-aways face the harbour, including the Snack du Port. Two recommended restaurants near the harbour are the Progrès and the Marine; both have large menus, including excellent fish, and need not be expensive.

*What to see*

The **Benedictine Museum**, which includes relics of the original **abbey** where the liqueur was invented, has a rather frustrating exhibition of the production process, because you don't see any Benedictine actually being made; but the display of large numbers of labels from imitations of the drink is fascinating. Visit the **Municipal Museum** for local history and collections of art and ceramics, and the modern fishing museum on the front. The **Holy Trinity Church** has many treasures inside, including a relic of the Holy Blood and the footprint of the angel who appeared there in 943. The tombs of Dukes Richard I and Richard II of Normandy are also here.

*Entertainment*

**Le Palace** in Rue Boufart has four cinema screens. There is also a municipal theatre and a casino.

*Excursions*

The well-furnished sixteenth-century **Château de Bailleul** set in a beautiful park, about seven miles from Fécamp, is a welcome diversion from the sea.

*Exercise*

Swimming from the beach is safe, and there is lifeguard surveillance. Walk round the inner harbour, alive with fishing boats, and follow the lanes up the hill to the north. From the hill the view stretches for miles towards **St Valéry-en-Caux** and you can walk in the fresh, cooler air from the sea. Southwards, make your way along the front, up past the casino and municipal campsite to the lanes towards **Yport** and **Etretat**. The former is a valley with holiday cottages leading to the beach, the latter a small seaside resort. You can walk back to Fécamp along the beach, though it can be a scramble near high water when you have to walk over the rocks.

## TRANSPORT AND TRAVEL

**Buses** From Avenue Gambetta to Le Havre and Dieppe
**Trains** To Rouen, Paris and Le Havre
**Taxis** From Avenue Gambetta

☎ 35.28.17.50
**Car hire** Rouen-locations P I Bigot
☎ 35.28.48.09
**Bicycle hire** From SNCF

*Further information* from tourist offices at the corner of the harbour on Quai Vicomté, open afternoons only, and in town near the post office.

# Port de Fécamp

| | |
|---|---|
| **Harbourmaster** ☎ 35.28.13.58 | **VHF Channel** 9 |
| **Callsign** Fécamp | **Daily charge** ££ (third night free) |

After the rather daunting entrance, Fécamp harbour is pleasant. It is a typical French port, with houses and cafés on the quays and the usual collection of yachts on the pontoons. The outer basin can be restless in a swell, but you can lock in on the tide to Bassin Bérigny, which is calmer, though nearer to the busy street traffic. The harbourmaster, whose office is part of the clubhouse complex, is a friendly anglophile.

## STEP ASHORE

**Nearest payphone** In the yacht club or at the south-west corner of harbour behind tourist office

**Toilets, showers** Below the clubhouse

**Clubhouse** It has a pleasant bar, with a good view along the coast towards Etretat, and also serves snacks; orders for duty-free goods can be placed here

**Shopping** All the amenities of a small town are here: most major banks are represented, plus a post office, a variety of shops and a covered fish market as well as stalls on the quayside. Large supermarket up the hill due south of the harbour – follow the back streets past the Benedictine Museum. On the quayside opposite the old fishing harbour is a well-stocked wine shop, which will deliver your order to your boat

## SHIPS' SERVICES

**Water and electricity** On pontoons

**Fuel** (petrol and diesel) From south-east corner of the outer basin

**Chandler, boatyard, engineer** In the marina

# Le Havre

Although Le Havre is the usual unprepossessing post-war reconstruction, it has hidden attractions. Among them is the church of St Joseph, made of dreary concrete, but with a 275-foot lantern. Go inside, take a tip-up seat, look up and become vertiginous.

The streets around the Bassin du Commerce are enlivened by the sails of tiny dinghies in the basin and an asymmetrical bridge. The Cultural Centre, shaped like a crown roast, is difficult to penetrate, the entrance being well hidden. To the north-east you will find the older town, Le Quartier St François, which retains its original character, and to the west the seaside resort of Ste Adresse.

## SHORE LEAVE

### Food and drink
Restaurants of every kind are plentiful in Le Havre. Few are near the marina but the restaurant in the Société des Régates clubhouse is reported to be first class.

### Entertainment
Of the several cinemas in Le Havre, the nearest is in Rue Louis Brindeau. There is also a municipal theatre and concert hall.

### What to see
Le Havre has much to offer in the way of museums, art galleries, concerts and other cultural events. The **André Malroux Museum of Fine Arts** has a collection of Dufy and some Boudin paintings. The **Old Havre Museum** in the old quarter is a restored seventeenth-century house with a collection of glass, pottery and documents relating to Le Havre's history (open Wednesdays to Sundays). There is a **natural history museum** near the harbour. Motor boat trips round the harbour start from the northern end of the marina.

### Excursions
Transport from Le Havre is prolific; you can travel in most directions by bus, or train. It takes only an hour to get to **Rouen**, a historic city of great interest; **Honfleur** is also very accessible. **Montgeon Forest**, on the outskirts of Le Havre, has 700 acres of woodland with a boating lake, games areas, campsite and zoo.

### Exercise
You can walk to the west along the cliffs to the lighthouse (not open to the public) on **Cap de la Hève**: take a Ligne 1 bus to **Ste Adresse** to the start of the walk. A magnificent view is yours from the terrace of the fort at Ste Adresse. Beaches for swimming and windsurfing are west of the harbour at Ste Adresse.

### TRANSPORT AND TRAVEL

**Buses** Ligne 1 bus stops near the marina and goes through the centre of town to the bus and railway stations; buses to Rouen, Caen, Deauville, Lisieux, Fécamp and Etretat run from the railway station
**Trains** To Rouen and Paris

**Ferries** From Quai de Southampton to Portsmouth, Cork and Rosslare
**Taxis** ☎ 35.25.81.81
**Car hire** Avis, 37 Avenue Général Archinard ☎ 35.41.74.11

**Further information** from tourist office in Hôtel de Ville in town centre.

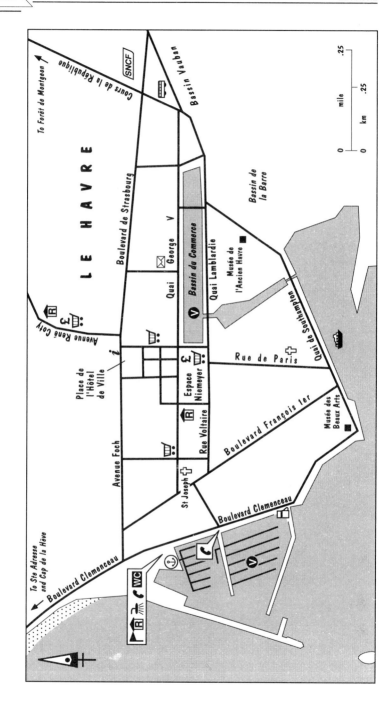

# Port du Havre

| Harbourmaster ☎ 35.21.23.95 | VHF Channel 9 |
| --- | --- |
| Callsign Le Havre | Daily charge ££ |

The entry to Le Havre is easy and a sharp turn to port just inside the pierheads quickly takes you out of the way of ferries and large ships. Visitors moor where they can find a space in the first basin; harbour staff are not likely to be around except when collecting harbour dues. If you are staying for a long time, the harbourmaster may be able to arrange for you to go into the Bassin du Commerce in the centre of town. It is possible to go up river to Rouen.

## STEP ASHORE

**Nearest payphone** At head of the pontoon ramps and in the clubhouses
**Toilets, showers, launderette** In both clubhouses
**Clubhouses** Two on the north quay: Société des Régates is smart, Sport Nautique Havrais is informal and friendly

**Shopping** A plan on a board at the road entrance to the marina shows where the nearest shops are. A quarter-mile walk due east via Rue Voltaire brings you to the market. More shops further on, including banks, post office and bureau de change.

### SHIPS' SERVICES

*Water and electricity* Available on the pontoons
*Fuel* (diesel and petrol) In the south-east corner of the basin

*Gas* (Camping and Calor) Available from the chandlers on the quay
*Chandler* Several near the marina
*Boatyard, engineer* In the marina

# Honfleur

A unique medieval French seaport full of beautiful old houses, still with a lived-in feeling, Honfleur is not preserved like a museum-piece. Take a walk round the poorer part of the town, such as the area uphill behind Quai Ste Catherine. Superb food is to be found in Honfleur, plus lots of arts and crafts shops and interesting museums. Don't miss Musée Eugène Boudin with famous local paintings and a collection of Norman costumes, rich in lace. The special quality of Normandy light inspired Boudin's paintings and drew other artists, such as Monet, to work here. If you want to avoid the tourists and get the French feeling, try visiting in late September when the last holidaymakers have left and the locals have time to idle again.

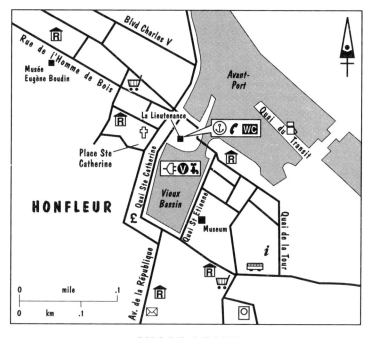

SHORE LEAVE

### Food and drink

Numerous restaurants are gathered around the old harbour and behind the Hôtel de Ville. L'Anchorage in the Vieux Bassin is recommended as having a very good menu, pleasant service and a view of the old harbour.

### What to see

The local **marine museum** is in the old church of St Etienne on the Quai St-Etienne; the **Museum of Norman Art** (Musée d'Ethnographie et d'Art Populaire Normand) in Rue de la Prison is worth visiting for the building, which is the old prison. The **Musée Eugène Boudin** in Rue de l'Homme de Bois (closed on

Tuesdays) is particularly recommended not only for Boudin, but for Courbet, Dufy and Monet too. **St Catherine's Church**, constructed of wood by shipwrights after the original was destroyed in the Hundred Years War, is very unusual: the roof resembles two inverted ships side by side, with a separate bell tower. Moored in the seventeenth-century **Vieux Bassin** you can enjoy the reflection of the narrow, slate-hung seven-storey houses on **Quai Ste Catherine** in the water and appreciate the floodlit two-storey stone houses on **Quai St Etienne**.

*Excursions*

A day trip to **Deauville** is easy to organise or you could visit the **Ferme St Siméon**, about a mile from Honfleur, where Boudin and his friends lived.

*Exercise*

Several walks are suggested in a tourist office leaflet. If you walk to the little chapel on the **Côte de Grâce**, you gain views of the sea, the Seine Estuary and the port of Le Havre. It was in this chapel of Notre Dame that navigators prayed before setting out on voyages of discovery; its beams are hung with various offerings of model boats. From **Mont Joli** you overlook the town, harbour and Seine Valley. There is a leisure centre with a swimming pool at Boulevard Charles V.

### TRANSPORT AND TRAVEL

**Buses** From coach station, Place Porte de Rouen to Le Havre, Deauville-Trouville and Caen

**Trains** The nearest railway station is at Lisieux, with connections for Paris

**Ferries** From Le Havre to Portsmouth

**Planes** From Deauville (St Gatien des Bois), six miles away, to Gatwick and Jersey

**Taxis, car hire** ☎ 31.89.44.73

**Bicycle hire** Mario Gregory, 12 Quai Le Paulmier

*Further information* from tourist office at 33 Cours des Fossés behind the coach station.

## Port d'Honfleur

| | |
|---|---|
| **Harbourmaster** ☎ 31.89.20.02 | **VHF Channels** 11, 16 |
| **Callsign** Port control | **Daily charge** ££ |

Visitors berth in the Vieux Bassin, lined up opposite the yacht club members' boats. Enter and leave smartly: ditherers are not indulged as a traffic jam quickly forms on the road when the bridge is open.

### STEP ASHORE

**Nearest payphone** Outside post office and in Boulevard Charles V

**Toilets** At La Lieutenance

**Showers** Nearest are those at the swimming pool at the leisure centre in Boulevard Charles V

**Clubhouse** Cercle Nautique behind Quai St Etienne, on the corner of Place Arthur Boudin

**Shopping** Good selection of shops; the best individual shops are in the area behind Quai Ste Catherine. Several banks in this area, most credit cards are accepted. Supermarket in Rue de la République, slightly set back on the right-hand side of the road leaving the harbour, opposite the post office. Fruit and vegetable market on Saturday mornings. Fresh fish is sold on the quay every day

## SHIPS' SERVICES

**Water and electricity** Available on the pontoons
**Fuel** (diesel and petrol) In the outer basin of the harbour on the Quai du Transit, near the entrance to the Bassin de l'Est, at high water only
**Gas** (Camping and Calor) From the supermarket
**Boatyard** In the outer docks

# Deauville-Trouville

The Normandy corniche is a nine-mile stretch of sand which runs from Deauville through neighbouring Trouville to Honfleur. The two towns, separated by La Touques River, are both fashionable resorts: Deauville is larger and more opulent, but that is not to decry Trouville, which has many interesting features. Deauville has all the fun of an upmarket seaside resort with horse racing and a casino, with a tinge of *fin de siècle*. The Planches, wooden boardwalks on the sand at the top of the beaches where the chic go to see and be seen, are a feature of both resorts.

The choice of where to berth is between the modern Marina de Port Deauville, on the western side of the outer harbour, and Port de Deauville, the old yacht basin further up the river.

## SHORE LEAVE

### Food and drink

Deauville has no fewer than 14 restaurants falling into the *'cuisine gastronomique'* category. Their names echo the preoccupations of the resort: Le Bistrot Gourmet, La Flambée, Le Royal, Le Spinnaker, Le Yearling and Ciro's sur les Planches. There is also a good selection of bourgeois restaurants. Trouville has a shorter list, but likewise includes a number of beach restaurants. Among the special recommendations is Les Vapeurs, a very popular fish restaurant opposite the fish market.

### Entertainment

Both resorts have cinemas, a municipal theatre, and casinos. Deauville is famous for racing, which takes place in July and August, and the international yearling sales in August. There are museums for wet days, and an aquarium in Trouville.

### Excursions

At **Bonneville-sur-Touques**, about two miles inland, the twelfth-century château is worth visiting, or take the bus to ancient **Honfleur** if you are not able to get there by sea.

### Exercise

Swim, windsurf or sand-sail on the wet sand. There are heated outdoor swimming pools in both Deauville and Trouville.

## TRANSPORT AND TRAVEL

**Buses** From Place de la Gare to Caen, Ouistreham, Honfleur and Lisieux
**Trains** To Paris and Lisieux
**Planes** From St Gatien airport to Gatwick and Channel Islands

**Taxis** Ranks in Place de la Gare and at casino; also radio taxi ☎ 31.88.02.43
**Car hire** Eurorent opposite railway station ☎ 31.88.08.40
**Bicycle hire** Pouchin, Quai de la Marine

*Further information* from tourist office at Place de la Mairie at the top of Rue Fossorier.

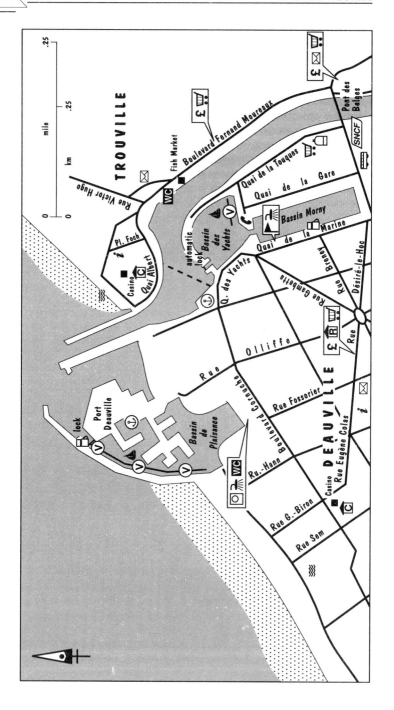

# Port de Deauville (Le Vieux Port)

| | |
|---|---|
| **Harbourmaster** ☎ 31.88.28.71 | **VHF Channel** 9 |
| **Callsign** Port de Deauville | **Daily charge** ££ |

The yacht harbour in the old basin on the west bank of the river, though called Port de Deauville, is sometimes referred to as being in Trouville. It is within easy reach of the shops in the centre of Deauville and those just over the river. The lock gate is automatically controlled and may not open at neap tides, when it would be wiser to use the marina.

## STEP ASHORE

**Nearest payphone** At south-west corner of basin and by harbourmaster's office
**Toilets** On quay and in yacht club
**Showers** In yacht club
**Clubhouse** Yacht Club de Deauville on Bassin Morny
**Shopping** Small supermarket in Quai de la Touques. If you continue up the road and turn left over the bridge into Trouville you will immediately find yourself in a main shopping area; alternatively cross over the lock gate to Bassin Morny and continue westward via Rue Gambetta to the main shopping district.

### SHIPS' SERVICES

*Water* On visitors' pontoon
*Fuel* Petrol from fuel berth in Bassin Morny; diesel has to be collected in a container from garage supplying fuel berth

*Gas* (Camping and Calor) From supermarket in Rue de la Touques
*Chandler, boatyard, engineer* On Quai Morny

# Marina de Port Deauville

| | |
|---|---|
| **Harbourmaster** ☎ 31.98.30.01 | **VHF Channel** 9 |
| **Callsign** Port Deauville | **Daily charge** ££ |

Port Deauville is a modern marina complex, but the entrance from the town still looks like the bomb-site it once was. It is usefully close to the town: a five-minute walk takes you to the market place, shops and pavement cafés, which are all very attractive. Mooring near the back of the basin is more convenient for the shops and toilet facilities, but there is quite a lot of traffic noise.

## STEP ASHORE

**Toilets, showers, launderette** Below ground level, under the pavement, on the south side of the marina

### SHIPS' SERVICES

*Water and electricity* On the pontoons
*Fuel* (diesel and petrol) From fuel berth to starboard by lock

*Gas, chandler, boatyard, engineer* All in marina complex

# Dives-sur-Mer — Port Guillaume

**Harbourmaster** ☎ 31.91.43.14                    **Daily charge** £££

This new marina at Dives-sur-Mer, between Deauville and Ouistreham, opened in June 1991. It is in a deep water basin with a lock. At the time of the inspection the pontoons were in position with water and electricity available and the shower and toilet block ashore was in operation. It was planned to bring other facilities into use shortly.

Dives-sur-Mer is a small industrial town and the shops and other facilities are some way from the marina. Its main claim to fame is that it was a major port for the launching of William's expedition to conquer England in 1066. Cabourg, on the other side of the River Dives, is an elegant holiday resort associated with Marcel Proust.

# Ouistreham

Ouistreham's main attraction is its proximity to other places. You can motor up the canal to Caen (watch bridge opening times) and stay in Bassin St Pierre right in the heart of the historic town, then go on by train to Bayeux (20 minutes) or even Paris if your holiday is long enough. The fine, sandy beach joins the beaches of Riva-Bella, a popular seaside resort. It is also a safe place to leave a boat and board the ferry to Portsmouth.

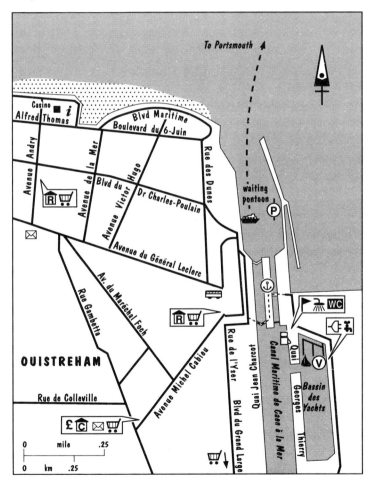

## SHORE LEAVE

*Food and drink*

There are take-aways and restaurants five minutes' walk across the lock area from the marina. Most restaurants are in the square on the west side of the locks. Le Roulis, popular with the French, is good value. The Hôtel Normandie has many awards but is expensive. Le Péniche on the canal provides a very good meal.

*Entertainment*

Le Cabieu cinema, in Avenue Michel Cabieu is in a turn-of-the-century half-timbered building; The casino in Riva-Bella has a night-club.

*What to see*

The only relic of the war is an intact German **blockhouse** between the Place Alfred-Thomas and the harbour. There is a **museum** at **Pegasus Bridge** with memorabilia of the events of June 1944. The bridge is famous because its capture was crucial to the success of the breakout from the beaches. The **church** in Ouistreham dates mainly from the twelfth and thirteenth centuries but has a window commemorating the D-day landings.

*Excursions*

Ouistreham is a good place from which to visit the historic city of **Caen**, either by bus or in your own boat, but check bridge opening times: convoys pass free through the bridges once or twice a day; at other times a charge is levied.

*Exercise*

You can walk along the canal path to the war cemetery and **Pegasus Bridge**, but it is quite a long walk. The sandy beaches of Ouistreham and Riva-Bella are safe for swimming. Windsurf from the beach near the marina.

### TRANSPORT AND TRAVEL

**Buses** From the ferry port to Caen; also a bus from the harbour to the church, which saves walking uphill

**Ferries** To Portsmouth four times a day
**Taxis, car hire** Falaize, 29 Avenue Général Leclerc ☎ 31.97.39.41

**Further information** from tourist offices at the ferry landing and Jardins du Casino.

# Port de Ouistreham

| Harbourmaster ☎ 31.97.14.43 | VHF Channels 16, 12, 68 |
|---|---|
| Callsign Ouistreham | Daily charge £££ |

Once you have managed to survive the crush at the floating pontoon in the outer port waiting area, and got through the lock with most of your varnish intact, you'll find Ouistreham a comfortable place in all weathers. You moor under the trees in a quiet yacht basin alongside the canal, a short walk from a selection of good eating places.

You can motor your boat to the barge restaurant Le Péniche and moor alongside the adjacent quay. There is a lovely view of the canal and the Pegasus Bridge from the restaurant.

## STEP ASHORE

**Nearest payphone** In yacht club; others near slipway on east side of marina, which is useful when the yacht club is closed

**Toilets, showers** At the yacht club, where you will be given the entrance code, which changes weekly

**Clubhouse** In marina, open 0800–1200 and 1430–1800

**Shopping** In the square across the locks including a late-night shop (open 0800–2200) which sells charcuterie. For other shopping areas: cross the lock, turn left and a 10-minute walk up Avenue Michel Cabieu will bring you to a village with a number of shops and a post office; one mile upstream you will find a supermarket near the campsite on the canal

### SHIPS' SERVICES

*Water and electricity* Available on the pontoons

*Fuel* (diesel and petrol) Available on the fuel jetty outside the marina, ask at yacht club for service

*Gas* (Camping and Calor) From the

*chandler* In the marina

*Boatyard* On Caen canal, opposite marina

*Engineer* PL Marine ☎ 31.96.29.92

*Sailmaker* Normandie Voiles
☎ 31.97.06.29

# Caen

Caen, the capital of Lower Normandy, was the favourite town of William the Conqueror. Caen stone from the quarries to the south of the city was used for Canterbury Cathedral and the Tower of London. People sheltered in these quarries during the 1944 bombardment.

Although devastated in the liberation, Caen has been sensitively rebuilt and many fine buildings survive. The castle and the two abbeys are well worth seeing; fortunately neither the Abbaye aux Hommes nor the Abbaye aux Dames was badly bombed and they remain among the most significant buildings in Caen.

There was a considerable English community here during the nineteenth century: Beau Brummel was consul briefly. Today Caen has all the sophistication of a large provincial city with restaurants, bars, night clubs, art galleries and museums.

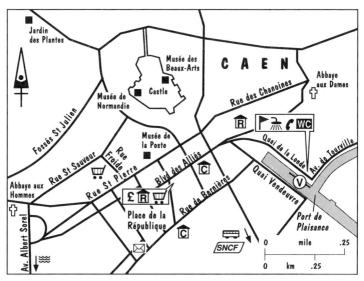

SHORE LEAVE

## Food and drink

From the large variety of restaurants you will have no trouble finding one to suit your taste and purse, especially in the lovely little squares of the Quartier du Vaugueux just north of the basin. La Bourride, 15–17 Rue du Vaugueux (closed Sundays and Mondays), has a reputation as the best restaurant in Normandy.

## Entertainment

La Halle aux Grange in Rue Pasteur is the home of a national ballet company. There are three cinemas, a municipal theatre and a casino.

## What to see

Rooted in 1,000 years of history, Caen has plenty of atmosphere and plenty to see. The castle was built in 1060 by William the Conqueror and he and his queen

Matilda founded the two abbeys. The City Hall is in the **Abbaye aux Hommes**, where William is buried; local government offices occupy the **Abbaye aux Dames** where Matilda is buried. William and Matilda were cousins and founded the two abbeys to earn papal dispensation for their marriage. The flamboyantly ornate Gothic church of St Pierre stands between the two.

The **Musée de Normandie** houses the folklore of Norman life – Romans, Vikings, agriculture and costume; the modern **Musée des Beaux Arts** has a large collection of paintings, including good Flemish and Italian Primitives, a beach scene by Boudin and water-lilies by Monet. The **Musée de la Poste** at 52 Rue St Pierre gives you a chance to play with French information technology. Lastly a world 'first', the **Musée pour la Paix** (museum for peace) in Esplanade Dwight Eisenhower, is a moving exposition of the effects of war, with the driving message that it must not happen again. Sixteenth-century half-timbered houses with steep gables line Rue St Pierre. The **botanical gardens** in Avenue de Creully are pleasant to wander in.

*Excursions*
**Bayeux**, another ancient town with plenty of interest, is only 17 miles from Caen, and easily reached by bus or train. It makes a very pleasant day's excursion. You could spend an hour or two looking at the famous Bayeux Tapestry and then explore the medieval streets. Lacemaking is also a feature of Bayeux, and the craft is demonstrated for tourists.

### TRANSPORT AND TRAVEL

**Buses** To Ouistreham and Bayeux
**Trains** To Cherbourg, Paris, Bayeux
**Planes** To Jersey from Caen airport in summer

**Ferries** To Portsmouth from Ouistreham
**Taxis, car hire** Abbeilles Taxis
☎ 31.52.17.89
**Bicycle hire** From SNCF station

*Further information* from tourist office at Hôtel d'Escoville in Boulevard des Alliés in the town centre.

# Port de Caen

**Harbourmaster** ☎ 31.52.12.88      **Daily charge** ££

The small marina in Bassin St Pierre, mainly for locals but adequate, is welcoming and not expensive. It is in a basin surrounded by busy roads which on a Sunday morning become part of the all-pervasive market.

### STEP ASHORE

**Nearest payphone** At north end of basin
**Toilets, showers, launderette** Behind the capitainerie

**Shopping** Small shops near the basin; the town centre is half a mile to the north-west

### SHIPS' SERVICES

*Water and electricity* Available on the pontoons
*Fuel* (diesel and petrol) Has to be

collected from the garage near marina in cans; it is easier to fill up in Ouistreham

# Courseulles

Courseulles is a simple holiday resort – a place to stop and potter. Sheltered by the mouth of the Seulles River, the port was used by British and Canadian forces before the Mulberry Harbour was established off Arromanches. Winston Churchill landed here on 12 June 1944 and Charles de Gaulle two days later. In settled weather you can sail along the coast to the Mulberry Harbour and anchor for lunch or a night.

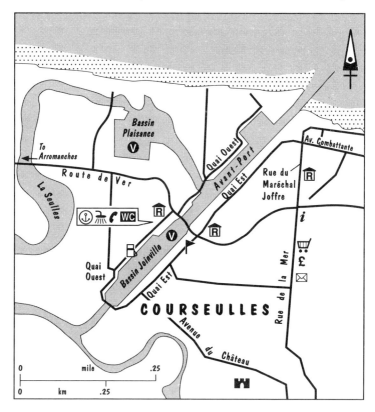

SHORE LEAVE

### Food and drink

Restaurants and take-aways are mainly situated at the seaward end of the main street. The Belle Aurore, by the lock, is well known and recommended for its seafood, particularly oysters.

### What to see

Courseulles, famous for oysters, offers guided visits of its **oyster farm**, where you can buy oysters; apply to Maison Hérault. The **aquarium** and **shellfish museum** on the east side of the harbour entrance has a display of oyster culture.

*Excursion*
Visit **Arromanches** to see the **D-Day Museum**.

*Exercise*
Courseulles beaches are good for swimming and windsurfing, and the heated seawater swimming pool is popular too.

### TRANSPORT AND TRAVEL

**Buses** From railway station to Caen and along the coast to Arromanches

**Trains** To Paris
**Taxis, car hire** ☎ 31.96.54.07

*Further information* from tourist office on corner of Rue de la Mer.

# Bassin Joinville

| | |
|---|---|
| **Harbourmaster** ☎ 31.37.51.69 | **VHF Channel** 9 |
| **Callsign** Courseulles | **Daily charge** ££ |

At busy times entrance to this little fishing port is very crowded, with everyone making for the lock into Bassin Joinville. The small yacht harbour is really intended for regulars, many of whom commute from Paris. Visitors are made very welcome, however, and if there is no room on the east quay, they are slotted into temporarily vacant berths on the west side. Part of the mooring fee is then credited to the permanent berth holder, a custom sadly unobserved elsewhere. The facilities are quite simple. If possible, avoid the new yacht harbour to starboard of the outer harbour: it is small, shallow and surrounded by blocks of flats.

### STEP ASHORE

**Nearest payphone** On quay opposite capitainerie
**Toilets, showers, launderette** In capitainerie
**Clubhouse** Société des Régates, on the east side of basin opposite the berths, is very welcoming

**Shopping** All shops are a quarter of a mile to the east over the bridge, where there is a good selection of small high-street shops plus banks and a post office. Markets on Tuesdays and Fridays in the main shopping street

### SHIPS' SERVICES

*Water, electricity, fuel* (diesel and petrol) Available on the quay
*Gas* (Camping and Calor) From the

*chandler* on Quai Ouest
*Boatyard, engineer* On Quai Ouest

# Grandcamp-Maisy

Grandcamp-Maisy is a fishing port that encourages tourists and is popular with yachtsmen. It is also a pleasant family seaside town with fairground fun for children of all ages, and beaches with rock pools.

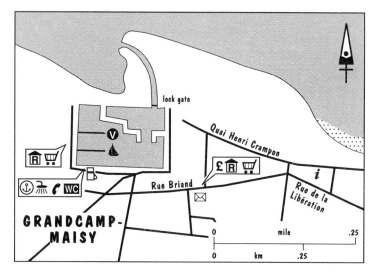

## SHORE LEAVE

There are several good restaurants and take-aways near the harbour and in town. Look out for seafood restaurants. This small resort is essentially a place where the sun and sea can be enjoyed. The beach at the other end of town is good for swimming and windsurfing and has rock pools at low tide. You can stretch your legs along the seafront and walk through the sand dunes.

### TRANSPORT AND TRAVEL

**Buses** To Bayeux and Isigny-sur-Mer     de Plaisance office or tourist office for
**Taxis, car and bicycle hire** Ask at the Port     details

*Further information* from tourist office on the east promenade in the summer; from the Mairie in winter.

## Port de Grandcamp-Maisy

| | |
|---|---|
| **Harbourmaster** ☎ 31.22.63.16 | **VHF Channel** 9 |
| **Callsign** Grandcamp | **Daily charge** ££ |

Approached over a long, drying foreshore, Grandcamp-Maisy offers several visitors' places on the long pontoons inside the lock gates. The harbourmaster is always pleased to see English visitors.

## STEP ASHORE

**Nearest payphone, toilets, showers, launderette** Behind office of Port de Plaisance

**Shopping** Late-night shop on the west quay, open till 2000, sells fruit and basic necessities. The main shops are on the east side of the harbour, a 10-minute walk away, where there are banks and a post office. A fish, fruit and vegetable market is held on the quayside on Saturday mornings

### SHIPS' SERVICES

**Water and electricity** Available on pontoons

**Fuel** (diesel and petrol) Both have to be collected in cans from the garage at the back of the harbour

**Gas** (Camping and Calor) From 3 Rue de Petit Maisy

**Chandler** Two near the marina

# Iles St Marcouf

St Marcouf was a sixth-century saint who lived on these islands; there are two, which look like ships at anchor, though a third appears at low water. The islands were occupied by the English from 1793 until 1802 and inhabited until 1914. It is fun to visit the islands for a picnic in good weather while on passage or on a day trip from one of the ports in this corner of the Baie de la Seine; they are not suitable for overnight stops. The best anchorage is between Ile de Terre (a bird sanctuary where landing is forbidden) and Ile du Large, but remember the tide runs fast in this channel and swimming is dangerous. Ile du Large has a navigation light and the ruins of a fort which can be explored. There are no facilities at all so take everything you will need for the day.

# Carentan

Carentan is a very pleasant town with all amenities at hand. The fifteenth-century church and ancient arches along one pavement in town convey the feeling of its medieval origins. Although at the heart of the dairy industry, it is a restful place and highly recommended as a change from St Vaast-la-Hougue, which is crowded on public holidays in summer, or Grandcamp-Maisy, which, being a fishing port, is often smelly and noisy.

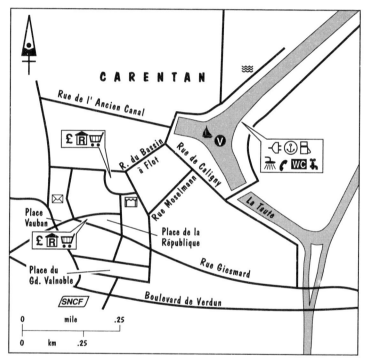

SHORE LEAVE

### Food and drink
Restaurants are not plentiful. The one nearest the marina is expensive and not particularly good; restaurants in town are better.

### Entertainment
There is a cinema and a theatre.

### What to see
The **church of Notre-Dame**, first built during the eleventh and twelfth centuries and rebuilt in the fifteenth century, has a dominating octagonal spire and chancel enclosed by a Renaissance screen and is worth close inspection. There are old houses with inner courtyards, seventeenth-century mansions, a medieval covered market and an attractive Town Hall, originally built as a convent.

*Exercise*

Walk along the banks of the canal or hire a bike and cycle through the lanes; it is all very flat. Carentan is developing as a tourist centre and caters for horse-riding and tennis. There is an open air swimming pool and a jogging trail near the marina.

## TRANSPORT AND TRAVEL

**Buses** From Rue du Dr Caillard to Cherbourg

**Trains** To Paris (two-and-a-half hours) and Cherbourg

**Car hire, taxis** ☎ 33.42.04.55

**Bicycle hire** Marcel Hardy, 33 Rue 101e Airborne

*Further information* from the Town Hall in Boulevard de Verdun.

# Port de Carentan

| | |
|---|---|
| **Harbourmaster** ☎ 33.42.24.44 | **VHF Channel** 9 |
| **Callsign** Carentan | **Daily charge** ££ |

The locked-in marina at Carentan is converted from an old cargo port and is about a quarter of a mile from the town. Berths are numerous, and usually visitors are placed near the town end of the marina. It is rustic and very sheltered and you feel as though you are in the country rather than by the sea. From the sea the approach is along a four-and-a-half-mile canal which dries out, for most boats, except for two and a half hours each side of high water. The passage along the canal, which was built by Napoleon, is pleasant, with pastoral banks on either side and, when the wind serves, is a treat to sail up, or down. Japanese weed floats up the canal on the flood and ends up in the lock; sometimes propellors are so fouled up that boats have to be towed and invariably propellors have to be cleared once berthed.

## STEP ASHORE

**Nearest payphone** Outside harbourmaster's office

**Toilets, showers, laundry facilities** Available 0600–2000; all free and very clean

**Shopping** The town, which is five to ten minutes' walk away, claims to have 160 shops; there are banks and a post office

## SHIPS' SERVICES

*Water and electricity* On pontoons

*Fuel* (diesel and petrol) Available in marina

*Gas* Camping Gaz can be bought in town

*Chandler, boatyard* In the marina

# St Vaast-la-Hougue

St Vaast, now a fishing port, was once a base of the French fleet. Evidence remains in the form of the seventeenth-century Fort de la Hougue at the end of the peninsula to the south and on the island of Tatihou to the east.

Although St Vaast is increasingly popular with English yachtsmen – indeed, it is the best port in the western half of the Baie de la Seine – there is no easy access to trains, planes or ferries for crew changes; transport by bus is of the twice-a-week variety. It is a pleasant but quiet town.

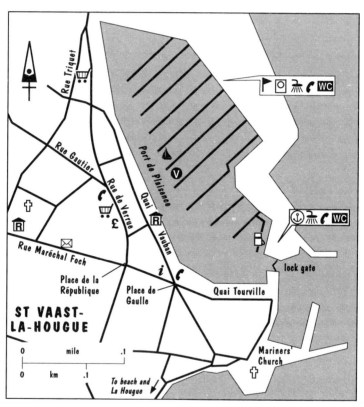

SHORE LEAVE

### Food and drink
Most of St Vaast's restaurants and bars are on the quayside. L'Escale, which specialises in seafood, is especially recommended. The setting of Les Fuchsias in Rue Maréchal Foch is very attractive, and if you choose carefully you can enjoy a good meal here.

*What to see/excursions*

Visit the **Chapelle des Pêcheurs** (the mariners' church) and the **church**. Between St Vaast and Barfleur is a beautiful sixteenth-century manor, **La Crasvillerie**, which is open to visitors. The bus to **Barfleur** goes there. Twice a week there is a bus to **Cherbourg** and back, which is useful for a day visit or to catch a ferry.

*Exercise*

Walk to and round the outside of **Fort de la Hougue**; walk to Tatihou at low tide or go by dinghy when there is enough water. There is a remand home on the island, but walking round the shore is not forbidden. The **Grande-Plage**, a mile-long beach to the south of St Vaast, is safe to swim from; you can also windsurf there. Hire a cycle and visit some of the villages inland or cycle along the coast road.

## TRANSPORT AND TRAVEL

**Buses** To Cherbourg and Barfleur stop on quay

**Car hire** From 34 Rue des Paumiers ☎ 33.54.40.29

**Taxis** 22 Rue de Choisy ☎ 33.54.58.08

**Bicycle hire** Garage Fesnien, 13 Rue Triquet ☎ 33.54.43.08

*Further information* from tourist office at the south-west corner of Quai Vauban.

# Port de St Vaast-la-Hougue

| | |
|---|---|
| **Harbourmaster** ☎ 33.54.48.81 | **VHF Channel** 9 |
| **Callsign** St Vaast | **Daily charge** ££ |

In the 1980s the old fishing harbour was enclosed to form a marina. Fishing boats moor in the west of the harbour and pleasure boats in the east. As you enter, a board is held up with the letter of your pontoon for berthing. The atmosphere is very welcoming and the marina itself is generally pleasant with good facilities.

## STEP ASHORE

**Nearest payphone** On sea wall, in yacht club and capitainerie

**Toilets, showers, launderette** In yacht club; also toilets and showers in capitainerie

**Clubhouse** On quay

**Shopping** One block back from quayside, about five or ten minutes' walk from the marina, is a 8-à-huit supermarket, baker and fish shop. M. Gosselin, on the corner of Rue de Verrue and Rue Gautier, runs a very superior, but not expensive, grocery; he roasts and grinds fresh coffee beans and has an awe-inspiring wine cellar from which he will deliver your duty-free purchases in a reproduction 1910 Rolls Royce van. Excellent oysters can be bought in Rue des Chantiers. Market on Saturday mornings in the main shopping streets

### SHIPS' SERVICES

*Water and electricity* On pontoons

*Fuel* (diesel and petrol) From fuelling berth on the pontoon under the capitainerie by lock entrance

*Gas* (Camping and Calor) By Chapelle des Pêcheurs where there are also basic *chandlery* and *boatyard* facilities

# Barfleur

Barfleur is an attractive town with a history going back to Roman times. It was an embarkation port for William the Conqueror's fleet in 1066, commemorated by a bronze plaque on a rock at the foot of the jetty. In 1120 a gallant company consisting of Henry I's young sons and daughter and 300 nobles perished in the *White Ship* which hit a rock and sank just offshore from here, having set sail with a crew which had celebrated too well earlier in the evening. Henry is said never to have smiled again after hearing the news.

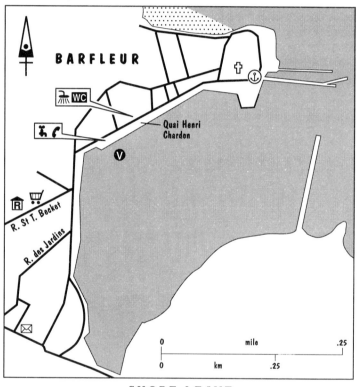

SHORE LEAVE

The rather sombre **seventeenth-century church** overlooking the harbour contains a notable sixteenth-century *pietà*. Walk to **Phare de la Pointe de Barfleur** at **Gatteville**, two-and-a-half miles from Barfleur; it is one of the tallest lighthouses in France, and is open to the public.

## TRANSPORT AND TRAVEL

**Buses** To Cherbourg and to St Vaast          **Car hire** 33.54.43.64
**Taxis** ☎ 33.54.58.08

*Further information* from the capitainerie.

# Port de Barfleur

| Harbourmaster ☎ 33.54.08.29 | VHF Channel 9 |
|---|---|
| Callsign Barfleur | Daily charge £ |

Once a busy fishing port, Barfleur is now increasingly dependent on tourists. It has a simple but large drying harbour with no modern developments. The harbourmaster may direct you to a suitable berth on the quay wall.

## STEP ASHORE

**Nearest payphone, toilets, showers** On the quay; shower and toilet facilities are fairly primitive

**Shopping** The shops in the street to the west of harbour, Rue St Thomas Becket, will supply most needs

### SHIPS' SERVICES

*Water and electricity* On the quay
*Fuel* (diesel and petrol) Can be collected in cans from the garage
*Engineer* M. Boudin

# Cherbourg

First-time visitors to Cherbourg are always impressed by its huge harbour, built during the eighteenth and nineteenth centuries to help keep the English away. Nowadays the town is geared to receive the English on passage to points south as well as day-trippers and sailors. There are many enjoyable shops and restaurants and for those interested in art and history much else to see, such as the friezes and column decorations in the Basilica of Trinity Church in the Place de la République or the paintings and sculptures in the Musée Thomas-Henry behind the theatre. The old town is pleasant to wander through or you can walk further afield – perhaps climb the Montagne du Roule for a commanding view of Cherbourg and its harbour and a visit to the Liberation Museum.

## SHORE LEAVE

### Food and drink
There is a restaurant in the marina complex and many others of all kinds in the town. Try Le Grand Cerf in Rue de l'Onglet for good value. Look out for the wide choice of local dishes: Normandy is renowned for its fish, cheese, cream, calvados and cider.

### Entertainment
Concerts and plays take place at the municipal theatre in the Place Général de Gaulle. There are four cinemas.

### What to see
As well as the **Thomas-Henry Museum** behind the theatre, with its sixteenth to nineteenth-century paintings and sculptures and collection of portraits by Millet, there is the **Fort du Roule Museum of Liberation** above the town. The **Parc Botanique Emmanuel-Liais** has a **Natural History Museum** and **botanical gardens**.

### Excursions
Out of town is the **Nez de Jobourg** – a wild promontory where you can walk and enjoy views of **Cap de la Hague** to the north and the Channel Islands to the west. Cap de la Hague itself can be explored or you could visit the La Hague **Atomic Power Station** exhibition which is open to the public 1400–1900 daily. The gardens of the **Château de Tourlaville** are worth a visit, as is the **Maritime Museum** three miles away; Ligne 1 bus goes there.

### Exercise
Cherbourg lacks beaches to swim from, but there is a swimming pool in the Chantereyne leisure centre close to the marina; you can windsurf from the Centre Nautique.

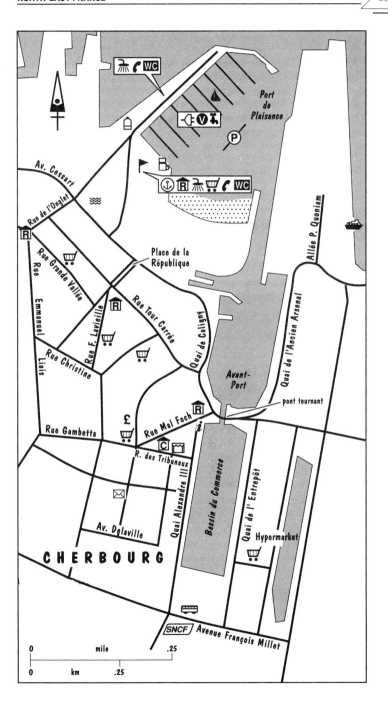

Port de Plaisance

Av. Cessart

Rue de l'Onglet

Rue Grande Vallée

Rue Emmanuel Liais

Rue

Rue F. Lavieille

Rue Christine

Place de la République

Rue Tour Carrée

Quai de Caligny

Rue Gambetta

Rue Mal Foch

R. des Tribunaux

Quai Alexandre III

Av. Delaville

Quai de l'Ancien Arsenal

Allée P. Quoniam

Avant-Port

pont tournant

Bassin du Commerce

Quai de l' Entrepôt

Hypermarket

**CHERBOURG**

SNCF  Avenue François Millet

0            mile            .25

0      km      .25

## TRANSPORT AND TRAVEL

**Buses** From Place Jaunes at head of Bassin du Commerce
**Trains** Frequent service to Paris, also to Carentan and Granville
**Planes** From airport at Maupertus to Bournemouth and the Channel Islands

**Ferries** From Gare Maritime to Portsmouth, Poole, Weymouth and Rosslare
**Taxis** Allo Taxi ☎ 33.53.36.38
**Car hire** Europcar, 4 Rue des Tanneries ☎ 33.44.53.85

*Further information* from Tourist Office, 2 Quai Alexandre III, at the south-west corner of the Avant-Port.

# Port de Chantereyne

| **Harbourmaster** ☎ 33.53.75.16 | **VHF Channel** 16 |
|---|---|
| **Callsign** Port Chantereyne | **Daily charge** ££ |

Cherbourg has a large, adequate but impersonal marina. Visitors are usually accommodated on the first three pontoons to starboard on entering the marina, but at busy times they are put on a detached pontoon, rafting up. From there it is necessary to go ashore by dinghy. Multihulls and bilge keelers can anchor in the marina clear of the pontoons. It is also possible to anchor just outside the marina in La Petite Rade or in La Grande Rade, Baie de Ste Anne.

## STEP ASHORE

**Nearest payphone** Near head of pontoon ramps
**Toilets** On quay, open 24 hours a day; **showers** 0900–1145 and 1400–1700; also toilets and showers in capitainerie, open 0800–2300
**Clubhouse** Over capitainerie
**Shopping** In the marina complex, including a duty-free shop and a small grocery selling bread, milk and fruit. For the main shopping area, walk due south

via Rue de l'Onglet to Rue de l'Union (about half to three-quarters of a mile) where there are all the facilities of a large town. There is a small supermarket in Rue de l'Union and a hypermarket on the east side of the Boulevard du Commerce which is popular with English holidaymakers. Local produce from the country can be bought in the markets held on Tuesdays, Thursdays and Saturdays in Place Général de Gaulle

### SHIPS' SERVICES

*Water and electricity* On every pontoon
*Fuel* (diesel and petrol) On the quay by the capitainerie

*Gas* (Camping and Calor) *chandler, boatyard, engineer, sailmaker* All available in the marina complex

# Omonville-la-Rogue

This small harbour between Cherbourg and Cap de la Hague often has a swell and it can be rough in winds east of north, in spite of which it is often crowded. There are two large white mooring buoys for visitors, who must secure bow or stern to a buoy. It is a useful place to spend a night in calm weather. Omonville does not offer a great deal to see or do ashore except stretch your legs. The thirteenth-century church has some mementoes of its ancient association with Canterbury and St Thomas à Becket.

There are few facilities ashore apart from a water tap near the public toilets, a telephone in the café, a bar and a restaurant; all are on the quay. About a mile along the road, past the church, is a village shop selling basic necessities such as bread, wine and cheese. It is safe to swim from the beach and pleasant to walk along the shore or inland.

# THE CHANNEL ISLANDS

# Alderney

Alderney is a flat-topped, grassy island, about four miles by two. Most of the 2,300 population live in St Anne, the capital of Alderney and its only town. Although more a village by English standards, this is the hub of the island's activities, the home of the administration and commercial centres. It is where you will find most of the hotels and the surprisingly wide range of shops. There is a church and a 'village green' called the Butes. The name suggests that it was once an archery ground where early protectors of the island may have practised their skills. Prehistoric burial sites, destroyed by builders in the last century, bore witness to the island's even earlier habitation by primitive man. An Iron Age site on Longis Common remains. Aurigny, the ancient name for Alderney, is remembered in the name of the airport and the island's airline.

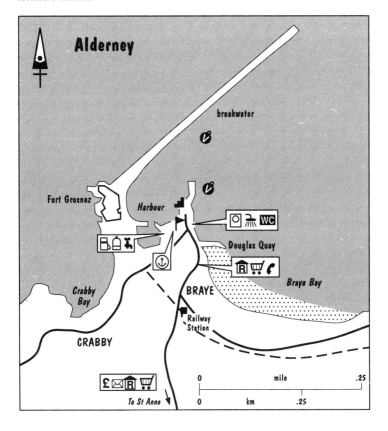

There are also houses and shops at Braye. Braye Harbour was built as a naval base in the nineteenth century to hold the whole British fleet. Two-thirds of the breakwater survive and shelter the moorings.

The island has a little industry and some agriculture, but its mainstay is tourism. Visitors always leave with a very high opinion of Alderney, its people and the services it offers. The islanders take a pride in helping you out of any difficulty.

## SHORE LEAVE

### Food and drink
Pubs are open from 1000 to midnight (Monday to Saturday). The Braye Chippy near the harbour is popular with starving crews. There are also several restaurants nearby: the Moorings Hotel and Bar, the First and Last Restaurant and the Sea View Hotel; however, it is worth putting an edge on your appetite by walking up the hill to St Anne and trying Nellie Gray's, which is recommended but expensive, or the Georgian House Hotel; both are in Victoria Street. Local crab and lobster are Alderney specialities. Unfortunately, it is not easy to find a simple, economical meal out unless you settle for fish and chips.

### Entertainment
Films are regularly shown at the small cinema in St Anne and there are occasional theatrical performances at local halls.

The first week in August is **Alderney Week**, the island's festival week, featuring a cavalcade, sailing regattas, windsurfing competitions, barbecues, fireworks and much more.

### What to see
The **Alderney Museum** in the Old School, Lower High Street, St Anne, is open every morning and on Tuesday and Sunday afternoons. It houses a well-displayed collection covering archaeology, geology and Alderney's domestic, marine and military history from Roman times to the present day. A natural history room displays flora and fauna.

**Alderney Pottery**, just off Royal Connaught Square, demonstrates not only pottery but spinning and weaving and has an attractive coffee and tea shop. St Anne has charming cobbled streets to explore and a well-designed modern church.

### Excursions
**Alderney Railway**, now a scenic railway, was built to haul stone from Mannez quarry to the harbour to build the breakwater. It has steam and diesel locomotives and runs on Wednesdays, at weekends and on bank holidays, from Easter until the end of September. The short trip is particularly enjoyable for its unusual views of the island.

On **Raz Island**, in the middle of Longis Bay, a Victorian fort houses the **Bird Museum** (closed on Mondays) – access is across a causeway when it is not covered by tide. Guided tours of Alderney are organised by Alderney Tours and Leisure Group, Braye Street ☎ (0481) 822611/822992 and Belle Vue Taxis, Victoria Street ☎ (0481) 822138.

Take an organised boat trip to visit bird sanctuaries at **Burhou** and **Little Burhou** and to see gannet and puffin colonies at **Les Etacs** and **Ortac**.

*Exercise*

No part of Alderney is much more than fifteen minutes' walk from a good beach. The beaches are rarely crowded and many are excellent for swimming. **Braye Bay**, with its long stretches of sand, is perhaps the best. **Saye Bay**, next to Braye, has a fine sandy beach and interesting rock outcrops.

**Corblets** and **Arch Bays** on the north coast are recommended for safe swimming; at Corblets sailboard, wet-suit hire and instruction are available. Longis Bay on the east coast is attractive for its seapools and shrimps, but beware of the strong tidal streams.

You can complete a circuit of Alderney on foot in a day. Walks along cliff paths, headlands and inland, where wild flowers, heather and gorse grow, are peaceful but there is a sense of sadness when one remembers that so much of the island has been a burial ground from neolithic times to the Second World War.

## TRANSPORT AND TRAVEL

**Buses** Daily round-the-island bus service and to main beaches in summer. Timetables are available from the Information Bureau at the harbour; services start from Marais Square

**Planes** Aurigny airport is one-and-a-half miles south of the harbour. Flights go to Cherbourg, Dinard, Guernsey, Jersey, Bournemouth, Southampton and Shoreham

**Ferries** Direct service to Torquay once a week during the summer. A hydrofoil service goes to Jersey, Guernsey, Sark, Weymouth and St Malo

**Water-taxi** Operated by Mainbrayce, fare £1 (more if only one person travelling); VHF channel M or 12, or wave

**Taxis, car hire** Alderney Taxis ☎ (0481) 822611/822992

**Bicycle hire** Pedal Power at the bottom of Victoria Street ☎ (0481) 822286

*Further information* from States Tourist Information Office on first floor of main States building in Queen Elizabeth II Street, open 0900–1230 and 1400–1700; also from Information Bureau at the harbour. A map and information about location of shops, and restaurants, including their opening hours, phone numbers and addresses are displayed on a noticeboard by the showers.

# Braye Harbour

| | |
|---|---|
| **Harbourmaster** ☎ (0481) 822620 | **VHF Channel** 74, 16 |
| **Callsign** Alderney Radio | **Daily charge** ££ |

Braye Harbour, on the north coast, is the only safe anchorage for small craft. You must have the harbourmaster's permission before beaching craft in Braye or Saye Bays or anchoring in Braye Bay. There is no marina or traditional harbour here for visiting yachts but a roadstead with some 70 visitors' mooring buoys, plenty of anchoring space and an efficient but expensive water-taxi service. The harbour is very uncomfortable in a north-easter but is quite secure if chain warps are used. The harbour staff are invariably helpful.

Do remember that it is necessary to fly a yellow flag when arriving in

Alderney, whether from the UK, France or another Channel Island. You are required to register within two hours of arrival at the Harbour Office just above the dinghy slip.

## STEP ASHORE

**Nearest payphone** Outside First and Last Restaurant in Braye Street, 50 yards from harbour steps

**Toilets, showers, launderette** In services building near Commercial Quay

**Clubhouse** Alderney Sailing Club above the harbour is very welcoming. Coffee is served in the morning, tea and cakes at tea time. There is a bar

**Shopping** Several shops in Braye Street, near the harbour, including a well-stocked grocery and a general store open on Sunday mornings. The main shopping centre is in St Anne, approximately three-quarters of a mile from the harbour and steeply uphill. Early closing Wednesdays. No shops stay open late. Alderney has a wide range of shops for its size, four UK clearing banks in St Anne and a post office (in Victoria Street). Banks are closed on the first Monday in May and the first Monday in August as well as on the usual UK bank holidays. Channel Jumpers Ltd, near the harbour, operates a bureau de change. Postbox near the harbour

### SHIPS' SERVICES

**Water, fuel** Although it is possible to tie up alongside, temporarily, two hours either side of high water in the inner harbour (Little Crabby Harbour) for fuel and water, conditions are often difficult and crowded, and arrangements to do so should be made with the Harbourmaster's Office. A charge is made for the use of the water hose. It is advisable to use carry-cans wherever possible and transport by water-taxi. Small quantities of water may be drawn, free of charge, from the stand pipe at the top of the dinghy slip.

**Fuel, gas** Diesel and Calor Gas can be obtained from Mainbrayce Marine Ltd by the inner harbour, as can **chandlery** and **boatyard** and **engineering** needs. Diesel, petrol and Camping Gaz are available from Riduna Garage, Braye Street. Petrol and Camping Gaz are sold by Alderney Stores & Bunkering Co, in Braye Street

**Rubbish** Refuse bins are provided at the top of the dinghy slip

# Guernsey

Further west and more exposed to south-westerly winds than the other Channel Islands, this seven-by-three-mile island seems much larger because of its hilly terrain. Many of the older houses are built from Guernsey stone, a warm, pink granite particularly attractive when glimpsed half-hidden in wooded valleys.

Like all the Channel Islands, Guernsey is very conscious of its allegiance to the Duke of Normandy – currently better known as Queen Elizabeth II. Many old customs survive, such as the *clameur de haro*, by which a guernseyais can, by standing in the street and calling for the aid of *'mon duc'*, stop whatever his neighbour is doing until a hearing can be arranged in court.

Guernsey shares with the other Channel Islands a history stemming from the remote past, as its neolithic remnants show. Remains of Roman buildings in St Peter Port and sunken Roman ships off the harbour have

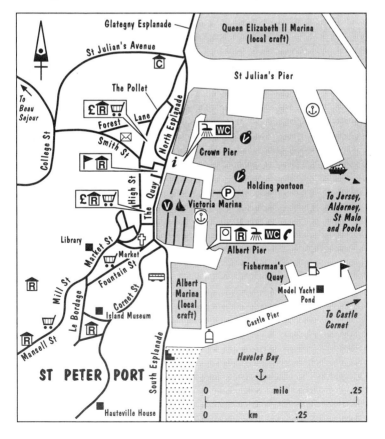

recently come to light and they should be on view after conservation. Several books on Guernsey's history have been published and are on sale in the bookshops. A quiet browse in the Guille-Alles Library in Market Street is particularly informative. St Peter Port, a safe harbour on the east coast established 900 years ago, is the main town.

## SHORE LEAVE

### Food and drink
Although concentrated in St Peter Port, there are restaurants to suit all tastes and pockets throughout Guernsey. Many specialise in locally caught seafood. L'Alchimie in Le Marchant House, Market Street, has a wide range of fish dishes, and is recommended for its very good set Sunday lunch. Café du Moulin in St Peter's Parish is a bit different from the usual run of restaurants: it is in a lovely valley setting away from the sea, and is suitable for a special occasion or a casual lunch (open for lunch and dinner from Tuesday to Saturday). A generous lunchtime buffet is served at the Wellington Boot in the Hotel de Havelet in Havelet, the road leading up the hill from the southern end of South Esplanade.

### Entertainment
Plays, films, concerts and discos all take place at Beau Sejour Leisure Centre.

### What to see
In St Peter Port, Victor Hugo's **Hauteville House**, 38 Hauteville, displays an intriguing record of the writer's partly self-imposed 15-year exile on Guernsey. **Castle Cornet**, with its view of the islands of Herm and Sark and museums of island history and military uniforms, provides an absorbing few hours. **The Guernsey Museum and Art Gallery** is in Candie Gardens, which are attractive to walk in. There is an **aquarium** at Havelet Bay.

### Excursions
Out of town, in St Martin's Parish, a short bus ride from St Peter Port, you can visit the **Guernsey Folk Museum** in the stables of **Sausmarez Manor**. Offshore, **Fort Grey** in **Rocquaine Bay** houses a maritime museum. Day trips are available to **Alderney, Herm, Sark, Jersey, St Malo** and, for that matter, the UK. There is so much to do in Guernsey that you should take a few minutes to read the excellent *Yachtsmen's Guide to Guernsey* which the friendly harbour staff will have given you.

### Exercise
Guernsey is an island of contrasts, with something for everyone, from beautiful beaches and countryside to a history which has left its marks from the stone age to the German occupation. Take walks on the cliffs or in the lanes (beware of traffic): everywhere you will find flowers, both wild and cultivated. For a start, take the walk along the cliffs southwards to **Jerbourg** and **Petit Port**. The way is through woods with views down into the bays, and the possibility of a dip or a cup of tea on the way at Fermain Bay. At this point, if your energy is flagging, you can return to St Peter Port in the Fermain boat or walk up the hill and catch a bus. The beaches are safe for swimming but it is wise to choose your beach according to the wind direction. In the south and east the beaches are shingle, the bays sheltered by high cliffs from prevailing westerlies, but the descent to them is steep. Sandy beaches and a flat, grassy hinterland on the long north-west coast can be enjoyed in settled weather and when the wind is in the east.

At Beau Sejour, a modern leisure centre, you can roller-skate, do aerobics, swim or luxuriate in a sauna.

## TRANSPORT AND TRAVEL

**Buses** Run all over the island from the terminus on South Esplanade; a timetable is available from the Piquet House
**Planes** From Guernsey airport (the bus takes about 20 minutes) to 16 UK airports including Heathrow, Gatwick, Southampton and Bournemouth as well as to Alderney, Jersey and Cherbourg
**Ferries** To Poole, Torquay, Cherbourg, Jersey and St Malo; hydrofoil to Weymouth, Alderney, Sark, Jersey and St Malo
**Taxis** From rank behind town church
**Car hire** Plenty of car hire firms and rates are cheap; the easiest to contact is Falles from freephone in amenity block lobby on Albert Pier; it is advisable to book in high season. Remember that there is no petrol or garage service on Sundays
**Bicycle hire** Moullins, St Georges Esplanade ☎ (0481) 21581

*Further information* from Tourist Office on Crown Pier.

# St Peter Port

| | |
|---|---|
| **Harbourmaster** ☎ (0481) 720229 | **VHF Channel** 12, 78 |
| **Callsign** St Peter Port Radio | **Daily charge** £££ |

On a sunny day the entry to St Peter Port is very inviting: with the islands of Herm and Sark in the haze behind you, the town comes clearly into view as you enter between the pier heads. You can either moor in the outer harbour, which is restless and entails going ashore by dinghy, or you can go into the Victoria Marina, which is convenient, but usually means being moored several deep with the attendant comings and goings and the traffic and crowds nearby. The marina staff are very welcoming and helpful.

St Peter Port marina is in the heart of the town, with old buildings rising up the hill behind and a mixture of modern shops and old ones in cobbled lanes to explore. Don't be too carried away by the shopping. Although prices are VAT-free they are very similar to those in mainland UK so you will lose out on some items if you take them home and have to pay duty. Spirits are a good buy, but wine is best bought in France.

## STEP ASHORE

**Nearest payphone** In amenity block on Albert Pier

**Toilets** In amenity block; open 0700–2200

**Showers** In amenity block; open 0700–2000

**Launderette** Beside marina office; open 24 hours

**Clubhouse** Royal Channel Island Yacht Club on the Quay opposite the Crown Pier and the Guernsey Yacht Club on Castle Emplacement both welcome visitors for drinks and snack meals

**Shopping** The main shopping area is on the Quay and in the streets just behind. There are shops of all types, from UK chainstores to local ones, such as Le Lievre for hardware, Gruts for cameras

and Marquands for chandlery. Le Riches in the High Street is the nearest supermarket to the harbour. In Glategny Esplanade a mini-supermarket is open till 2000 every day. Les Halles is a very large covered market behind the town church which sells every kind of food, local and imported. On Thursday afternoons the market closes and the streets fill with stallholders in Victorian dress selling local arts and crafts. There is another fish market on Castle Emplacement, particularly good for buying cooked local crabs. Shops cannot sell alcohol on Sundays

**Food and drink** Several take-aways as well as a wide choice of restaurants

### SHIPS' SERVICES

*Water* On pontoons or quayside

*Fuel (diesel and petrol)* From fuelling berth at Castle Emplacement during office hours Monday to Saturday and on Sunday mornings

*Gas (Camping and Calor)* from Herm Seaway, and from Boatworks +, both on Castle Emplacement

*Chandler* Herm Seaway and Boatworks +

*Boatyard, engineer, sailmaker* Boatworks +

# Beaucette Marina

| Harbourmaster ☎ (0481) 45000 | VHF Channel 80, M |
|---|---|
| Callsign Beaucette Marina | Daily charge £££ |

Beaucette Marina was created from a disused quarry by blasting the narrow barrier of rock which separated it from the sea to make the entrance. The result is a small, attractive and well-sheltered marina. Facilities are good and the staff helpful and friendly – anything not on-site will be sent for. In itself the marina is a pleasant spot, although a little bleak in bad weather or north-west winds. However, it is out of the way of all the island activities and interests and a hire car (remarkably cheap in Guernsey) or bicycles are essential if you are staying any length of time. The main attractions are the quietness, compared with a berth in St Peter Port, and its position in the north-east corner of the island so that on departure the best advantage can be taken of the north-running tide for Alderney and England.

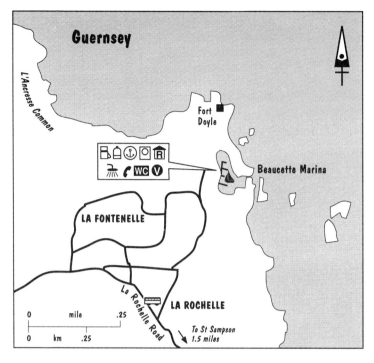

## STEP ASHORE

**Nearest payphone** On pontoon or at marina office

**Toilets and showers** In block to north of restaurant; open 24 hours a day

**Launderette** (with drying area) At bottom of the main gangway on to pontoons

**Shopping** The marina shop stocks groceries and is licensed. The nearest main shopping is in St Sampson, a two-and-a-half-mile walk from the marina along a busy road. Buses J1 or J2 run hourly from the bus stop in La Rochelle Road half a mile from the marina. St Sampson is Guernsey's second port and replicates most of St Peter Port's facilities

**Food and drink** The marina restaurant, specialising in seafood dishes, is open seven days a week for lunch and dinner

**Taxis, car and bicycle hire** Arrange through harbourmaster's office

### SHIPS' SERVICES

*Water and electricity Available on every pontoon*

*Fuel Diesel only is available from the fuel barge*

*Gas (Camping and Calor) Can be bought from the harbourmaster's office, which will also give you any assistance you need in obtaining the services of an **engineer**, **sailmaker** or **boatyard** facilities*

## SHORE LEAVE

From the marina you can follow the coast path north to **Fort Doyle**. Built in the eighteenth century on Guernsey's north-east extremity, the charm of the old stone has largely been covered by concrete adaptations to this century's wartime needs. A longer walk, along the coastal path to the south, will bring you after half a mile or so to Le Parcq Lane which passes close to 3,000 year old **Le Déhus dolmen**, one of the island's finest, with side chambers and a just-discernible face cut into one of the capstones.

# Herm

Herm is not an easy place to visit in your own boat. There are landings at the harbour and La Rosière Steps, both of which dry, and on the east coast at Belvoir Bay. All other landings require local knowledge. In fact, delightful though Herm is, it is probably best visited on a day-trip by one of the ferries from St Peter Port. There are no facilities or supplies for yachts.

Like Guernsey, Herm has high land in the south and low-lying grasslands in the north but it is only one-and-a-half miles long by half a mile wide. Herm is best known for its unspoilt beaches and peace and quiet. Surprisingly, the climate is warmer than in Guernsey: spring flowers are ready for market earlier and sub-tropical plants flourish. **Herm Common**, on the northern part of the island, is a flat sandy expanse rich in megalithic remains and bounded by sandy beaches which run on down the east side of the island. **Shell Beach** is famous and some of the shells are said to be brought from the Gulf of Mexico by the Gulf Stream. Further south, **Belvoir Bay** is a favourite spot for yachts to anchor for picnics.

There are farm buildings and grazing land in the centre of the island: Herm supplies three per cent of Guernsey's milk requirements. The fields have peculiar names: Monku, Frying Pan, Little Seagull and Top Valley Panto are a few. The origins of the names are lost in history, as is the name Herm itself. In the more hilly south of the island walks through lanes and along cliff paths are delightful. The one hotel, the White House, has a reputation for good food. The café, inn and village shop for souvenirs near the harbour supply a variety of needs but the best way to enjoy Herm is to set out on a walk around the cliffs or to a beach, taking a picnic with you.

Launches arrive from St Peter Port at regular intervals; the trip takes 20 minutes.

# Sark

Sark is the highest of the Channel Islands, with a plateau 300 feet high. The harbours most suitable for anchoring are La Maseline and Le Creux on the east side. The first is small and likely to be a rolly anchorage. The second is tiny and involves drying out. Both require you to keep clear of the ferry landings. Havre Gosselin, on the west of the

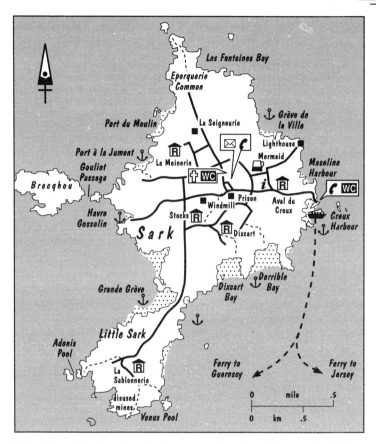

island, has a landing jetty but is very small and can be crowded. There are also bays all round the island where it is possible to anchor and go ashore from the beach. Dixcart and Derrible Bays are good for bathing. The island should only be visited by yachts in settled weather and the anchorage chosen according to the direction of the wind.

There are no quayside facilities apart from water and public toilets at Creux Harbour, so it is best to arrive fully provisioned. Fresh food can be bought in the village in the centre of the island, as can gas bottles, but it is a mile's walk away up a very steep hill. A tractor-drawn bus will take the less energetic to the top of the hill, where a horse-drawn carriage will meet you, if booked in advance. A church, the few shops, two banks and a post office, a pub and a café make up the village. Bicycles can be hired at Jackson's Stores but at the height of the season should be booked in advance. A tourist map and guide can be bought from the Tourism Office at the top of Harbour Hill.

Sark has none of the sophistications of modern life. There are no cars, and apart from a few tractors, the only traffic noise you will hear is the clip-clop of horses' hooves and the odd bicycle bell. This is a ramblers' paradise, with masses of wild flowers, particularly in spring, a magnificent coastline with high cliffs, and bays with caves and clear waters.

If you walk to **La Coupée**, the narrow road connecting Sark and Little Sark, you will find Little Sark is even less developed, with wild shores and a superb coastline. The **Bath of Venus** and **Adonis Pools** are spectacular rock formations and recommended for rock and skin diving. On the plateau are gorse-clad commons, leafy lanes and wooded valleys for attractive walks with glimpses of the sea and views to the other islands and to France.

Sark has been inhabited from earliest times and is still a feudal holding, dating back to the days of Elizabeth I, who appointed Helier de Carteret as the first Seigneur. His court can still confine you to the tiny prison for up to three days. **La Seigneurie** is a manor house in the French style with parts dating back to the seventeenth century. The attractive gardens are open to visitors from Tuesday to Friday in the height of summer. There are cafés and restaurants to suit all tastes all over the island, the best of them are attached to hotels. Dixcart Hotel and La Sablonnerie are well spoken of and are convenient from the west or south anchorages.

Launches from and to St Peter Port run regularly, and take about 40 minutes. A hydrofoil and other boats come from Jersey in the summer months.

# Jersey

Jersey, the most southerly Channel Island, slopes gently from high granite cliffs in the north to sandy beaches in the south. It has a green and fertile interior, much of it arable. Plant life flourishes in the warm climate (1900 hours of sunshine a year on average) and hedgerows and gardens are colourful with exotic flowers and shrubs. Small villages, cliffs and beaches are there to be explored. The island is nine miles by five and nowhere are you much more than two miles from the sea. The sandy beaches are one of Jersey's great attractions, from the very safe St Aubin to the challenging surf of St Ouen. A glimpse of pre-history emerges at low tide at St Ouen when stumps of trees show through the

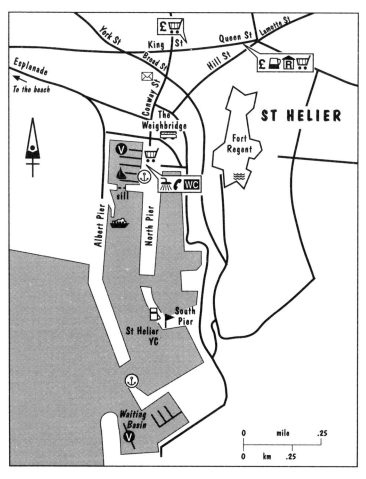

sand: they were once part of the vast French forest of which Jersey was a rocky outcrop. Habitation goes back a very long way and La Cotte de St Brelade is one of the most important palaeolithic sites in Europe. Evidence of Roman remains in Jersey is slight but St Helier, sixth-century hermit and martyr to Saxon pirates, gave his name to the capital.

## SHORE LEAVE

### Food and drink
Most restaurants use local produce, such as Jersey Royal potatoes, courgettes and tomatoes, and menus feature locally caught fish and shellfish. Restaurant de la Poste, 59 King Street, is a cheerful place with good Italian cooking. It is in the main pedestrian precinct, about five minutes' walk from the marina. There is no need to dress up and it offers good value. The Old Court House, St Aubin's Harbour, known to viewers of *Bergerac* as the 'Barge Aground', is next to the Royal Channel Islands Yacht Club, overlooking the harbour. The food is good, and the restaurant frequented by local youth. The leisure pages of the *Jersey Evening Post*, on sale from mid-afternoon, give details of where to eat and what to do in St Helier each evening.

### Entertainment
There are several cinemas in St Helier, including Ciné de France and Lido de France in St Saviours Road, and the Odeon in Bath Street. Live entertainment is usually on offer in Fort Regent and often in restaurants too. There are several discos. Fort Regent is a vast leisure complex: it has a 2,000 seat auditorium where concerts and exhibitions are held, and a permanent fairground.

### Excursions
**Elizabeth Castle**, a sixteenth-century fortress once occupied by Sir Walter Raleigh and named by him after his queen, is open to the public. Gerald Durrell's **Jersey Wildlife Preservation Trust** (Jersey Zoo) houses many rare animals and is very popular. You could happily spend half a day at **Samarès Manor** in the parish of St Clement enjoying the largest garden in Jersey, noted for its herbs, as well as seeing the house itself, the home of Seigneurs for many centuries – the eleventh-century dovecote testifies to its origins as only Seigneurs were allowed to own one. Within the grounds is a typical Jersey dairy farm, with guided tours twice a week.

### Exercise
For the energetic there is badminton, squash and bowls at Fort Regent and swimming or surfing from the beaches – windsurfing is good at St Clement's Bay at high water, but beware of the dangerous current at low water. The States of Jersey Public Works Committee publishes a free guide to coastal walks. The three miles from St Helier to St Aubin's Harbour make a pleasant evening walk. Longer walks can easily be begun or ended by bus.

## TRANSPORT AND TRAVEL

**Buses** From the Weighbridge bus station to most coastal areas; infrequent at night
**Planes** To Guernsey, Alderney, Bournemouth, Southampton, Gatwick, Heathrow, Manchester and to Paris, Dinard, Cherbourg
**Ferries** To Guernsey, Sark, Poole, St Malo and Granville; hydrofoil service to

Guernsey, Alderney, Sark, Herm and St Malo
**Taxi** Weighbridge cab rank
☎ (0534) 32001
**Car hire** Hallmark Rent-A-Car, The Weighbridge
**Bicycle hire** Kingslea, 70 The Esplanade

*Further information* from tourist office at The Weighbridge, by the harbour.

# St Helier Marina

| | |
|---|---|
| **Harbourmaster** ☎ (0534) 79549 | **VHF Channel** 14 |
| **Callsign** Pierhead Control | **Daily charge** £££ |

On arrival off St Helier you must report to Pierhead Control. You will probably be sent to the holding basin to wait for the marina gate to be opened. The marina is crowded but it is right in the centre of the town and convenient for all shops and facilities. St Helier is a busy cosmopolitan resort, popular with holidaymakers from the United Kingdom and the continent.

## STEP ASHORE

**Nearest payphone** In lobby of amenity block (open 24 hours a day) at the head of the landing ramp
**Toilets, showers** In amenity block at head of ramp
**Clubhouses** Royal Channel Island Yacht Club at the Bulwarks, St Aubin, and the St Helier Yacht Club on South Pier; both offer a cordial welcome to visitors.

Drinks and meals are available
**Shopping** The marina shop near the amenity block sells basic supplies. Jersey has a reputation for good shopping and many UK chain stores are there to cheer you up if you feel homesick for a shopping spree. Duty-free prices are not much lower than mainland duty-paid and if you exceed your allowances the customs duty will make your purchases seem expensive

### SHIPS' SERVICES

**Water and electricity** On pontoons
**Fuel** (diesel and petrol) From fuel berth on South Pier
**Gas** (Camping and Calor) From the Marina Shop

**Chandler** Channel Island Yacht Services, Old Harbour
**Boatyard, engineer** D K Collins, South Pier (Cruising Association Boatman)
**Sailmaker** Island Yachts, La Folie
☎ (0534) 25048

# Gorey Harbour

| | |
|---|---|
| **Harbourmaster** ☎ (0534) 53616 | **VHF Channel** 74 |
| **Callsign** Gorey Port Control | **Daily charge** £ |

Gorey harbour dries completely and it is best to contact the harbourmaster beforehand to check that a berth is available. Anchorages are also available outside the harbour. The harbour is in an attractive setting with old houses lining the sweep of the bay and Mont Orgueil Castle dominating the scene as it has done for more than 500 years.

## STEP ASHORE

**Nearest payphone** At 'root' of pier
**Toilets and showers** On pier

**Shopping** Small shops around the harbour and in the village

### SHIPS' SERVICES

*Water, fuel At end of pier*

*Gas From chandler in village*

## SHORE LEAVE

### Food and drink
There are several pubs and restaurants round the harbour. The Drive-in-Barbecue, Coast Road, is about five minutes' walk from the harbour. It caters well for families and provides good alfresco eating, with cover in case it rains. The home-brewed cider is excellent.

### What to see
**Mont Orgueil**, a well-preserved fortress with a museum and tableaux of Jersey history, offers a terrific view from the battlements. **Jersey Pottery**, the largest pottery in the Channel Islands, is on the main road north of Gorey Village, set in three acres of attractively laid-out gardens. You can watch work in progress as well as buy the pottery, and eat – indoors or out – at the very good restaurant. A mile or so to the north-west is **La Hougue Bie**, a renowned prehistoric burial chamber in a state of complete preservation – Bus 3a from Gorey stops there.

### Excursions
Gerald Durrell's **Jersey Wildlife Preservation Trust** (Jersey Zoo), with many rare species rescued from extinction, is within easy reach of Gorey Village at Les Augres Manor, Trinity.

### Exercise
Walks along the coast and over Gorey Common are pleasant and so is swimming from Grouville Beach.

## TRANSPORT AND TRAVEL

**Buses** Around the island and to St Helier
**Taxis, car and bicycle hire** All available in the village

**Ferries** To Carteret and Portbail on the Normandy coast

---

*Alternative moorings*

There are several small harbours round the coast of Jersey which can be visited if you can take the ground or anchor off, notably **St Aubin**, where the **Royal Channel Island Yacht Club** has its headquarters. At **Bonne Nuit**, a small town on the north coast, is a bay protected by cliffs and a sheltered anchorage. The annual Sark to Jersey rowing race in July finishes there. **Rozel** and **Bouley Bays** on the north-east coast offer attractive anchorages.

---

*Note*

It is mandatory to clear Customs inwards at St Helier or Gorey before entering any other harbour in Jersey or its offshore islands.

---

# Les Ecrehou

A visit to Les Ecrehou, a tiny island with a handful of houses set in the middle of a reef to the east of Jersey, is an unusual experience. A priory was built here in the thirteenth century; in the eighteenth century it was used for smuggling; in the nineteenth century it had a 'king'. Recent excavations have revealed evidence of man living there 5,000 years ago. Visits with fishermen from Gorey can be arranged.

# NORTH-WEST FRANCE

# Carteret

Ten miles east of Jersey, on the Gerfleur estuary, Carteret is one of the most popular seaside resorts on the Cotentin Peninsula. Like all the harbours on this coast, Carteret dries right out and is little frequented by yachts. However, it is a pleasant place and worth a short visit in the right conditions. By English standards this is a quiet seaside resort; the main attraction is the vast area of sand dunes stretching away to the north.

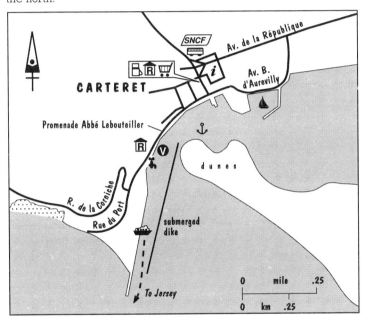

## SHORE LEAVE

There are several restaurants – l'Hermitage on the quayside is good value, serves excellent seafood, and is very welcoming. Walking on the cliffs and dunes is very pleasant. If you follow the **Sentier des Douaniers** (Customs Officers' Path) to the north you can visit the lighthouse, open 1000–1200 and 1400–2000, then continue to Carteret's second beach, about a half-hour walk. The fine, sandy beaches are safe to swim from. You could take a bus, or walk, to **Barneville** to see the eleventh-century church.

### TRANSPORT AND TRAVEL

**Buses** From Place Flandre-Dunkerque to Coutances and Granville
**Trains** From Place Flandre-Dunkerque to Carentan
**Ferries** To Gorey, Jersey, daily in summer; take 30 minutes
**Taxis** M Pilot, Avenue des Douits
☎ 33.53.81.96
**Car hire** Sport-Marine, 18 Rue de Paris
**Bicycle hire** Ask at tourist office

*Further information* from tourist office in Place Flandre-Dunkerque.

# Port de Carteret

**Harbourmaster** ☎ 33.04.70.84                    **Daily charge** £

You can dry out alongside the harbour wall east of the Hôtel de la Marine by arrangement with the fishing boat owners, or sound for a flat spot away from the quay if you have legs or bilge keels. Further up the harbour is the Port de Plaisance – a row of mooring buoys – but you will still lie on the mud at low water. It is for berth holders only, but you might find a place by arrangement.

## STEP ASHORE

**Nearest payphone** On quay by sailing school
**Shopping** Simple shops, a bank and a post office one block inland from the end of the quay. The main area for shops and banks is Barneville-Bourg, two miles away

### SHIPS' SERVICES

**Water and electricity** On the quayside
**Fuel** (diesel and petrol) In cans from the garage in town

**Gas** (Camping and Calor) From Carteret Marine, Avenue de la République

# Portbail

The little town of Portbail is a mile away from the harbour along the causeway. Two fine sandy beaches are all that enable it to call itself a seaside resort but it is a pleasant place for a short stay and the town and countryside are worth exploring. Portbail has no fewer than five Roman roads converging on it, suggesting a past more lively than the present.

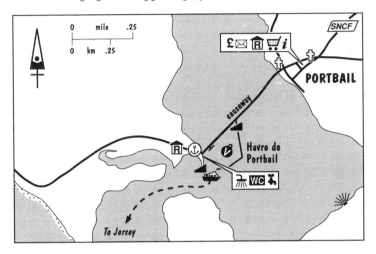

## SHORE LEAVE

You will find a bar and crêperie in the dunes behind the harbour and several restaurants in Portbail. Walk in the dunes and marshes; swim and windsurf from the beaches to the west. The fifteenth-century **Notre-Dame church** has an ancient baptistry.

### TRANSPORT AND TRAVEL

**Buses** From centre of town by church to Carteret and Carentan

**Ferries** Daily to Gorey, Jersey, in summer; take 30 minutes

*Further information* from tourist office, 26 Rue Philippe Lebel.

## Havre de Portbail

| | |
|---|---|
| **Harbourmaster** ☎ 33.04.83.48 | **VHF Channel** 9 |
| **Callsign** Portbail | **Daily charge** ££ |

Approached over drying flats, this small harbour is very welcoming. It consists of a small, drying basin, more sheltered than Carteret, but with few facilities – just some huts and a café tucked away in the dunes. The harbourmaster will find you a mooring.

## STEP ASHORE

**Nearest payphone, toilets, showers** On quay

**Shopping** Small shops, a bank and a post office

### SHIPS' SERVICES

**Water and electricity** *On quay*
**Fuel** *(diesel and petrol) From town in cans*

**Gas** *From small supermarket in town*

# Granville

Granville is dominated by its Gibraltar-like rock which is topped by a walled town complete with military barracks. This old, fortified part of the town, Haute Ville, with its sixteenth and seventeenth-century houses, has an air of being left 200 years behind the times. It is quite detached from the popular, bustling resort below, which is partly built on reclaimed land.

Long beaches stretch away northwards, while to the south can be seen Mont St Michel like a ship at sea. The town is a great centre for thalassotherapy (this consists of being hosed down by a water cannon, but here you pay good money for the privilege); the 'Centre' dominates the narrow neck of land at the foot of the rock, on which the casino also stands.

The town was captured and fortified by the English in 1439, who dug a huge moat (Tranchée des Anglais) at the north end of the rock, but this did not prevent recapture by the French three years later.

## SHORE LEAVE

### Food and drink
Restaurants and take-aways abound, but for seafood try in particular those by the old fishing harbour in Rue du Port.

### Entertainment
There is a three-screen cinema in the casino in Place Maréchal Foch.

### What to see
The old town on the hill (**Haute Ville**), approached over a drawbridge through the ramparts, will take half a day to explore. There are some interesting model ships in the old church of **Notre Dame.** The **Musée d'Ancien Granville** is full of local history and some fine examples of regional head-dresses. The **aquarium**, which has sealions and turtles, is also in the old town.

### Excursions
Every day vedettes leave Granville on day trips to **Iles Chausey** and **Jersey**. Also on offer are tours inland to see the 1944 invasion headquarters at **Avranches**. Coaches run twice a week to **Mont St Michel** and while the abbey, fortress and village on the rock are fascinating to explore, Mont St Michel proclaims itself France's foremost tourist attraction and as such is sometimes so crowded in summer that tourists who are not part of an organised tour are refused entry. It may be better to admire the spectacle of the island, with its towering buildings, as you sail on passage from Granville to the Channel Islands or St Malo.

Buses run north along the coast to **Coutances.** The eleventh-century cathedral set on a hill above the town is the best example of Norman-Gothic architecture in the Cotentin peninsula.

### Exercise
Swimming is safe from the excellent sandy beaches or you could use the indoor pool; windsurfing, tennis, golf and riding are all catered for. Walks, especially **Le Tour du Roc** round the old town to the cliffs and the lighthouse at the far end, are recommended.

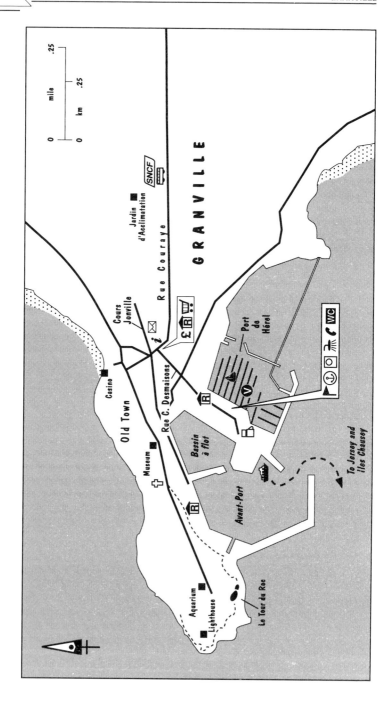

## TRANSPORT AND TRAVEL

**Buses** From Cours Jonville to Coutances and Carteret
**Trains** To Paris (2 hours), Cherbourg (1 hour) and St Malo
**Ferries** Vedettes run daily to Iles Chausey and Jersey (75 minutes)
**Planes** From Bréville-Granville airport, 10 miles from Granville, to Iles Chausey, Mont St Michel, Jersey, Guernsey and Alderney
**Taxis** From rank in Cours Jonville or ☎ 33.50.01.67
**Car hire** Europcar, Avenue des Vendéens
**Bicycle hire** From SNCF

*Further information* from tourist office at Cours Jonville in the town centre.

# Port de Hérel

| | |
|---|---|
| **Harbourmaster** ☎ 33.50.20.06 | **VHF Channel** 9 |
| **Callsign** Port de Hérel | **Daily charge** ££ |

The last and largest of the harbours on this difficult coast, Granville is approached over a long drying bay. The modern marina is to starboard of the old harbour, the entrance signalled by an illuminated indicator showing the depth over the sill. The visitors' pontoon is straight ahead on entering. The marina is completely protected and has all modern facilities.

## STEP ASHORE

**Nearest payphone, toilets, showers** By harbour office
**Clubhouse** Yacht Club de Granville on quay
**Shopping** Basic shops in the marina, but the main shops, post office and banks are in the town a quarter of a mile to the south along Rue Lecampion. Small Comod supermarket in Rue Clément Desmaisons and a Codec that stays open late in Rue Lecampion.

## SHIPS' SERVICES

**Water and electricity** *On pontoons*
**Fuel** *(diesel and petrol) From fuelling pontoon*
**Gas** *From chandler*
**Chandler** *Granvil'eole on quay*
**Engineer** *Lecoulant Marine*
**Sailmaker** *Voilerie Mora, 17 Rue Clément Desmaisons*

# Iles Chausey

Two hours' sail from Granville are the Iles Chausey, an almost unspoilt archipelago of small islands. Find a visitors' mooring in the Sound (they are laid by the Yacht Club de Granville) or anchor nearby. Dry out in the small bay if you can take the ground.

Iles Chausey are as near as one can get to a desert island in these parts. Unfortunately half the population of Granville and Jersey thinks so too, but don't be put off. The trippers arrive late and leave early and there is plenty of room for the sailors and campers who remain for the night. There are no ships' supplies but there is a water tap (intended for residents) on **Grande Ile**, plus two hotels with restaurants, a café or two and a small shop. The one public telephone kiosk is tastefully draped in honeysuckle.

At high water the archipelago is a vast cluster of rocks and small islands, sparkling in the sun if you are lucky. At low water it becomes a sandy plateau over which you can wander and explore.

# Cancale

Cancale is a pleasant little fishing harbour-cum-resort in the corner of
the Baie du Mont St Michel, renowned for centuries for its oysters.
Cancale has no facilities or provision for yachts and is not a good place
to leave your boat and go off on long trips ashore.

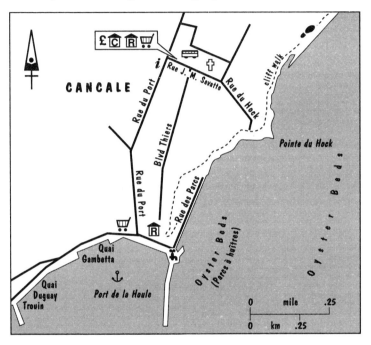

## SHORE LEAVE

Films are shown in the old church which also houses a museum devoted to
regional arts and traditions. There is a panoramic view of the bay from the
church tower and in clear weather you can see Iles Chausey and Jersey. Walks
along the cliffs are pleasant, and so is a visit to the oyster beds at low water – you
can buy and eat half-a-dozen on the spot for elevenses. Visit the **oyster-culture
museum** on the corniche.

### TRANSPORT AND TRAVEL

**Buses** From Place de l'Eglise to St Malo

*Further information* from tourist office, 44 Rue du Port.

## Port de Cancale

Find a place to anchor among all the oyster barges, if you can dry out, or a long way further out if not. Off the beach at Port-Mer, two miles to the north, is another anchorage for yachts.

### STEP ASHORE

**Nearest payphone** On quay
**Toilets, showers** Municipal facilities behind tourist office
**Shopping** Several shops along the quay, up Rue du Port and into town where there are more, also banks, a post office and bureau de change

### SHIPS' SERVICES

**Water** On quay
**Fuel** In cans from garage

**Gas** (Camping and Calor) From supermarket in town

## Rothéneuf

Rothéneuf is a village four miles east of St Malo but in effect a suburb of the city. Once through the difficult entrance – not for beginners – you arrive in a large, well-sheltered, drying basin, but with room for only a couple of visiting yachts because most of the space is taken up by moorings. There is also a good anchorage outside the harbour entrance, sheltered except from the north, but you are left with a three-quarters-of-a-mile row into the village, which offers few facilities to reward your efforts. The village and yacht club are in the south-west corner where there is also a payphone, plus a few shops and an excellent restaurant. This is a quiet little resort with good access to St Malo by bus.

# St Malo

Few towns contain so much of their country's adventurous history as St Malo. Approached through a maze of islands, the mighty walls, topped by the roofs of rows of rich merchants' houses and the spire of the cathedral, look much as they did in the seventeenth century. Sadly almost the whole of the town inside the walls was razed by fire in the last days of the German occupation in 1944. It has been rebuilt with great skill and dedication, and whilst the buildings are now fireproof and

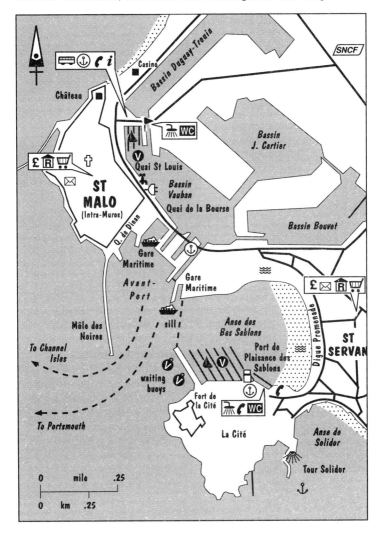

modern, much of the atmosphere of a cramped medieval city has been recaptured.

The great days of St Malo began with the discovery of the New World, and the names of explorers and privateers are commemorated at every turn. Jacques Cartier, who went to look for gold in Newfoundland in 1534, found the St Lawrence River. Duguay-Trouin and Surcouf were privateers and slavers in the seventeenth and eighteenth centuries and thorns in the flesh of the English, Dutch and Spanish. A less aggressive son of St Malo was the French poet Chateaubriand.

There is a choice of moorings: you can lock into the old basin close to the old town or go to the marina at St Servan in the Anse des Sablons. It is also possible to anchor in the Anse de Solidor near to the tower, land on the beach and walk up into St Servan.

## SHORE LEAVE

### Food and drink

There are restaurants and take-aways to suit all tastes in the walled city, especially just inside the walls facing the harbour. Street entertainments often enliven meals at the outside tables of restaurants such as A La Duchesse Anne, 5–7 Place Guy La Chambre, which is always popular with the English for its fine seafood. Le Petit Bedon, 3 Rue Gouin de Beauchesne, is a bright little restaurant where the food is of a good standard and not expensive. La Pomme d'Or in the Place du Poids du Roi, just inside the walls, is also recommended.

### Entertainment

There are four cinemas, a theatre in Place Bouvet, St Servan, a casino with theatre productions and several nightclubs and discos.

### What to see

A walk round the almost complete walls of the town will reveal glimpses of the few remaining old buildings as you look inwards, and views over the vast docks, the Baie de St Malo and the islands to seaward. In the north-east corner is the fourteenth and fifteenth-century **château** with museums of the town's history in the keep and the waxworks in the **Quic-en-Groigne Tower**. On summer evenings there are often displays of dancing and performances of folk music in the square outside the castle gate, which you can enjoy sitting outside a café with a coffee and calvados.

The **cathedral of St Vincent**, built between the eleventh and eighteenth centuries, has been beautifully restored over the last forty years. The fine modern stained-glass windows, muted in the transept, brighter in the side aisles, give life and colour to the interior. **Fort National** was built by Vauban in the seventeenth century to defend St Malo from the English and Dutch. Visit the dungeons for an authentic sense of the seventeenth century.

If you have moored in the Anse des Sablons you will have a long, possibly hot and dusty, walk through the dock area to get to the walled city. Nearer St Servan is the **Corniche d'Aleth** with views over the bay and upstream to the hydro-electric barrage on the Rance. The thirteenth-century **Solidor Tower** houses the **International Museum of Cape Horners**. The history of the sailing ships and men who have braved this legendary cape is described with the aid of models and photographs – you may be privileged to have an ancient mariner as your guide. See the model of *Victoria*, the first ship to sail round the world between 1519 and 1522.

*Excursions*

Visit **Grand Bé Island** in the bay, where Chateaubriand's tomb lies, to see the plain tombstone and heavy cross, as well as the superb view of the Emerald Coast. It is also possible to visit the Rance **hydroelectric barrage** – find out about its workings from the harbour office at St Malo or Bas Sablons.

A ferry crosses the Rance to **Dinard** at frequent intervals throughout the day, useful if you want to explore there; day trips by hovercraft or ferry to the **Channel Islands** are available. Vedettes go to **Dinard**, **Dinan**, **Cap Fréhel**, **Cézembre**, **Chausey**, the **Rance River** and **Mont St Michel Bay**. Day trips by coach are arranged to Cancale to see the oyster beds and fishing harbour and to **Mont St Michel**.

The sixteenth-century **manor house of Jacques Cartier** near **Rothéneuf** has been restored and has contemporary furnishings.

*Exercise*

You can swim from beaches to the west and north of the city, or use the olympic-size swimming pool at St Servan. Windsurfing, tennis and golf are all part of the summer scene here.

## TRANSPORT AND TRAVEL

**Buses** From bus station by tourist office, Esplanade St Vincent on the north side of Bassin Vauban, to Rennes, Rothéneuf, St Servan, Cancale and Dinan
**Trains** To Rennes, change for Paris and Brest
**Planes** From Dinard-Pleurtuit (the St Malo airport) to Channel Islands and England
**Ferries** From Gare Maritime du Naye, roughly half-way between the two yacht harbours, twice a day to Portsmouth;

ferries and hydrofoils leave frequently for Jersey, Guernsey, Sark and Alderney. The ferry to Dinard runs between 0930 and 1900 and takes 10 minutes from Cale de Dinan, near the Gare Maritime
**Taxis** ☎ 99.81.30.30
**Car hire** Europcar, 16 Boulevard des Talards (near railway station)
☎ 99.56.75.17
**Bicycle hire** From SNCF

*Further information* from tourist office at Esplanade St Vincent on the north side of Bassin Vauban.

# Bassin Vauban

| | |
|---|---|
| **Harbourmaster** ☎ 99.56.51.91 | **VHF Channel** 9 |
| **Callsign** Bassin Vauban port de plaisance | **Daily charge** ££ |

Reached through a large lock, the end of this old basin has been transformed into a pleasant marina with modern facilities. There is a certain romance to being moored near the walls of this ancient stronghold; the only drawback is the bustle and noise of traffic.

## STEP ASHORE

**Nearest payphone, toilets, showers** In clubhouse
**Clubhouse** Yacht Club de St Malo on quayside
**Shopping** Through the gates into the walled city there is a full selection of shops, banks and bureaux de change. Market inside the walls on Tuesdays and Fridays

### SHIPS' SERVICES

*Water and electricity* On pontoons
*Fuel* (diesel and petrol) Can be obtained from a nearby garage but it would be easier to get fuel from St Servan marina in Anse des Sablons
*Gas, chandler, boatyard, engineer, sailmaker* All at St Servan marina

# Bas Sablons (St Servan)

| | |
|---|---|
| **Harbourmaster** ☎ 99.81.71.34 | **VHF Channel** 9 |
| **Callsign** Bas Sablons | **Daily charge** ££ |

This is a modern, impersonal marina at St Servan in the Anse des Sablons. You will find all facilities there, but it is a long walk into St Servan, an unexciting suburb, for shopping or to St Malo for sightseeing.

## STEP ASHORE

**Nearest payphone** Near harbour office
**Toilets, showers** Near harbour office
**Launderette** 19 Rue des Bas Sablons
**Shopping** A good range of shops and banks in St Servan, a half-mile walk from the marina. Markets on Tuesdays and Fridays
**Food and drink** A café-bistro in the marina

### SHIPS' SERVICES

*Water and electricity* On pontoons
*Fuel* Alongside at south end of marina
*Gas* From chandlers on quay
*Chandler, boatyard, engineer, sailmaker* All in marina

# Dinard

| | |
|---|---|
| **Harbourmaster** ☎ 99.46.65.55 | **VHF Channel** 9 |
| **Callsign** Dinard | **Daily charge** £ |

Dinard is the queen of north Brittany's resorts, with sweeping yellow sands, a superior casino and the air of the fine old Edwardian watering place it once was. If you can moor off the yacht club you will appreciate Dinard's imposing architecture and the views of the estuary of the Rance. However, it is very crowded and it is likely that you will end up a long way out. Facilities such as fuel and water are on the quay, but you would be better advised to go a mile across the bay to the St Servan marina. Moor in St Malo and visit Dinard by vedette if you want to experience the contrast between St Malo and a modern luxury resort.

---

*The Breton Flag*

The Breton flag is made up of five black stripes representing the former bishoprics of High Brittany: Rennes, Nantes, Dol, St Malo and St Brieuc. Four white bands represent the bishoprics of Low Brittany: Léon, Cornouaille, Vannes and Tréguier. The ermine tails recall the ancient Duchy of Brittany itself. The Bretons started the pleasant custom of wearing regional flags as courtesy ensigns which is now seen in many parts. Patriotic Bretons sometimes fly it as a national ensign, but you should always wear it with and *below* the Tricolore if you want to avoid an awkward moment with the French authorities, who may not be natives of Brittany and can fine you for getting it wrong. Don't forget to change it when you cross boundaries: it will not have the same effect in Normandy or the Vendée.

# Dinan

This delightful medieval city has many old streets and fine buildings, but is rather crowded in the season. The quayside is lined with old merchants' houses and stores. The approach to the town is up a steep and winding lane with more fine old houses, most of which are now given over to restaurants and craft shops with colourful displays adding an air of gaiety.

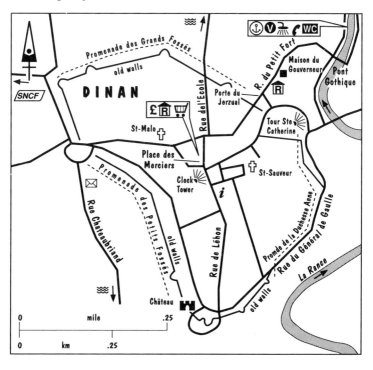

## SHORE LEAVE

There are many restaurants, bars and crêperies by the river, in the Rue du Petit Fort and in town. The Restaurant Gastronomique des Terrasses by the bridge is very good. Explore the old town, famous for its château, walls, old houses and gardens. Climb the **Tour de l'Horloge** (Clock Tower) for a grand view over the surrounding countryside. If you are nervous, don't go up when the clock is about to strike. You'll get plenty of exercise walking up the hill into Dinan. If you need a swim, try the swimming pool in Rue du Champ Garel.

## TRANSPORT AND TRAVEL

**Buses** From Place 11 Novembre 1918 to St Malo and Dinard
**Trains** To Paris via Rennes and to Dinard
**Planes** Dinard-Pleurtuit airport to Channel Islands and England
**Taxis** Place Duclos ☎ 96.39.06.00
**Car hire** Europcar, 48 Rue de Brest
**Bicycle hire** From SNCF

*Further information* from tourist office, 6 Rue de l'Horloge.

# Port de Dinan

Harbourmaster ☎ 96.39.56.44          Daily charge ££

The 14-mile voyage up the Rance to Dinan has its excitements, with the passage through the barrage and the sudden changes in water level. (You should get information about the workings of the hydroelectric station from the harbour office at St Malo or Bas Sablons.) Several rural anchorages line the way up the river and there is a quayside mooring in the old port below Dinan town. If you are fortunate enough to draw sufficiently little to be able to go on through the canals to the Vilaine, this is where you will have to take your mast down (if you have not already done so at St Servan). There is a crane on the quayside for the purpose.

### STEP ASHORE

**Nearest payphone** On quayside opposite fuel pumps
**Toilets** Public WC on quay
**Shopping** Small shops in the Rue du Petit Fort, the road up to the town, and all the facilities of a large town at the top of the hill

### SHIPS' SERVICES

*Water and electricity* On pontoons          *Fuel* (diesel and petrol) On quayside

# St Cast-le-Guildo

St Cast is in three parts stretched over two miles: St Cast Bourg is the town and seaside resort; a mile to the north is the port at l'Isle St Cast; the yacht club is at Pointe de la Garde a mile to the south. The whole is coupled with the neighbouring village of Le Guildo further south. L'Isle is famous for scallops and clams.

St Cast was first visited by Britons when they fled from the Saxon invasions in the fifth century. It is still welcoming.

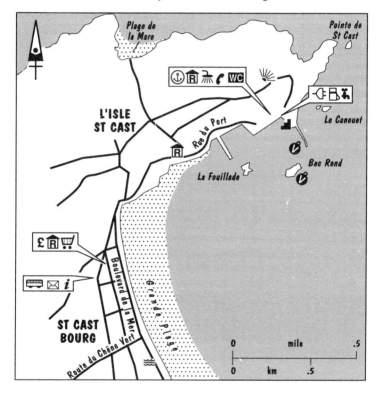

## SHORE LEAVE

### Food and drink
The port runs to a snack bar and crêperie, but most restaurants are in Le Bourg. Hôtel l'Etoile de Mer at the top of Rue du Port is the nearest. It is a friendly place, with a restaurant and bar.

### Entertainment
There is a cinema, Eden, Rue de la Vallée de Besnault.

### What to see
The chief point of interest is the column crowned by a hare stamping on the

British lion, erected in 1858 to commemorate the centenary of a battle in the bay when the English lost 2,400 men.

### Excursions

Go to **Fort de la Latte**, an ancient stronghold on the end of a rocky peninsula, either by land or in your own boat. Boat trips leave from the harbour for **Cap Fréhel**, the most impressive cape on the Breton coast. Red, grey and black cliffs rise vertically 229 feet above sea level – they are at their most beautiful with the evening sun on them. Coach trips to **Mont St Michel** and **St Malo** leave from Le Bourg.

### Exercise

Walk to the top of the hill behind the harbour for fine views and carry on westwards along the waymarked footpaths to **Plage de la Pissotte**. Swimming and waterskiing are popular on St Cast beach in the bay between Pointe de la Garde and Pointe de St Cast. There is an indoor swimming pool by the beach in Salle d'Armor.

## TRANSPORT AND TRAVEL

**Buses** From Place A. le Braz to Erquy and Dinard, plus a twice-daily coach service to Lamballe railway station in July and August
**Taxis** M Renault, Rue du Champ Gauron

☎ 96.41.86.16
**Car hire** Enquire at tourist office
**Bicycle hire** M Page, Rue de L'Isle
☎ 96.41.87.71

*Further information* from tourist office in Place Charles de Gaulle.

# Port de St Cast

**Harbourmaster** ☎ 96.41.88.34          **Daily charge** first day free then ££

The harbour is sheltered from the prevailing winds but would not be a good place to leave a boat. It is enjoyable for a break but is really only suitable for an overnight stop. Visitors moor to buoys at the end of the breakwater; the facilities are quite basic.

## STEP ASHORE

**Nearest payphone, toilets, showers,** At the harbour office
**Clubhouse** Yacht Club de St Cast is at Pointe de la Garde
**Shopping** Small shops at the top of Rue du Port; the main shops, banks and post office are in Le Bourg a mile from the harbour. Market in Le Bourg on Monday and Friday mornings

### SHIPS' SERVICES

*Water and electricity, fuel* (diesel and petrol) On the quay

*Gas* (Camping and Calor) From the chandler
*Chandler* LMB Marine ☎ 96.41.80.23

# Erquy

This little harbour is mainly used by small fishing boats (it is a busy scallop-fishing port), but visitors are welcome. Erquy is also a thriving seaside resort. The main attractions of the area are the sandy beaches, sheltered by dunes and pine trees and the cliff walks, especially over the wild heathland to the north towards Cap d'Erquy.

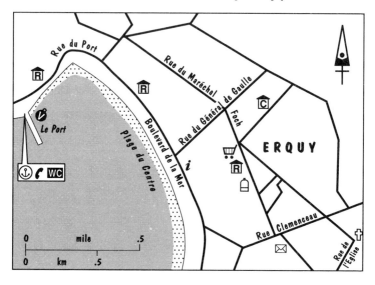

## SHORE LEAVE

### Food and drink
Several restaurants and a crêperie line the seafront in Rue du Port and Boulevard de la Mer; there are bars and restaurants in town as well.

### Entertainment
The cinema is in Rue Chemin Vert.

### What to see
The fifteenth-century church in the centre of the town is noted for a carving of Romulus and Remus and their wolf-mother.

### Excursions
About three miles south of Erquy is **Château de Bienassis**, a fifteenth to seventeenth-century mansion with collections of porcelain and furniture. The bus to **Le Val André** goes past it. Vedettes go from Erquy to **Le Val André**, **Dahouët** and **Bréhat**.

### Exercise
Beautiful beaches with fine sand line the coast at Erquy, with views of **Cap d'Erquy** and **Cap Fréhel**. A half-hour walk along a well-maintained footpath through a nature reserve brings you to Cap d'Erquy. Directions for longer walks are available from the tourist office.

## TRANSPORT AND TRAVEL

**Buses** From Rue de la Corniche to Le Val André and Sables d'Or-les-Pins

**Taxis, car hire** Thomas ☎ 96.72.30.37
**Bicycle hire** Loca-Loisirs ☎ 96.72.06.97

*Further information* from tourist office, Boulevard de la Mer.

# Port d'Erquy

| | |
|---|---|
| **Harbourmaster** ☎ 96.72.19.32 | **VHF Channel** 9 |
| **Callsign** Erquy | **Daily charge** 2 days free of charge, then £ |

You can anchor in the lee of the jetty or use one of the four red visitors' buoys. In a strong south-west wind the harbour is untenable as there is no real shelter. A boat should not be left except in settled weather, when you might prefer to be sailing.

## STEP ASHORE

**Nearest payphone, toilets, showers** By capitainerie
**Clubhouse** Cercle de la Voile, Le Port

**Shopping** Walk inland a block or two along Rue du Port to shops, banks and post office. Street market on Saturdays

### SHIPS' SERVICES

*Water* On quay
*Gas* (Camping and Calor) From Ets Collet,

*Rue Foch*
*Chandler* Loop Marine, Rue du Port

# Dahouët

The wind here is predominantly westerly and Dahouët claims an exceptionally warm climate due to a diversion of the Gulf Stream, resulting in an abundance of plant life usually found much further south. The surrounding area is fertile, hilly and offers lovely walks among trees and shrubs to the north, especially towards Erquy. Dahouët is the fishing port and pleasure-boat harbour for Le Val André, a popular resort with excellent restaurants, shops, beaches, walks and windsurfing. There are lots of campsites tucked away, and a large number of summer villas, which accounts for the good facilities.

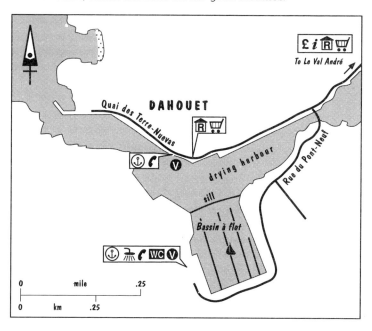

SHORE LEAVE

### Food and drink
From a good choice of restaurants in Dahouët, Hôtel de la Mer is particularly recommended and so is Café Zef.

### Entertainment
There is a municipal casino in Le Val André with a disco and two cinemas

### What to see
Trips are organised to the bird sanctuary on the **Verdelet archipelago** and to the submarine grottoes at **La Cotentin** at low tide.

### Excursions
Car hire is worthwhile for a trip to **Cap Fréhel**, which is very attractive with views extending from Grouin Point to Ile de Bréhat with an occasional sighting

of the Channel Islands. **Fort de la Latte** to the east is also within visiting range. Vedettes for **Ile de Bréhat** leave from Dahouët.

*Exercise*
The beach at Le Val André is good for swimming and for every kind of water sport. Walks along cliffs and wooded valleys are particularly pleasant.

### TRANSPORT AND TRAVEL

**Buses** From Le Val André to Erquy, Lamballe and St Brieuc
**Trains** From Lamballe, eight miles away

**Planes** From St Brieuc, 22 miles away
**Taxis** Bivel ☎ 96.72.22.20
**Car and bicycle hire** From Le Val André

*Further information* from tourist office in the casino on the sea front at Le Val André ☎ 96.72.20.55.

# Port de Dahouët

| | |
|---|---|
| **Harbourmaster** ☎ 96.72.82.85 | **VHF Channel** 9 |
| **Callsign** Dahouët | **Daily charge** first night free, then ££ |

Dahouët is a small port with a new marina on the estuary of the Flora River to the east of the Baie de St Brieuc but the west-facing entrance is narrow and rocky and dries out. The outer harbour is reserved for fishing boats, though in good weather you can anchor in the *rade* (roads) and off the beach at Le Piégu. There are buoys outside the marina which can be used by visiting yachts, but they dry. The new marina is well constructed, secure and has good facilities. There is a very helpful chandler's shop by the quay and several other shops. Le Val André is about a mile away and has all provisions. The yacht club moorings off Le Val André are, again, suitable only in settled weather.

## STEP ASHORE

**Nearest payphone** By Hôtel du Port on quay, near harbourmaster's office
**Toilets, showers** (cold only) On quay
**Shopping** Dahouët has village shops only but there is a bank, bureau de change and post office. Le Val André and Pléneuf are both about a mile away and have a variety of shops, but they are closed in both places from 1230 till 1500 Monday to Friday, Saturday afternoons and all day Sunday.

### SHIPS' SERVICES

*Water and electricity* On pontoons
*Fuel* (diesel and petrol) Through harbourmaster
*Gas* (Camping and Calor) From chandler

*Chandler* Côte Ouest, Bassin des Salines
*Boatyard* Réparations Navales, Rue Bouquet
*Engineer* M Rondeau ☎ 96.72.95.46

# Binic

In the past Binic was a cod-fishing port; now its commerce is tourism and shellfish. There is one long quayside street where everything happens, with some good restaurants. The surrounding area is most attractive with lovely villages and cheap places to stay. It is popular with tourists in the height of summer.

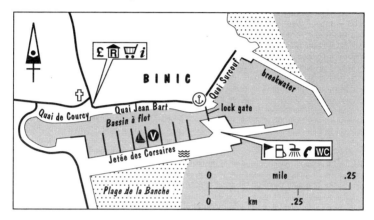

SHORE LEAVE

### Food and drink
The selection of small traditional restaurants is good, particularly Le Galion and Le Printania hotels. There are specialist seafood restaurants, a crêperie, pizzeria and several snack-bars.

### What to see
There is a **war memorial museum** and a **regional crafts museum** where you can browse among local costumes and display models of Newfoundland fishing expeditions.

### Excursions
In summer this area is very apt to be congested with holiday traffic and secondary routes for excursions by car or bike are probably best.

Try to visit the village of **Kermaria**, some six miles to the north-west, where there is a chapel with fifteenth-century frescoes portraying a *danse macabre*: skeletons dance and caper, beckoning after them 47 figures such as pope and emperor, monk and ploughman. The **Moulin de Richard zoo** and **safari park** is five miles away at **Trégomeur**. Vedettes for **Ile de Bréhat** leave from Binic.

### Exercise
There are extensive beaches to swim and windsurf from and good coastal walks, including a path to **Pointe de la Rognouze**.

## TRANSPORT AND TRAVEL

**Buses** To St Quay-Portrieux and St Brieuc
**Trains, planes** From St Brieuc
**Ferries** Local, to Ile de Bréhat

**Taxis, car and bicycle hire** Enquire at tourist office

*Further information* from tourist office on Esplanade de la Banche.

# Port de Binic

| | |
|---|---|
| **Harbourmaster** ☎ 96.73.61.86 | **VHF Channel** 9 |
| **Callsign** Binic | **Daily charge** ££ |

Binic is not difficult to reach by sea, given sufficient rise of tide – at low water the harbour dries out, as does the surrounding shoreline. The marina is locked in, but the gates don't open at neaps. It is very sheltered from westerly winds. This medium-sized marina has facilities well up to the best of French standards, security is good and it is easy to leave the boat in the marina in the care of the helpful harbourmaster.

## STEP ASHORE

**Nearest payphone** By marina quay
**Toilets, showers, launderette** In marina
**Clubhouse** Small sailing club by quay
**Shopping** All the shops are within 200 yards; they are village shops only, but include banks, bureau de change and post office. Everything closes 1230–1500

## SHIPS' SERVICES

*Water and electricity* On pontoons
*Fuel* (diesel and petrol) On quay
*Gas* (Camping and Calor) From chandler

*Chandler* Jean Bart Marine by quay
*Engineer* Refer to harbourmaster

# St Quay-Portrieux

Portrieux is the harbour of the seaside resort of St Quay. The harbour itself is rather featureless, but over the hill is St Quay, set in lovely surroundings. It is a popular town with fine beaches and every kind of sport available. The cliffs are excellent for walking with maintained paths and good views. A few miles north is Plage Bonaparte, from which Allied pilots shot down during the war were taken off by submarine in the middle of the night for return to the United Kingdom, having been smuggled to the beach by the Resistance. St Quay, though a tranquil resort, marks the start of rugged cliffs, isolated hamlets and the bleak and rocky shores of the coast to the west.

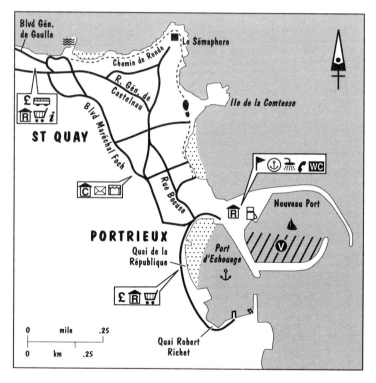

## SHORE LEAVE

There are restaurants in Portrieux round the harbour and in St Quay. You will find a cinema and a theatre in Boulevard M. Foch in St Quay and also a lively casino. However, water sports are the main occupation: there are five sandy beaches where swimming is possible at all states of the tide, a seawater swimming pool and windsurfers for hire; riding or cycling are alternatives. Organised boat trips go to the little islands off St Quay and to **Ile de Bréhat**.

### TRANSPORT AND TRAVEL

**Buses** From Place Verdun to Paimpol and St Brieuc

**Trains** From St Brieuc to St Malo, Brest and Paris

**Planes** From airport at St Brieuc

**Taxis** Batard ☎ 96.70.59.46

**Car and bicycle hire** Ask at tourist office

*Further information* from tourist office at 17 bis, Rue Jeanne d'Arc in St Quay.

# Nouveau Port de St Quay

| | |
|---|---|
| **Harbourmaster** ☎ 96.70.49.51 | **VHF Channel** 9 |
| **Callsign** Nouveau Port de St Quay | **Daily charge** ££££ |

Portrieux is an old drying harbour to which a large new marina has been added. The old harbour was crowded and little used by visitors, though for yachts able to take the ground it was, and still is, possible to go right in to the beach. The new marina charges are almost as great as in some English marinas and are higher than any others found on the Normandy and Brittany coasts. Full facilities are not yet in operation.

### STEP ASHORE

**Nearest payphone** By capitainerie

**Toilets, showers** In 1991 these were in portacabins and already tatty; cold water showers only

**Launderette** Not yet open (summer 1991)

**Clubhouse** Not yet open (summer 1991)

**Shopping** Several shops round the harbour, but most are in St Quay, one mile up the hill to the north

### SHIPS' SERVICES

*Water and electricity* On pontoons

*Fuel* (diesel and petrol) From fuelling berth

*Gas, chandler, boatyard, engineer, sailmaker* None available summer 1991, but these services will appear in time

# Paimpol

This busy commercial port was once the centre of the cod-fishing industry, but competition from Iceland and Newfoundland has resulted in fishing being confined to the coast and has placed the emphasis on oyster cultivation. Over the last 10 years Paimpol has developed considerably as a holiday resort. There are several streets of old houses worth exploring, and the town is surrounded by some wild and attractive country.

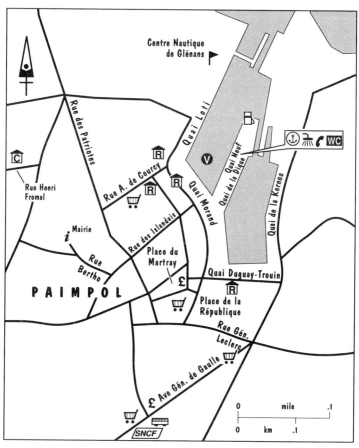

SHORE LEAVE

### Food and drink
On the quayside are salons de thé, bars and restaurants to suit all tastes. Try Café-Restaurant du Port, 17 Quai Morand, for a good all-round menu.

### Entertainment
There is a cinema in Rue Henri-Fromal, and an abundance of discos.

*What to see*
**Museum of the Sea** in Rue de Labenne vividly portrays the history of the Icelandic fishing fleet; on Quai Duguay-Trouin *Mad Atao*, a restored Camaret-built fishing vessel berthed in the harbour, is fitted out as a museum with information on sand-dredging. In Rue R. Pellier there is a museum of local costume.

*Excursions*
Two-and-a-half miles to the south in **Kerity**, a pretty village, is **Abbaye de Beauport**, a thirteenth and fourteenth-century monastery now largely in ruins. About five miles to the north is **Pointe de l'Arcouest** with a view over **Ile de Bréhat**. Buses go to both these places. Paimpol is a good base from which to visit Bréhat; boats leave every hour.

*Exercise*
Walk out on the peninsula to the east, to **Pointe de Guilben**, about a mile-and-a-half from Paimpol, where you get a good view of the many islands and reefs that lie off this rugged coast.

## TRANSPORT AND TRAVEL

**Buses** From the railway station to St Brieuc
**Trains** To Guingamp, change for Brest, St Malo and Paris
**Planes** From St Brieuc

**Taxis** Cab rank in Place de la Gare
**Car hire** Europcar, Garage Poidevin, Route de Lanvollon ☎ 96.20.96.96
**Bicycle hire** Quenec'h Du, Route de Lanvollon ☎ 96.20.75.94

*Further information* from tourist office in the Mairie, off Rue S. Bertho.

# Port de Paimpol

| | |
|---|---|
| **Harbourmaster** ☎ 96.20.80.77 | **VHF Channel** 9 |
| **Callsign** Port de Paimpol | **Daily charge** ££ |

The locked-in harbour at Paimpol is at the top of a long and beautiful drying inlet. The yacht harbour is surrounded by busy streets and is close to the centre of the town.

## STEP ASHORE

**Nearest payphone, toilets, showers** All by the capitainerie (called *Maison des Plaisanciers*) on the quay
**Launderette** Laverie 717 on the quayside
**Clubhouse** Centre Nautique des Glénans, Quai Pierre Loti
**Shopping** The shops are across the road that surrounds the harbour and extend back into the centre of the town, including the usual banks and a bureau de change in the post office. Weekly market on Tuesday mornings in the streets south of the basin. The Comptoir Coopératif, 46 Avenue Général de Gaulle, sells a wide range of sailing clothing

## SHIPS' SERVICES

*Water and electricity* On pontoons
*Fuei* (diesel and petrol) At the end of Quai de la Digue
*Gas* Camping Gaz from Supermarché

*Festival facing the port*
*Chandler, engineer* Le Lionnais Marine on the quayside
*Boatyard* Dauphin, Quai de Kernoa

# Ile de Bréhat

About two miles long by a mile at its widest, Bréhat is in fact two islands joined by Pont ar Prat, a causeway built by Vauban in the eighteenth century. The southern, more cultivated part of Bréhat has tiny fields bounded by dry stone walls, while the northern end is more wild and rugged. There are two main anchorages. Port-Clos, where the vedettes come in, is very busy and crowded. La Chambre, a little to the east, is crowded with yachts but much more peaceful and pleasant. Although the tide runs hard at times, at the turn it is very gentle and you will find your boat doing a complicated dance, probably out of step with the others.

Ile de Bréhat is a place to visit once you're settled in France, with victualled boat and a desire to visit an out-of-the-way, pleasant and relaxing place. The climate is even milder than the rest of Brittany; mimosa, oleander, myrtle and fig trees, palm trees and flowers usually found further south grow well.

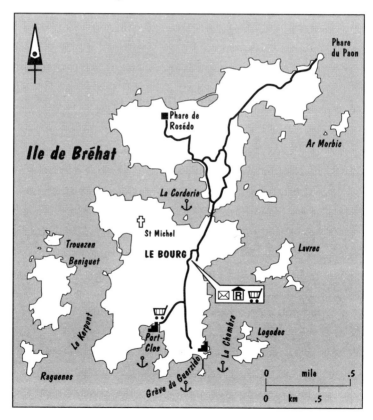

There are some facilities on Bréhat: **Le Bourg** has a couple of small shops, a small market and a number of family restaurants. The bread from the bakery is fresh and delicious as only French bread can be in such places. In the small shady square is an ancient church with a rose granite spire, and a Town Hall.

Vedettes from a number of ports on the Brittany coast come into **Port-Clos**, the only other settlement, where there is a shop, a hotel and a few cottages. It has a dinghy landing place and there is another at **La Chambre**. It is a 10-minute walk from both landings to **Le Bourg** along labyrinths of paths bordered by low houses and walls overhung with flowering creepers. The island is much-visited by day-trippers, most of whom leave at night because there are only two or three hotels on the island.

Cars are not allowed on Bréhat, but a taxi service, in the form of a tractor-trailer, is offered by local farmers. The island can be explored easily in a morning although it is better to take a day or more to investigate the many hidden coves and well-protected harbour of **La Corderie**, once used as a port by many ships, but now only suitable for shallow draught boats. You could walk to the **chapel of St Michel** in the west on the highest point on the island and admire the beauty of the **Kerpont Channel** at sunset. At the northernmost point there are wonderful coastal views from the **Phare du Paon** lighthouse on the rose granite rocks. The lighthouse-keeper will also show you over the **Phare de Rosédo** lighthouse on the north-western shore. Swimming is safe in **La Grève du Guerzido**.

## STEP ASHORE

**Nearest payphone** In Le Bourg

**Water** Tap close to path from la Grève du Guerzido

# Lézardrieux

The River Trieux has a spectacular entrance and there is a great sense of achievement as you pass between the rocky islets off the mouth of the river into the wooded valley beyond. Lézardrieux is about two miles up the river on the north bank. The sleepy village is separated from the equally sleepy port by a steep hill.

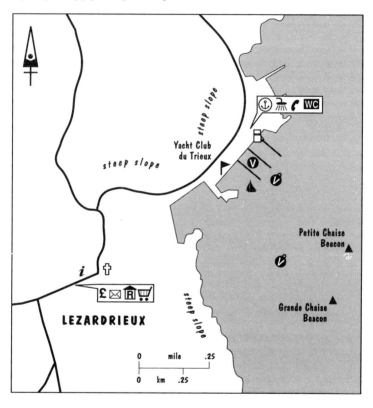

## SHORE LEAVE

### Food and drink
There are a couple of bars in the port opposite the quay and several more, as well as a restaurant or two, in the village up the hill.

### What to see
The **eighteenth-century church**, its pierced spire, with bells in the arcades, rising between two turrets, is typical of churches in this region.

### Excursions
**Sillon de Talbert** is a long narrow spit of land running out towards **Les Héaux**, a wild stretch of coast with magnificent views of the reefs. On the way to Sillon de Talbert, take a right turn off the road to see the ruined tide mill on the Trieux.

If you visit **Bodic lighthouse** near the mouth of the river, you will find a path on the left that leads through fields to a belvedere with a view of the estuary and offshore islands.

Ferries for **Ile de Bréhat** leave from Lézardrieux.

### TRANSPORT AND TRAVEL

**Buses** From Place du Boucy to Tréguier and Paimpol

**Car hire** Europcar ☎ 36.65.02.22

*Further information* from tourist office in Place du Boucy in the village.

# Port de Lézardrieux

**Harbourmaster** ☎ 96.20.14.22      **Daily charge** ££

The marina has every facility but is very crowded – it is the nearest French harbour to the Channel Islands and always popular with British sailors. You may be lucky enough to find a pontoon berth but are more likely to be put on a swinging mooring out in the river. Half a mile downstream there is room to anchor, free of charge, out of the strong current, a dinghy ride from the village.

### STEP ASHORE

**Nearest payphone** By capitainerie
**Toilets, showers** By capitainerie on quay
**Clubhouse** On the quay

**Shopping** Half a mile uphill to the west in the village are basic shops, a bank with bureau de change and a post office

### SHIPS' SERVICES

*Water and electricity* On pontoons
*Fuel* (petrol and diesel), *gas* (Camping

and Calor), *chandler, boatyard, engineer* All in marina

# Pontrieux

After the big marinas and crowded harbours on the coast, the sheer peacefulness of Pontrieux will strike you. Here you are quite removed from the vagaries of the sea – even the water is fresh and will clean the weed off your hull. You are warned against feeding the ducks lest they return in the small hours and ask for more. Geraniums grow in window boxes on almost every cottage. Half a mile above the moorings is the small town, a few bars and restaurants, and more geraniums, some filling a floating dinghy moored below the bridge. Pontrieux is a good, cheap and safe place to leave your boat and explore inland Brittany by car for a few days.

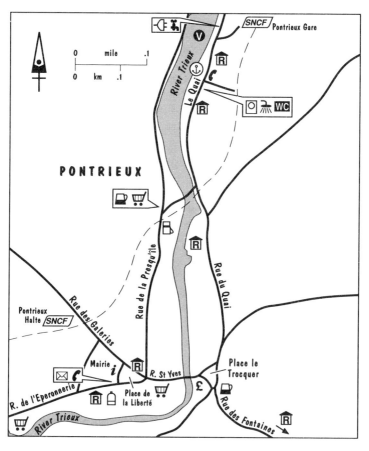

## SHORE LEAVE

*Food and drink*
Pizzeria Moulin du Richel, Rue du Quai, also has a traditional menu and is recommended. There are several bars near the quay and other restaurants and bars in town.

*Entertainment*
Films are shown on Friday evenings at the cinema in the town.

*What to see*
A **medieval house** in Place le Trocquer is being restored and looks attractive and colourful. There is also a charming old granite fountain.

*Excursions*
**Château de la Roche-Jagu** is a well-restored fifteenth-century castle which has not been lived in for some 300 years and so has never been 'modernised'. There is a good restaurant in the courtyard and another just down the road towards Lézardrieux. Vedettes for **Ile de Bréhat** leave from La Roche-Jagu.

Three miles west of Pontrieux at **Runan** is a large and richly decorated fourteenth and fifteenth-century church which belonged to the Knights Templar. It has a Renaissance ossuary and an outside pulpit dating from 1400.

*Exercise*
You can walk along the river bank to Château de la Roche-Jagu; it takes about an hour. Canoeing on the river is popular.

### TRANSPORT AND TRAVEL

**Trains** Pontrieux-Gare is a few minutes' walk from the moorings. Do not confuse it with Pontrieux-Halte which is in the town. Trains run to Paimpol and Guingamp; change for Brest, St Malo and Paris
**Planes** St Brieuc

**Ferries** St Malo
**Taxies** Michel Milon, 2 Rue des Fontaines
☎ 96.95.60.43
**Car hire** Garage du Viaduc
**Bicycle hire** Alain Marchal, 2 Rue du Quai

*Further information* from tourist office in the Hôtel de Ville in Place de la Liberté.

# Port de Pontrieux

| | |
|---|---|
| Harbourmaster ☎ 96.95.64.66 | **VHF Channel** 12, 16 |
| **Callsign** Port de Pontrieux *or* Ecluse de Pontrieux (lockmaster) | **Daily charge** £ |

Pontrieux is five miles upstream from Lézardrieux. The river runs through a steep-sided, wooded valley with glimpses of the railway high up on its viaducts and the impressive but friendly-seeming Château de la Roche-Jagu, below which there are visitors' buoys awaiting the tide up to the lock. Try to arrive one hour before high-water St Malo, which is also high-water Pontrieux, in spite of what the almanacs say. Call up the lockmaster if in doubt. There are no lights and the river is hazardous with manoeuvring sandboats at night. Once through the lock, continue for about a mile to the beginnings of the village and the moorings on the east bank. The harbourmaster will make you very welcome.

## STEP ASHORE

**Nearest payphone** Beside capitainerie
**Toilets, showers, laundry facilities** Near capitainerie (there is a service laundry in town)
**Shopping** Bread from the bar Chez Jacqueline and a limited selection of groceries are available from the Bar du Viaduc; otherwise the shops, bank (with cash dispenser) and post office are a half-mile walk up the road under the railway viaduct (Rue du Quai). The harbourmaster will lend you a trolley for fuel and heavy shopping

## SHIPS' SERVICES

*Water and electricity* On quayside
*Fuel* (diesel and petrol) From Garage du Viaduc; they will deliver in cans
*Gas* (Camping and Calor) From the wine shop in Place de la Liberté; they, too, will deliver

*Chandler* In Paimpol (a short trip by train) opposite the railway station, and on the quay
*Engineer* Alain Marchal will service outboard motors

# Tréguier

One of the few hill towns in Brittany, Tréguier is built in terraces overlooking the estuary of the Jaudy and Guindy Rivers and has a port which can receive big ships. The old cathedral is one of the main attractions of this former episcopal city. There is a large monastery dating back to 848 and many other interesting and historical buildings. It is a lively market town with very good shops, and some good restaurants. With its attractive river and lovely scenery, Tréguier is certainly a place to visit.

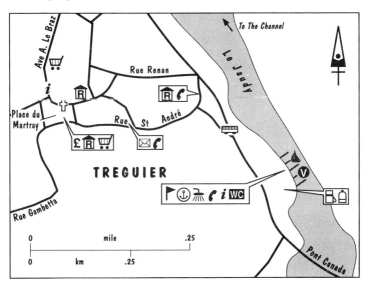

## SHORE LEAVE

### Food and drink
There are bars, pubs and restaurants on the quay and in town. The Hôtel l'Estuaire in Place Général de Gaulle is recommended. Le Canotier, 5 Rue Renan, is highly recommended for both food and service.

### Entertainment
Regular art exhibitions are held in the town.

### What to see
**St Tugdual's cathedral** dominates the square in the heart of the town. Its thirteenth to fifteenth-century Gothic architecture, some of the finest in Brittany, contrasts with the romanesque Hastings tower, which is all that remains of the twelfth-century building. The 202-foot-high perforated stone spire is very fine. A sixteenth-century half-timbered house in the square has been turned into a **museum** to celebrate the life of philosopher Ernest Renan. Notice the old town gates at the corner of Rue du Port and Rue Renan.

*Excursions*

The fifteenth-century **Château de la Roche-Jagu** six miles away is worth a visit (see under Pontrieux). Another excursion would be to **Sillon de Talbert**, the two-mile-long sand spit out towards **Les Héaux** (see under Lézardrieux). **Plougrescant** is a small village to the north with some interesting rock formations at **Le Gouffre**, a deep cleft in the rocks into which the sea roars.

*Exercise*

There are several beaches on the coast for swimming and windsurfing and a swimming pool in Tréguier. Follow the pleasant walk through **Bois du Poète** overlooking the Guindy River.

## TRANSPORT AND TRAVEL

**Buses** From the port to Guingamp and St Brieuc

**Trains** From Guingamp, 25 miles away

**Planes** From St Brieuc

**Ferries** From St Malo or Roscoff

**Taxis** ☎ 96.92.23.92

**Car hire** ☎ 96.48.00.10

**Bicycle hire** From the shop 200 yards along the road towards town

*Further information* from tourist offices in the marina and behind the cathedral.

# Port de Tréguier

| | |
|---|---|
| **Harbourmaster** ☎ 96.92.42.37 | **VHF Channel** 9 |
| **Callsign** Tréguier | **Daily charge** ££ |

The marina and quay facilities are good and the staff who run the harbourmaster's office as well as the sailing club are helpful and very welcoming. There are strong currents at half-ebb and flood-tides running through the pontoons which makes careful berthing necessary. There is no problem in leaving a boat here by arrangement.

## STEP ASHORE

**Nearest payphone** On the quay

**Toilets, showers** In clubhouse

**Launderette** Half-way up the hill into town

**Clubhouse** Club Nautique du Trégor on quay

**Shopping** In central square

### SHIPS' SERVICES

*Water and electricity* On pontoons

*Fuel* (diesel and petrol) On quay

*Gas* (Camping and Calor) At chandlery

*Chandler, boatyard, engineer* On quay

# Port Blanc

**Harbourmaster** (at Ecole de Voile)          **Daily charge** £
☎ 96.92.64.96

Port Blanc is an attractive harbour, with some forbidding-looking rocks
in the entrance. Once you have passed them the roadstead opens up
with grassy islands on either hand and a wooded shore ahead. Above
the lighthouse the **Moulin de la Comtesse** can be seen peeping through
the trees, if they have been cut back sufficiently. The bay is full of tiny
dinghies sailed by even tinier children, who are sometimes not in full
control and bump into the moored yachts. Anchor or pick up a visitor's
buoy. The moorings are some way from the shore, to which there is little
to draw one except the chance to stretch the legs. The village, for basic
supplies only, is a mile-and-a-half inland, a dusty walk. The hotel on the
seafront serves meals to non-residents.

This picturesque natural harbour, on the edge of the Côte de Granit
Rose, is popular for family holidays with its rocks and sandy bays and
busy sailing school.

## STEP ASHORE

**Nearest payphone** At the sailing school          **Toilets, showers** At the sailing school
or hotel

# Perros-Guirec

Perros-Guirec is a large holiday resort, the most lively on the Côte de Granit Rose. The main town is on a hill, and a steep climb from the harbour; the beaches, too, are a little distance from the marina. It is a good place to stop for a break from sailing and to visit such places as the Satellite Telecommunications Centre and Planetarium at Pleumeur-Bodou. (This is the site of the Radôme antenna, as tall as the Arc de Triomphe,which is such an outstanding landmark as you sail westward.) Inland there are several châteaux and churches well worth a visit. In the town centre the fine, partly twelfth-century, red-granite church has a richly carved south porch.

The beaches and other leisure attractions are very popular in the height of summer. The hotels and restaurants are expensive.

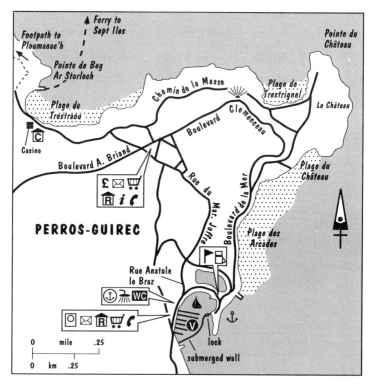

## SHORE LEAVE

### Food and drink
There are several restaurants, bars and take-aways within 100 yards of the marina. Le Levant on the quay is recommended by one visitor as are La Bonne Auberge in Place de la Chapelle, and the Homard Bleu and Excelsior.

*Entertainment*

There is a cinema at the Palais des Congrès on the seafront at Plage de Trestraou and a casino nearby.

*What to see*

The **Waxworks and Historical Documents Museum** is opposite the yacht club. The Table d'Orientation in Boulevard Clemenceau has magnificent views.

*Excursions*

A vedette leaves twice a day from Trestraou beach for a cruise around **Les Sept Iles** to see the bird sanctuary on **Rouzic** and the lighthouse on **L'Ile aux Moines**.

There is an **aquarium** near Trégastel Bay; at Pleumeur-Bodou you might be interested by the **planetarium** and exhibition of mounted sea-birds; guided visits to the bird wildlife sanctuary are organised from here. There is also a guided visit to the **Radôme**, the first antenna directed to satellites to receive world-wide communications.

**Lannion**, set amid plummeting hills and with even steeper stairways, is an attractive reminder of an older Brittany. Streets of medieval architecture line both banks of the Léguer River – it is well worth visiting.

*Exercise*

There are three or four very good beaches within a mile or so of the marina, all suitable for windsurfing. The leisure centre in Rue de Kerabram has a swimming pool. Play golf or tennis in the Parc des Sports.

The tourist guide has a list of walks along the attractive and often spectacular coastline. **Le Sentier des Douaniers**, leading to the rocks around Ploumanac'h, is the best. Eastward, **Pointe du Château**, with beaches on either side, gives a particularly fine view towards Les Sept Iles and Ile Tomé.

### TRANSPORT AND TRAVEL

**Buses** Three buses a day leave the centre of the town for Lannion, eight miles away
**Trains** From Lannion to Brest, Paris, Roscoff and St Malo via Plouaret
**Planes** From Lannion airport to Paris and Jersey
**Ferries** To Les Sept Isles, Roscoff,
St Malo, Jersey and Guernsey
**Taxis** By gendarmerie in Boulevard Aristide Briand ☎ 96.37.02.40
**Car hire** Europcar, Place de l'Hôtel de Ville
**Bicycle hire** Le Coant, Rue Ernest Renan, opposite quay

*Further information* from tourist office, 21 Place de l'Hôtel de Ville.

## Perros-Guirec Marina

| Harbourmaster ☎ 96.23.37.82 | VHF Channel 9 |
| --- | --- |
| Callsign Perros-Guirec | Daily charge ££ |

The marina is in a sheltered bay on the north side of the town. It is possible to anchor off and dry out, but it would be a long walk to get ashore. The marina is well run with helpful staff. It is easy to leave a boat there by arrangement.

## STEP ASHORE

**Nearest payphone** On the quay by capitainerie opposite Pontoon P

**Toilets, showers** In capitainerie across the road from the marina; open during office hours

**Launderette** Laverie du Port opposite quay

**Clubhouse** Association des Plaisanciers near lock

**Shopping** Small collection of very adequate shops and restaurants near the marina, but the main shops are half a mile away up the hill to the north, with banks and a post office. Late-night shopping Thursdays; shops closed every day 1200–1500. The nearest supermarket is Rapid, off Rue du Maréchal Joffre; Intermarché is in Rue Lejeune. Market in the Place du Marché on Friday mornings

### SHIPS' SERVICES

*Water and electricity* On pontoons
*Fuel* (diesel and petrol) On quay near lock
*Gas* (Camping and Calor) From chandler

*Chandler* On quay
*Boatyard, engineer* In Chaussée du Linkin

# Les Sept Iles

Guidebooks in English call them 'The Seven Islands', which sounds far less romantic – more like a salad dressing than a group of desert islands. There is a mooring buoy in the bay south of Ile aux Moines for the vedettes which bring hordes of tourists; you can anchor nearby and land at the slip. At lunchtime or in the late afternoon you will have the place to yourself. Of the four main islands, **Rouzic** and **Ile de Bono** are bird sanctuaries with a large and interesting population ranging from puffins and guillemots to various gulls and oyster-catchers. Landing is permitted only on **Ile aux Moines**, where the lighthouse can be visited and a walk over the island will reveal derelict fortifications and many wild flowers. The islands are best visited as a break on passage.

# Ploumanac'h

Ploumanac'h is a little fishing port at the mouth of the Grand and Petit Traouïéro Rivers. The bay is outstandingly attractive with its spectacular rose granite rocks and boulders that look as though they are tumbling into the sea. On one of the islands in the bay is the nineteenth-century Château Costaérès, another picturesque addition to the landscape, while further west is La Pendante, a very impressive rocking stone.

As a resort Ploumanac'h is very popular with the French at the height of summer, even more so than Perros-Guirec, and the restaurants are apt to be booked up. Nevertheless, they are very well run and have excellent food. The shops are rather touristy. Drive or walk around the nearby area to enjoy the hilly countryside and attractive villages.

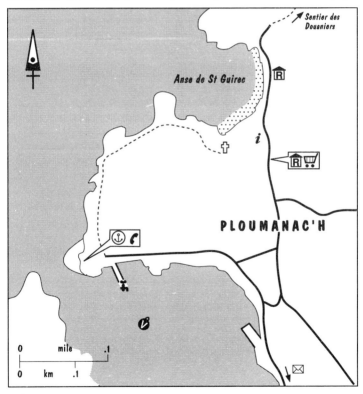

SHORE LEAVE

### Food and drink

Hôtel des Rochers, L'Albatros and Bistro du Port are all on the quay. Mao-Snack Bar is very good value and the Hôtel Roch Hir recommended. Le Relais is up the hill in La Clarté village.

### What to see

You can hardly avoid noticing the rocks and boulders on the shore: waves and weather have worn them into fantastic shapes, many of which have been given names like witch, whale, corkscrew, umbrella, skull, clog and foot — see if you can find others. They are best seen from **Château du Diable** and **Pointe de Squewel** or best of all from the **lighthouse** at **Pors Kamor**, especially at sunrise and sunset when the rocks seem to change colour. All these are on the **Sentier des Douaniers** path to Perros-Guirec.

On the beach there used to be a wooden statue of St Guirec into the nose of which girls seeking a husband would stick pins. The poor man's nose was worn away by the girls' headlong rush on their fate and a new statue of granite has been erected in its place, so they have had to find other means of attaining the married state.

### Excursion

Visit **Trégastel** which rivals Ploumanac'h for the beauty and strangeness of its rocks.

### Exercise

There are plenty of safe beaches and attractive walks along the coastal shoreline. From Ploumanac'h to Perros-Guirec by the **Sentier des Douaniers** coast path takes three hours there and back. For the most dramatic views go in the afternoon at high tide.

### TRANSPORT AND TRAVEL

**Buses** From village centre to Perros
**Taxis** Dauphin, Boulevard des Traouïéros
☎ 96.91.62.00

**Car hire** Vallart, Boulevard du Sémaphore
☎ 96.91.43.76

**Further information** from tourist office in Rue St-Guirec.

# Port de Ploumanac'h

Harbourmaster ☎ 96.23.36.51                    Daily charge ££

There is a simple harbour with only basic facilities. In the channel opposite the Anse de St Guirec are three visitors' buoys, or you can go on into the floating basin, where visitors moor to the first line of buoys beyond the fishing boats. It is a very sheltered spot and a suitable place to leave a catamaran or craft that takes the bottom easily.

### STEP ASHORE

**Nearest payphone** Near bureau du port
**Toilets, showers** On quay
**Launderette** In village to north
**Shopping** Some shops in village to north

or one-and-a-half miles east towards Perros-Guirec. The post office is about one mile along the Perros road

### SHIPS' SERVICES

*Water* On quay
*Gas* (Camping and Calor) From supermarket in town

*Chandler, boatyard, engineer* Ask at bureau du port

# Primel

| | |
|---|---|
| **Harbourmaster** ☎ 98.72.38.76 | **VHF Channel** 9 |
| **Callsign** Primel | **Daily charge** £ |

This small harbour at the entrance to the Baie de Morlaix is crowded but there are a few visitors' buoys and a little space for anchoring. Primel is a pleasant rural resort with facilities for day-sailing. Not really oriented to visiting cruisers, it is a good sheltered place to spend a night. There are some facilities and shops at Le Diben but they are all too far away to be convenient. It is nearly two miles to the town of Plougasnou.

## STEP ASHORE

**Nearest payphone** At root of jetty
**Toilets, showers** At Le Diben, which is well up the harbour in the south-west corner
**Shopping** A few shops near the harbour at Le Diben and a small village half a mile up the hill from Le Diben. It is nearly two miles to the town of Plougasnou

### SHIPS' SERVICES

**Water** On quay

## SHORE LEAVE

If you need to stretch your legs, walk to the **Pointe de Primel**, a jumble of rocks comparable to those at Ploumanac'h and Trégastel and very impressive from seaward. The point is connected to the rest of the peninsula by an isthmus which can be crossed at low tide.

**Further information** from tourist office in Plougasnou ☎ 98.67.31.88.

# Morlaix

Situated seven miles from the sea where the deep valleys of the Jarlot and Queffleuth join to form the Morlaix River, Morlaix is approached up a pleasant wooded valley. After the last turn in the river the town opens up with buildings climbing the hills on either side and the huge railway viaduct dominating the scene.

Morlaix's connection with England goes a long way back, to tit-for-tat raiding in the Middle Ages. In 1522 the English sacked the town while the locals were away at a fair; having drunk too much free French wine, the raiders were asleep when the enraged townsfolk returned and duly dispatched them. The Château du Taureau was built in the estuary to

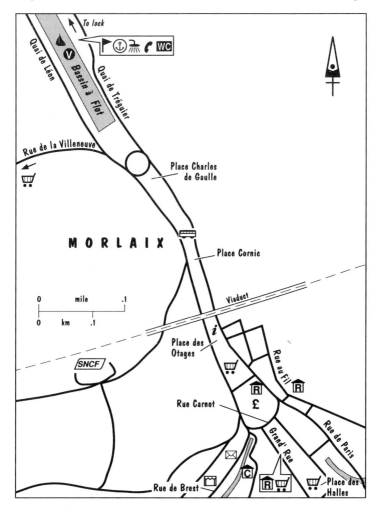

prevent further raids; it took 21 years to complete, so builders were not known for speed even then.

On your way into or out of Morlaix you may have to wait out a tide. There are several attractive places where you can anchor or pick up a buoy. Pen Lann is one, tucked in behind Ile Louet, with its lighthouse and garden sheltering behind the rock, and just the lantern peeping to seaward over the top.

## SHORE LEAVE

### Food and drink
Many good eating places can be found in town, especially in the Rue du Mur district. La Table de Rabelais, 9 Rue au Fil, is highly recommended. Brasserie Lof, 1 Rue d'Aiguillon, is also good.

### Entertainment
There are theatres in Rue de Brest and Rue Gambetta, cinemas in Chemin de l'Hospice and La Boissière.

### What to see
At first sight the town seems just a busy thoroughfare, with traffic and people rushing about, but look further. Find the steep old back streets like Rue du Mur and the ancient houses in **Rue Ange de Guernisac**, **Grand'Rue**, and **Place des Halles** where the staircase in **Maison de la Reine Anne** is a masterpiece of medieval craftsmanship. Visit the **museum** in Place des Jacobins which depicts the history of Morlaix from prehistoric times as well as housing a collection of modern art.

### Excursions
Ten miles inland are the **Arrée mountains**, a region of desolate heathland with superb views, and wooded valleys with small hamlets. This is also the region of the **parish closes:** these are a combination of church, charnel-house and triumphal arch built round a courtyard. They developed during the Renaissance and are peculiar to Brittany. Rivalry between villages led to ever richer and more elaborate constructions being built, and a day tour would be very interesting.

### Exercise
There is an indoor swimming pool at La Boissière.

### TRANSPORT AND TRAVEL

**Buses** From Place Cornic
**Trains** To Brest, Roscoff and Paris
**Planes** From Morlaix-Ploujean airport, two miles from Morlaix, to Gatwick and Cork

**Ferries** from Roscoff
**Taxis** At Place des Otages
☎ 98.88.36.42
**Car hire** Europcar, Rue des Lavoirs
**Bicycle hire** From SNCF

**Further information** from tourist office in Place des Otages, under the viaduct.

# Port de Morlaix

| | |
|---|---|
| **Harbourmaster** ☎ 98.62.13.14 (at lock ☎ 98.88.54.92) | **VHF Channel** 9 |
| **Callsign** Morlaix | **Daily charge** ££ |

The harbour is in a locked basin in the heart of a busy town – a safe and secure place to leave a boat. The harbourmaster is friendly and helpful and facilities are adequate, although there is not much boating activity on weekdays.

## STEP ASHORE

**Nearest payphone** By yacht club
**Toilets, showers** In clubhouse on quayside
**Launderette** Rue des Lavoirs, off Rue Carnot in town centre
**Clubhouse** Yacht Club de Morlaix on quay by pontoons

**Shopping** All the shops you would expect in a medium-sized French town are about 10 minutes' walk from the basin. There is a Euromarché hypermarket two miles away, uphill, at St Martin des Champs

### SHIPS' SERVICES

**Water and electricity** On pontoons
**Fuel** On quay
**Gas** From **chandler** on west side of basin

**Boatyard, engineer** Rio, downstream near lock

# Penzé River

Between the Morlaix River and Roscoff, this is a pleasant river with quiet anchorages suitable for an overnight stop. There are no facilities. The nearest town, **St Pol de Léon**, a mile inland, has a fine cathedral and a chapel with another of the region's magnificent belfries, visible from the sea. The name is a corruption of St Paul the Aurelian, a Roman who disposed of the dragon at Ile de Batz.

# Roscoff

Roscoff is a rugged granite town, representative of the rugged coast on which it lies. It has an air of hardy seagoing tradition about it and is still a busy fishing port in spite of the modern holiday crowds. Mary Queen of Scots landed here as a five-year-old child on the way to her betrothal to the Dauphin in 1542; the house where she rested still stands on the quayside. Two centuries later Bonnie Prince Charlie arrived in the port just ahead of the English pursuit when escaping after the '45 rising.

The climate here is surprisingly mild, given the wild weather offshore to the west, and the land is correspondingly fertile.

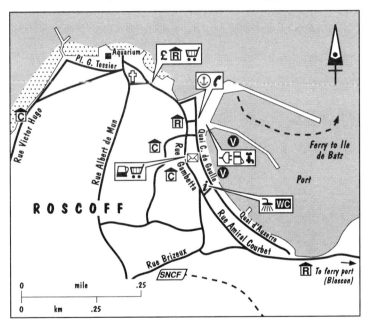

## SHORE LEAVE

### Food and drink
You get the impression that every other building is a snack-bar or crêperie, especially round the harbour. There are a dozen or more hotels in Roscoff, many of which have restaurants, and if you choose with circumspection you might find one to your taste, but don't expect a gourmet's *expérience gastronomique*.

### Entertainment
There is a cinema in Rue Victor Hugo and another off Rue Gambetta.

### What to see
The town is small and soon explored, but visit the church of **Notre Dame de Kroaz-Batz**, which dominates the skyline with its outstanding openwork belfry.

Visit also the **aquarium** and **oceanographic museum**, connected with the University of Paris. Between Roscoff and Bloscon, on the coast, is a garden with exotic plants. There is a small beach to the east of the town, with *viviers* (floating fish tanks), stocked with sea trout, salmon, lobster and crab. To the west are more beaches and a three-mile walk will bring you to the fine beaches at **Dossen** and **Ile de Sieck** for swimming and windsurfing.

*Excursions*
Vedettes leave frequently for **Ile de Batz**.

## TRANSPORT AND TRAVEL

**Buses** To St Pol-de-Léon and Morlaix
**Trains** To Paris and Brest, change at Morlaix
**Planes** From Morlaix-Ploujean (21 miles away) to Gatwick
**Ferries** From Bloscon to Plymouth

(six hours) and Cork
**Taxis** Boulay, 5 Rue Ropartz-Morvan
☎ 98.69.70.67
**Car hire** Kreisker-Voyages, St Pol-de-Léon
☎ 98.69.00.93
**Bicycle hire** Desbordes, Rue Brizeux

*Further information* from tourist office in Rue Gambetta.

# Port de Roscoff

| Harbourmaster ☎ 98.69.76.37 | VHF Channel 9 |
|---|---|
| Callsign Roscoff | Daily charge £ |

It is possible to lie afloat off Roscoff but it is uncomfortable because of the swell and a long way from shore. It is best to go into the inner harbour and dry out against the wall if there is room. Alongside, the wall is steep and rough in parts and you may need your own ladder.

Bloscon, the ferry terminal, is an alternative place to moor, with a few visitors' buoys. It is strictly utilitarian with only a landing slip and few facilities. If the terminal is open, toilets and snacks may be found there, and it is only a brisk 10-minute walk into Roscoff.

## STEP ASHORE

**Nearest payphone** On quay
**Toilets, showers** Municipal conveniences close to the lighthouse on the promenade

**Shopping** All the shops in this small town are near the harbour, as are banks, the post office and bureau de change

### SHIPS' SERVICES

*Water* Available on quay
*Electricity* On quay

*Fuel, gas* From Coop Maritime

# Ile de Batz

Separated from Roscoff by a narrow channel, the Ile de Batz enjoys a surprisingly mild climate. It is treeless and largely devoted to market gardening. Moor in the picturesque drying harbour or anchor just outside near the ferry landing. There are no facilities or supplies but the village has shops to provide essential stores and cafés and restaurants for refreshments. Bicycles can be hired at the landing stage. There are pleasant walks over the island to see the lighthouse and the north coast where you will find the rock from which St Paul the Aurelian threw out the dragon which had terrorised the island.

# Les Abers (Finistère)

This is where Brittany looks out to the Atlantic. From Roscoff westward and through the Chenal du Four as far as Le Conquet, the coastline is grey, rocky and forbidding, carved into dramatic shapes by the huge seas which crash down on it. Inland it is mainly flat, farming country with crops of artichoke and cauliflower and small villages of granite houses and churches, often with the parish closes typical of this area.

The *abers* (estuaries) – the same word as in Welsh – dwindle to little streams. The villages are small, built to serve small fishing or farming communities; nowadays they are often afflicted by the blight of shuttered up holiday homes and abandoned farms. Dolmens and menhirs abound in this ancient Celtic land. Ten miles inland is the village of **Le Folgoët**, with its fine basilica and one of the best belfries in Brittany. There is also an attractive fifteenth-century manor house, **Le Doyenné**, in the village. On the first Sunday in September there is a Pardon, when crowds of pilgrims come to drink from the spring under the altar. Frank Cowper, the Victorian sailor, author of *Sailing Tours*, and founder-member of the Cruising Association, suggests you may like to walk the twenty-mile round trip to and from L'Aber Wrac'h.

There are many small harbours, mostly with little to offer visitors and needing very careful pilotage, but if you are feeling intrepid or ready for a break in pleasant rural surroundings, you might like to put in to some of them. A small shop, restaurant or bar can usually be found after a healthy walk, but L'Aber Wrac'h is the only place with fuel on this coast.

### Moguériec
A drying harbour just west of Roscoff.

### Pontusval
It is possible to anchor in the entrance of this harbour but it would be better to go right in and dry out. There is a tabac-bar in the south-west corner, from which a short walk will bring you to Brignogan village with small shops.

### L'Aber Wrac'h
This is the staging post for crossing the Channel or venturing westward through the Chenal du Four. It is the only place for fuelling alongside before Brest. See detailed entry on page 376.

### L'Aber Benoît
A sheltered deep-water anchorage, more peaceful and beautiful than L'Aber Wrac'h; there are a few shops and crêperies to be found in the lanes if you are really determined.

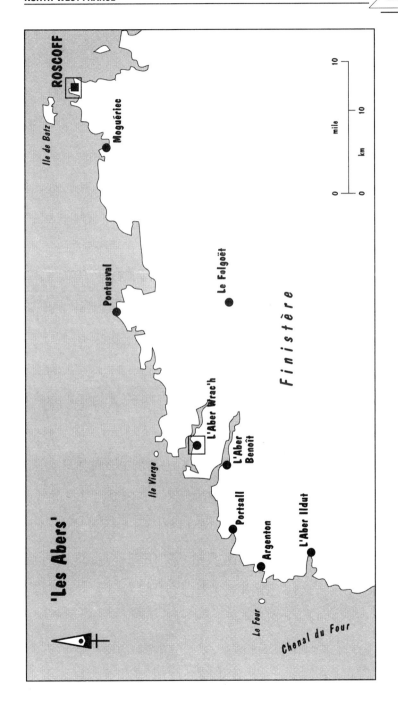

### Portsall

A pretty fishing harbour where you can lie off in deep water behind the rocks which sank the *Amoco Cadiz* and fouled the whole coast with oil. You can also dry out further in, close to the village. There are only basic shops here, a crêperie and a couple of bars. At the top of the hill to the south, along Rue du Port, there is a restaurant in the Hôtel de Bretagne.

### Argenton

A dinghy sailing harbour; it is possible to anchor off or dry out closer in.

### L'Aber Ildut

This is a useful, sheltered harbour half-way through the Chenal du Four. It is very crowded with small boats. There are small shops and cafés. The large granite quarries on the starboard hand supplied stone for French harbours in the nineteenth century and also for the Thames Embankment.

# L'Aber Wrac'h and Paluden

| | |
|---|---|
| **Harbourmaster** ☎ 98.04.91.62 | **VHF Channel** 16, 9 |
| **Callsign** L'Aber Wrac'h | **Daily charge** ££ |

L'Aber Wrac'h is the westernmost French harbour to provide facilities for stocking up before going through the Chenal du Four, so it is very popular with British yachts. Once inside the rocks guarding the entrance, you will find that it is completely sheltered. Mooring is to buoys – with a free water-taxi service to the shore – or to the crowded pontoon. There is little to do ashore except for walking.

For more peace and quiet, either anchor nearer the entrance (avoid the oyster beds), or go further up the river towards **Paluden** where you can either anchor or find a mooring. The restaurant on the quay at Paluden is well spoken of and you will be nearer to Lannilis for the shops.

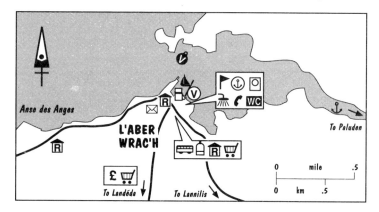

## SHORE LEAVE

There are small bars and restaurants near the marina; grander meals can be had at Hôtel Baie des Anges in high season only.

### TRANSPORT AND TRAVEL

**Buses** To Brest several times a day

**Taxis** ☎ 98.89.81.58

*Further information* from capitainerie.

## STEP ASHORE

**Nearest payphone, toilets, showers, launderette** In clubhouse on the quay. Also sauna

**Shopping** Simple needs can be met by the mini-market south of the entrance to the marina; the post office is close by to the north. Village shops and a bank one mile up the hill at Landéda or a larger selection two miles inland at Lannilis.

### SHIPS' SERVICES

**Water** On pontoon
**Electricity, fuel** (diesel) On the quay
**Gas** (Camping and Calor) From bar at the entrance to marina

**Chandler** Comptoir Maritime des Abers
**Boatyard, engineer** Tech-Marine in south-west corner of harbour

# Le Conquet

Le Conquet is a good staging point if the Chenal du Four is rough or you need a rest, but it is a crowded fishing harbour. Once your boat is secure, go ashore to the little town. Although it is not a place for more than an overnight stop, the streets are pleasant to wander in and the cliff walks to both north and south of the harbour afford views of the port and out to the islands of Ushant and Molène.

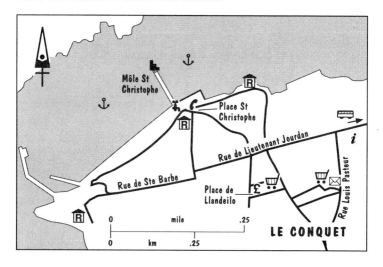

SHORE LEAVE

### Food and drink
The Crêperie du Drellach is near Môle St Christophe and saves walking up the hill. The Bar-Restaurant la Taverne du Port in Rue St Christophe is recommended, as is the very good restaurant in Hôtel St Barbe.

### Excursions
It is an easy and pleasant two-mile walk along the corniche road to **Pointe de St Mathieu**, where there are the imposing ruins of the abbey founded in the sixth century by St Tanguy. The head of St Matthew was said to have been brought back from Ethiopia and kept here. The Breton name for Pointe de St Mathieu is **Pen Ar Bed**, meaning 'world's end', which expresses just how it feels to stand there and look out to the west.

### TRANSPORT AND TRAVEL
**Buses** To Brest
**Trains, planes** From Brest

**Taxis** Jean le Ray ☎ 98.89.32.28
**Car Hire** ☎ 98.80.43.98 (in Brest)

**Further information** from tourist office in Parc de Beauséjour.

# Port du Conquet

**Harbourmaster** ☎ 98.89.00.05    **Callsign** Le Conquet

The moorings are private, but you may be invited to use one; anchoring is possible but difficult due to lack of space. If you can dry out, go upstream of the north-south Môle St Christophe, which is the main landing point.

## STEP ASHORE

**Nearest payphone** On Môle St Christophe
**Shopping** The town with usual range of shops, banks and post office, is at the top of the steep hill leading up from the harbour. The Rallye supermarket in the town centre is open 0900–1215 and 1430–1915

### SHIPS' SERVICES

*Water* On Môle St Christophe
*Gas* From Rallye supermarket

*Chandler* Coop Marine on Môle St Christophe

# Brest

The city of Brest is overwhelmingly large after the fishing villages of the coast or the river ports of the Rade. It is a large modern city, rebuilt after the bombing of 1944 – only a few old buildings survive – with every kind of shop and entertainment: nightlife, museums, markets, parks and gardens.

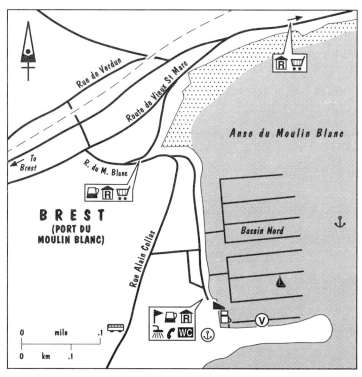

SHORE LEAVE

### Food and drink
The cafés and restaurants in the marina itself are offhand and uninspiring. In Rue du Moulin Blanc, the street behind the marina, is a bar and restaurant – part of the village shop – where you can buy a newspaper and have a continental breakfast of coffee and croissants; otherwise sample the wide choice in the city.

### Entertainment
There are several cinemas: two are Le Club, 136 Rue Jean-Jaurès and Le Mac Orlan, 65 Rue de la Porte.

### What to see
There are art galleries, a marine museum and a fine arts museum. The **Pont de Recouvrance** over the Penfeld River, near the entrance to the dockyard, is the largest lifting-bridge in Europe. The naval dockyard looks interesting but

cannot be visited by foreigners. The **Château de Brest**, on the east bank of the mouth of the Penfeld, houses the **marine museum**. On the opposite bank is **Tanguy Tower**, also open to the public, in the old district of **Recouvrance**, itself an interesting area to wander through. **Océanopolis**, alongside the marina, is a large new **aquarium** which offers many adventures, rather like a marine safari park. It is a scientific research centre and the largest aquarium in Europe – 500,000 litres.

*Excursions*
Vedettes leave from the Port de Commerce for many of the rivers of the Rade, as well as the **Crozon peninsula** and the island of **Ushant**.

*Exercise*
All water sports are catered for, including several swimming pools. If you need a change from these, riding is a popular alternative.

### TRANSPORT AND TRAVEL

**Buses** From outside marina into Brest (2–3 per hour)
**Trains** To Roscoff, Rennes, St Malo, Paris
**Planes** From Brest airport
**Ferries** From Roscoff

**Taxis** ☎ 98.80.43.43
**Car hire** Europcar, 43 Rue Voltaire ☎ 98.44.66.88
**Bicycle hire** From SNCF

*Further information* from tourist office, 8 Avenue Georges Clemenceau.


# Port du Moulin Blanc

| | |
|---|---|
| **Harbourmaster** ☎ 98.02.20.02 | **VHF Channels** 9, 16 |
| **Callsign** Moulin Blanc | **Daily charge** ££ |

The marina in the Anse du Moulin Blanc is a vast place with all facilities for yachts, but it is impersonal and divorced from both the city and countryside by fast roads and its distance from the city centre – three miles. It is a useful place to stay if you want to explore Brest, leave your boat, or have crew joining or leaving you; otherwise victual up and take off from Moulin Blanc to explore the Rade de Brest.

### STEP ASHORE

**Nearest payphone** By capitainerie
**Toilets, showers, launderette** In toilet block under yacht club
**Clubhouse** On quay
**Shopping** Convenience shops in the marina and small villages shops in the street at the back of the marina. Everything else you could possibly want can be found in Brest

### SHIPS' SERVICES

*Water and electricity* On pontoons
*Fuel* (diesel and petrol) From fuelling berth

*Gas* From chandler in marina
*Chandler, boatyard, engineer, sailmaker* All in marina

# La Rade de Brest

La Rade de Brest, a lagoon providing nearly 60 square miles of sheltered water, makes a grand cruising ground away from the open sea. Apart from Brest itself and the naval base opposite, the surrounding land is pleasantly rural with wooded slopes and fields. Three rivers — the Elorn, the Daoulas and the Aulne — run into the Rade. The Elorn dries but the seven miles to **Landerneau** are navigable. However, the town is very disappointing: you will lie in smelly mud in the middle of a busy town centre. The River Daoulas also dries out, but is rural, with a small town, also called **Daoulas**; a typical Breton parish close by is well worth a visit. The Aulne dries too but is navigable for a greater distance and runs between wooded banks to **Port Launay**. Here you can lock in and lie against a stone quay backed by grassy banks and a quiet village street, with water meadows opposite. There are small shops and a restaurant nearby. You can carry on up stream to lie below the larger town of **Châteaulin**.

Back in the Rade, there are numerous small bays, some with landing stages and pretty villages behind them. There may be a bar or restaurant, but the main pleasures are the peace and lovely surroundings. **Lauberlach** and **Tinduff** are two such villages. There is also a sheltered anchorage among the hulks of old naval ships at the mouth of the Aulne, with a climb through the trees to the village of **Landévennec** and its charming restaurant.

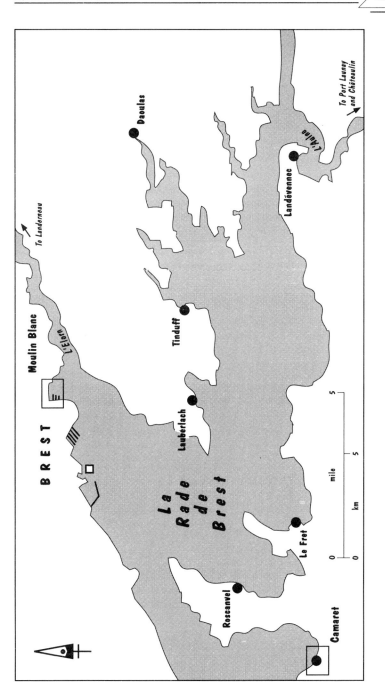

# Camaret

Camaret is on the Presqu'île de Crozon, a name which gives a good indication of the isolation of the town. It lies in a well-protected bay, which, for yacht crews, is conveniently situated at the southern end of the Chenal du Four and at the south-west entrance to the Rade de Brest.

The Anse de Camaret is famous for the first underwater test of a submarine made in 1801. Fortunately the unsuspecting British ship, the target of the experiment, weighed anchor and left before the oar-powered submarine reached it with a load of explosives.

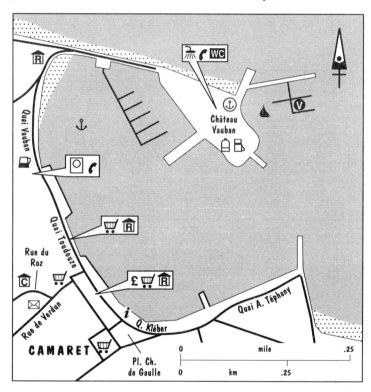

## SHORE LEAVE

### Food and drink

There are many bars, snack-bars, take-aways and restaurants around the harbour and in the neighbouring streets. Several have very good seafood menus. Hôtel de France is very welcoming and so is La Voilerie, a small restaurant specialising in seafood. Both are recommended and both are on Quai Toudouze.

### What to see

Near the marina is a fishermen's church, **Notre Dame de Rocamadour**, on the

Sillon Dyke. The tower on Sillon Point is **Vauban Castle**. Built in the seventeenth century to keep the English at bay, it now houses a **maritime museum** devoted to the town's history.

*Excursions*
**Pointe de Penhir**, two miles from Camaret, is the finest of the four headlands of the Crozon peninsula, with panoramic views of St Mathieu and Toulinguet points and, on a clear day, the islands of Sein and Ushant.

*Exercise*
A pleasant evening walk can be taken along the cliffs looking northwards into the Rade de Brest as well as westwards over the rocks of Toulinguet. It is from here that Admiral Cornwallis besieged the port of Brest, preparing detailed pilots through the rocks and the promontories of this beautiful coastline. Looking out to sea, you can still imagine the square-rigged ships of the line standing off and on in all weathers watching for the French fleet to come out.

### TRANSPORT AND TRAVEL

**Buses** To Morgat, Châteaulin, Brest and Quimper
**Trains** From Brest and Quimper
**Planes** From Brest-Guipavas and Quimper-Pluguffan
**Bicycle hire** Bar La Flibuste, Quai Toudouze

*Further information* from tourist office, Quai Kléber.

# Port de Camaret

| Harbourmaster ☎ 98.27.95.99 | Daily charge ££ |
| --- | --- |

This typical, picturesque, French fishing port has most of the facilities required by yachtsmen: a small visitors' marina, a town with a market, supermarket, bakeries and many small restaurants around the port. The marina is a bit of a hike from the town – about a mile. For those with shallow draught vessels and who do not mind taking the ground, the beach near the old fishing hulks is a good clean place to dry out; it is also convenient for shops, restaurants and the beach.

## STEP ASHORE

**Nearest payphone** In toilet block (coin-operated); two card phones outside launderette
**Toilets, showers** Near the landing pontoon, under the Tour Vauban
**Launderette** Quai Vanban

**Clubhouse** Club Léo Lagrange on Quai Téphany
**Shopping** All the usual shops, banks and post office are on the Quai Toudouze, which runs along the harbour, or in the streets behind

### SHIPS' SERVICES

*Water and electricity* On pontoons
*Fuel* (diesel and petrol), *gas* (Camping and Calor) From Mecamar on Quai Téphany

*Chandler* Uship, on Quai Téphany
*Boatyard* Close to marina and on Quai Téphany
*Engineer* On quay

# Morgat

Morgat is a small seaside resort a mile from Crozon, the town which gives its name to the peninsula enclosing the southern side of the Rade de Brest. There is very little to Morgat beyond a few shops and cafés. There are grottoes in the cliffs just south of the harbour to which boat trips can be taken. The churches at Crozon and Roscanvel are modern, the latter having some fine stained glass.

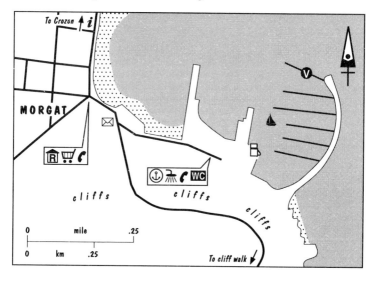

## SHORE LEAVE

### Food and drink

There are several bars and restaurants. Visit the crêperie in the thatched barn where the display of dolls, lace, pictures, bygones and general bric-à-brac will keep you amused while you eat.

### What to see

In **Crozon** there is a permanent exhibition of regional geology.

### Exercise

Swim from the very good beaches: there is a small uncrowded beach at the root of the mole, a wide sandy stretch to the south. Walk up through the woods and out on to the heathland towards **Cap de la Chèvre**, or westwards across the peninsula to look out to sea and to the Tas de Pois rocks off Pointe de Penhir. In all directions the walks lead over heathlands to impressive cliffs and promontories. Northwards, a longer walk will bring you to a view over the Rade de Brest and the village of **Le Fret** with a ferry to Brest itself. The Crozon peninsula is rich in menhirs and *alignements* (standing stones).

## TRANSPORT AND TRAVEL

**Buses** From village centre to Crozon, Camaret, Brest and Quimper
**Trains, planes** From Brest and Quimper

**Bicycle hire** Pizzeria Bella Spiaggia, 50 Boulevard de la Plage

_Further information_ from tourist office, Boulevard de la Plage.

# Port de Morgat

| | |
|---|---|
| **Harbourmaster** ☎ 98.27.01.97 | **VHF Channel** 9 |
| **Callsign** Morgat | **Daily charge** ££ |

Mooring is to the first pontoon in this large marina, making it a half-mile walk to the shore facilities. It should be possible if you can dry out, and are bold enough, to anchor off the beach just west of the fish quay. It might be noisy but is likely to be free.

### STEP ASHORE

**Nearest payphone** At capitainerie
**Toilets, showers** At capitainerie
**Launderette** Near the town end of quayside
**Shopping** Small village at the root of the quay with food shops, banks and a post office. The town of Crozon is one mile up the hill to the south, with a wider range of facilities

### SHIPS' SERVICES

_**Water and electricity**_ On pontoons
_**Fuel**_ (diesel and petrol) From fuelling berth
_**Gas**_ (Camping and Calor) From Uship, the _**chandler**_ on the quay
_**Boatyard, engineer, sailmaker**_ Ask at Uship

# Douarnenez

Like the Rade de Brest, the Baie de Douarnenez covers some 60 square miles and offers sheltered sailing. In settled weather, overnight anchorages can be found off sandy beaches and in little coves. Douarnenez, in the south-east corner of the bay, offers moorings in the old **Port du Rosmeur** on the east side of the town – yachts are not allowed in the new fishing harbour – and in the modern **Tréboul Marina** on the west bank of the mouth of the Pouldavid River. You can also moor, or anchor, in the estuary of the river, on the east side of **Ile Tristan**, but that is not so sheltered. The Pouldavid River dries but is navigable on a rising tide for most yachts as far as **Port-Rhu**, where you can lie alongside the quay. Water is available on the quay and fuel from the nearby garage.

Douarnenez is one of the busiest fishing ports on the Brittany coast. The steep, narrow streets of the old quarter and the colourful harbour of Port du Rosmeur create an attractive atmosphere.

This is the last port in this guide. Another day's sail to the south, and you will be in a land where the mists fall away and the sun comes out: South Brittany.

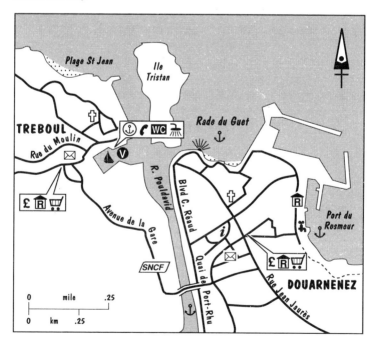

SHORE LEAVE

*Food and drink*
There is a good selection of restaurants in Douarnenez, many specialising in seafood.

*What to see*
Visit Douarnenez old town, and the harbour, especially if you are there when there is a fish auction.

*Excursions*
**Locronan**, six miles inland, is an old town worth visiting. Very picturesque with its Renaissance houses and church, it was once a centre for sailcloth manufacture, but now flourishes as an arts and crafts centre. A trip by land to the **Pointe du Raz**, especially in rough weather, will enable you to see this impressive headland from the safety of the shore.

### TRANSPORT AND TRAVEL

**Buses** From Tréboul and Douarnenez to Quimper
**Trains** From Tréboul and Ploaré to Quimper
**Planes** From Quimper-Pluguffan to Brest, Paris and Gatwick
**Taxis** ☎ 98.74.14.14
**Car hire** Ask at Tréboul Marina office or at tourist office
**Bicycle hire** From SNCF

*Further information* from tourist office, Place Edouard Vaillant, Douarnenez.

# Tréboul Marina

| | |
|---|---|
| **Harbourmaster** ☎ 98.92.18.18 | **VHF Channel** 9 |
| **Callsign** Tréboul | **Daily charge** ££ |

Tréboul, at the mouth of the Pouldavid River, is the seaside resort for Douarnenez. The modern marina, with all the usual facilities, is about half-a-mile from the resort and is completely sheltered from all winds. There are visitors' buoys outside the marina, useful when it gets very crowded in August.

STEP ASHORE

**Nearest payphone, toilets, showers** By capitainerie
**Shopping** Shops, banks and post office are just to the west of the marina

**Food and drink** Not much of a selection in the way of restaurants; more choice in Douarnenez, which entails a two-mile walk to the bridge above Port-Rhu

### SHIPS' SERVICES

*Water and electricity* On pontoons
*Fuel* (diesel and petrol) At fuelling berth
*Gas* From chandler

*Chandler, boatyard, engineer, sailmaker* All in the marina

SHORE LEAVE

There are good bus and train connections from Tréboul which makes inland excursions easy. A pleasant path along the ridge between the pier and the beach offers good views of the bay.

# INDEX

# The Good Food Guide® 1992

## 40th anniversary edition

edited by Tom Jaine

In 1951 Raymond Postgate published a pocket-size volume that strongly criticised the mass of British restaurants while bringing the best of them to wider public knowledge. Forty years on **The Good Food Guide** is a national institution ('the finest restaurant guide around,' according to *The Independent*), and still campaigning hard on behalf of the consumer. The *1992 Guide* draws on over 10,000 accounts of meals eaten by consumers and *Guide* inspectors during the previous 12 months, searching out high quality and good-value cooking in restaurants of every kind, from the temples of haute cuisine to humble fish and chip shops. This edition features 1,300 recommendations from the Scilly Isles to the Shetlands, guiding the food-lover to the best on offer.

Paperback    210 x 120 mm    720pp

# Out to Eat

All of us at some time look for places to eat a
straightforward, good-value meal: somewhere to
have lunch with friends or family; a pub or hotel
just off the motorway; somewhere to have supper
when staying overnight in an unfamiliar town. This
new book, edited by Elizabeth Carter, features
over 1000 restaurants, cafés and pubs where the
quality of food is reliable and prices are
reasonable. Like *The Good Food Guide*, it's based
on reports received by Consumers' Association
from thousands of readers, backed up by
hundreds of anonymous inspections conducted
in the months before publication. A book to keep
at the ready in the glove compartment or on the
hall table – or right next to all your pilots and
almanacs.

Paperback   198 x 129 mm   416 pages

# Holiday Which?
# GOOD WALKS GUIDE

The original *Good Walks Guide* contains 212 walks in outstanding surroundings in England, Scotland, Wales and the Isle of Man – from Kent to Cumbria, Cornwall to Orkney, each with some special feature of interest. Details of sights to watch out for, snippets of fascinating historical information, or comments on the area's wildlife, architecture or archaeological remains are provided in the descriptions for each walk together with a route map. The walks themselves vary from short strolls along canal towpaths to walks within easy driving distance of London or other large cities, and routes in areas in classic walking country such as the Lake District, the Yorkshire Dales, Dartmoor and the Welsh National Parks.

Paperback    210 x 120 mm    556 pages

# Holiday Which?
# TOWN AND COUNTRY WALKS GUIDE

With 180 walks in England, Scotland and Wales, from remote country trails to part-urban/part-rural routes and tours of historic cities and charming country towns, this compact guide is the ideal companion for days out and weekend breaks. Whether your mood is for exploring an ancient archaeological site, contemplating the majesty of nature or strolling in dramatic mountainous terrain, you'll find something to suit you, for all walks are graded for difficulty and their length ranges from two to 12 miles. Each has some particular appeal, such as outstanding views or intriguing architecture, uncommon flora and fauna to look out for or surprising natural features. The guide is carefully researched to ensure suitability for a wide range of ages, energy levels and enthusiasm, and route maps for each walk guarantee ease of use.

'A three-star job which should last for years to come.' John Hillaby, *Yorkshire Post*

Paperback    210 x 120 mm    656 pages

All Consumers' Association's books are available from: Consumers' Association, Castlemead, Gascoyne Way, Hertford X, sɢ14 1ʟʜ tel: (0992) 597773, as well as from the Which? Shop at 359-361 Euston Road, London ɴw1 3ᴀʟ (on the corner of Conway Street between Great Portland Street and Warren Street tube stations; open 9–5.30 Monday to Friday), and from other book shops.

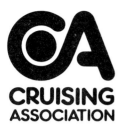

# CRUISING ASSOCIATION

# Join now . . .
# Make friends with the
# Cruising Association

The Cruising Association is a non-commercial international organisation run by and for yachtsmen and women to encourage safe, pleasurable cruising in yachts, under sail or power, and to protect the interests of yachtsmen in general.

The Association was founded in 1908 and now has some 6,000 members worldwide. The headquarters is located in the beautifully restored Ivory House in St Katharine Dock, by the Tower of London, and is manned by professional office staff. Within the headquarters, and available to members for reference or borrowing, is the large and comprehensive nautical library. This is complemented by a well-equipped chart room, providing pilots, charts and reference material for passage planning anywhere in the world.

A bar is available for members and their guests, and many social functions and technical lectures are organised throughout the year. During the winter, local groups also meet in various parts of the country: in summer members attend rallies around the coast.

Honorary Local Representatives and Boatmen, at home and overseas, welcome and assist visiting yachtsmen. All members are kept in touch with a bi-monthly Bulletin, the quarterly "Cruising" magazine and the annual yearbook. Non-boatowners are equally welcome and particularly enjoy the benefits of the computerised crewing service which introduces owners requiring crew and vice versa.

# Complete the form overleaf –
# or telephone 071-481 0881

# APPLICATION FOR MEMBERSHIP
# OF THE CRUISING ASSOCIATION

Surname_____ Forenames_____

Title_____

Address _____

_____

_____

Telephone: Home_____ Other_____

Profession/Occupation_____

Your Yacht (if any) Name_____ Home Port_____ LOA_____

Class_____ Rig_____ Part of Full owned_____

I/We apply to become (a) Member(s) of the Cruising Association and hereby agree, if elected by the Council, to abide by the Rules and Regulations of the Association and the Code of Conduct.

I/We undertake to pay the entrance fee and first year's subscription on election (by the enclosed cheque) and thereafter to pay the yearly subscription by means of the attached Banker's Direct Debit form.

Signed by applicant_____

Signed by spouse (if also applying)_____

Date_____

| Subscriptions for 1991 | Entrance Fee | Annual Subscription | | Annual Subscription |
|---|---|---|---|---|
| Full Ordinary Member | £10.00 + | £48.00 | Spouse Member | £12.00 |
| Full Overseas Member | £10.00 + | £24.00 | Spouse of Overseas Member | £10.00 |
| Young Member (under 25) | | £20.00 | Cadet Member (under 18) | £10.00 |
| Date of birth_____ | | | Date of birth_____ | |

Please circle appropriate amounts. (There may be a small annual change. Please telephone for current rates)

National Westminster Bank plc, 1 Mincing Lane, LONDON EC3 M3JH. Account 1138963. Sort Code 60-70-01. The Association undertakes not to debit any amount other than annual subscriptions, as agreed in General Meeting.

Direct Debit Mandate

To the Manager,_____Bank plc  Branch_____

Postal Address_____ Post Code:_____

I/We authorise you, until further notice in writing, to charge my/our account on or immediately after 1st January in each year unspecified amounts which the Cruising Association may originate by Direct Debit.

Full name of account to be debited_____

Bank Account No:_____ Sort Code:_____

Signature_____ PRINT Member's Name_____

Date_____

(Banks may decline to accept instructions for direct debits to other than current accounts)
After completion, please return this form to The Cruising Association, Ivory House, St Katharine Dock, London E1 9AT.